PRAISE FOR
The Psilocybin Connection

"The book's blend of scholarship, erudition, and imagination makes a compelling argument that human evolution, even the enlargement of our brains, has been due in part to psilocybin mushrooms and their effects on perception, cognition, and imagination. Central to Khamsehzadeh's analysis is that this evolution is continuing to this day and that the future is already visible. His scholarly perspective is persuasive, optimistic, and a pleasure to read."

—JAMES FADIMAN, PhD, microdose researcher and author of *The Psychedelic Explorer's Guide*

"*The Psilocybin Connection* explores how the psychedelic renaissance impacts lives across the planet. Jahan compiles compelling scientific research, provocative theories, and bold visions for the evolutionary role of psychedelics. He guides readers through what this means for us now, how it affects our views of the past, and what amazing possibilities may unfold in our future. He does all this through using integral theory, the most sophisticated and comprehensive set of ideas, frameworks, and practices for making sense of complexity. The integral map helps readers navigate the multifaceted terrain of psychedelics applied to self, culture, and nature. Reading this book will expand your mind without any chemical compounds. And it just might inspire you to engage the territory yourself."

—ADAM B. LEONARD, coauthor of *Integral Life Practice*

"At the outset, Dr. Khamsehzadeh makes clear his book is the result of an intense, two-decade-long journey of integration that was kicked off by his own transformative psychedelic experiences. His story alone inspires. But through his efforts to continue exploring, learning, and integrating, we all may benefit. *The Psilocybin Connection* is an extensive survey of complex and sometimes controversial ideas about the role psilocybin mushrooms have played throughout human history, with an eye not only on the distant past and our present times but also possible futures. Having been trained in both worlds, Dr. Khamsehzadeh weaves psychedelic Western cultural history with Indigenous wisdom traditions. This book demonstrates a clear integration of passion, scholarship, and a healthy dose of wonder—an elixir for those seeking to connect with the mystery that's woven into not only our human lives but also the very fabric of the cosmos."

—KILE ORTIGO, PhD, author of *Beyond the Narrow Life*

"This book is *the single most comprehensive* on the subject of psilocybin mushrooms that I've come across in twenty-plus years of exploring the subject. I found answers to questions I didn't even know I had. Regardless of your level of knowledge or experience, Jahan's book is accessible, inviting, inspiring, and incredibly informative. This will be my go-to recommendation when anyone asks me any question about the history, use, science, or potential of psilocybin mushrooms."

—MICHAEL ROESSLEIN, MS, FDN-P, holistic health
and wellness educator and founder of Inaura

"Beautifully complex, yet perfectly comprehensible. From cave paintings to singularities wrapped in the holonic nature of the universe, *The Psilocybin Connection* weaves the profound nature of the conscious universe through the lenses of the anthropological, the social, and the technological. It invites the reader along humanity's historic journeying with psychedelics from the prehistoric through to the modern day. The perfect story for anyone trying to more deeply understand the role of psychedelics in human civilization, myth, and the future of human evolution—absolutely brilliant!"

—MATT MCKIBBIN, cofounder of the Crypto-
Psychedelic Summit and founder of DecentraNet

"Within our current social conversation about psychedelics and their therapeutic use Jahan Khamsehzadeh offers a comprehensive overview of sacred mushrooms and psilocybin, their history, and their meaningful place in our lives as a species. *The Psilocybin Connection* reads like a transmission anchored in the historical, philosophical, and societal facets of sacred mushrooms and psilocybin, while bringing us closer to Jahan's personal views on life, existence, and the transcendent. His own inner journeys clearly permeate this narrative; and just like the mycelium's intelligence runs in the heart of Earth herself, the spore prints of Khamsehzadeh's broad connectivity of body, mind, spirituality, the collective, and Nature shine through the title of this book."

—FRANCOISE BOURZAT, author of *Consciousness Medicine*

"A unique overview of the rare knowledge that can be obtained through deep inner journeys, reflective meditations, and a careful study of the science and history of the sacred mushroom. Rooted in a foundation of humanistic and transpersonal psychology, Khamsehzadeh weaves together a beautiful alchemical tapestry—overflowing with treasured revelations and valuable psychological insights. A philosophically-intriguing, personal story, as well as a mythic adventure into the collective, self-organizing mind of nature, *The Psilocybin Connection* inspires a spirit toward healing and self-realization. Most highly recommended."

—DAVID JAY BROWN, author of *The New Science of Psychedelics*

THE
PSILOCYBIN
CONNECTION

THE
PSILOCYBIN
CONNECTION

PSYCHEDELICS, THE TRANSFORMATION OF CONSCIOUSNESS, AND EVOLUTION ON THE PLANET

JAHAN KHAMSEHZADEH, PhD

North Atlantic Books
Huichin, unceded Ohlone land
aka Berkeley, California

Cover images © gettyimages.com/ARTYuSTUDIO, gettyimages.com/Berya113, Forager/Shutterstock.com
Cover design by Jasmine Hromjak
Book design by Maureen Forys, Happenstance Type-O-Rama

Published by North Atlantic Books
Huichin, unceded Ohlone land
aka Berkeley, California

Printed in the United States of America

The Psilocybin Connection: Psychedelics, the Transformation of Consciousness, and Evolution on the Planet is sponsored and published by North Atlantic Books, an educational nonprofit based in the unceded Ohlone land Huichin (aka Berkeley, CA) that collaborates with partners to develop cross-cultural perspectives, nurture holistic views of art, science, the humanities, and healing, and seed personal and global transformation by publishing work on the relationship of body, spirit, and nature.

North Atlantic Books' publications are distributed to the US trade and internationally by Penguin Random House Publishers Services. For further information, visit our website: www .northatlanticbooks.com.

Library of Congress Cataloging-in-Publication Data
Names: Khamsehzadeh, Jahan, 1984- author.
Title: The psilocybin connection : psychedelics, the transformation of consciousness, and evolution on the planet—an integral approach / by Jahan Khamsehzadeh, Ph.D.
Description: Berkeley, California : North Atlantic Books, [2022] | Includes bibliographical references.
Identifiers: LCCN 2021038768 (print) | LCCN 2021038769 (ebook) | ISBN 9781623176549 (trade paperback) | ISBN 9781623176556 (ebook)
Subjects: LCSH: Psilocybin—Psychological aspects. | Mushrooms, Hallucinogenic.
Classification: LCC BF209.H36 K43 2022 (print) | LCC BF209.H36 (ebook) | DDC 154.4—dc23
LC record available at https://lccn.loc.gov/2021038768
LC ebook record available at https://lccn.loc.gov/2021038769

1 2 3 4 5 6 7 8 9 KPC 27 26 25 24 23 22

This book includes recycled material and material from well-managed forests. North Atlantic Books is committed to the protection of our environment. We print on recycled paper whenever possible and partner with printers who strive to use environmentally responsible practices.

*Imagination is the
goal of history.*

TERENCE MCKENNA

LIST OF FIGURES

Figure 1. Maslow's Hierarchy of needs. This is the updated version of Maslow's famous model. Before he passed, Maslow revised his theory to include Self-Transcendence at the top. **Page 9**

Figure 2. Quadrants. **Page 51**

Figure 3. Holons. **Page 55**

Figure 4. Autonomy. The picture shows energy going inward toward the self. **Page 60**

Figure 5. Communion. In the image we see a holon moving to connect with other holons of the same depth. **Page 63**

Figure 6. Transcendence. In the image we see a holon expanding toward that of the greater holon. **Page 66**

TABLE OF CONTENTS

List of Figures **x**

Preface: The Story of How Psilocybin Changed My Life **xiii**

Introduction **1**

PART I: The Present

CHAPTER 1: The State of (the) Union **7**
Peak Experiences **8**
Science: Evidence of Transformation **22**
Modern History **35**

CHAPTER 2: An Integral Approach to Psychedelics **49**
The Quadrants **50**
Holons **52**
Instincts of Consciousness **57**
Autonomy **59**
Communion **63**
Transcendence **66**
Dissolution **69**

CHAPTER 3: An Ecology of Synergy **75**
Gaia and Living Systems Theory **76**
Symbiosis **78**
Revisioning Evolution **80**
Fungi and Plants **83**
Animals and Psychedelics **88**
The Ecological Self **94**

PART II: The Past

CHAPTER 4: Emergence of Humanity   **103**
Big Bang to Primates   **104**
Life in the Trees   **106**
From the Trees to Planting Seeds   **109**

CHAPTER 5: The Mycelial Mind   **123**
Group Dynamics   **127**
Spirituality   **132**
The Expansion of the Mind:
Art, Logic, and the Perception of Time   **137**
Language   **149**
Psilocybin and Brain Development   **158**
Contrasts with Other Theories of Human Evolution   **166**
Humanity's Long Psychedelic History   **173**

PART III: The Future

CHAPTER 6: Creativity, Healing, and Economics   **189**
Psychotherapy and Guides   **190**
Visionary Art and Culture   **214**
Philosophy and Science   **231**
Psychedelic Economics: Cryptocurrency, Blockchain, and Psychedelics   **245**

CHAPTER 7: Strange Attractors   **265**
Complexity of Novelty   **265**
Teleological Visions   **276**
The Psychedelic (Re)Evolution   **289**

Bibliography   **299**

Index   **321**

About the Author   **347**

PREFACE

The Story of How Psilocybin Changed My Life

L ike so many people that become focused on healing and self-growth, I had a rough childhood. My parents were both immigrants—my mother from Mexico and my father from Iran. They met in California while trying to learn English. After my sister and I were born, we moved to the Arizona desert. Because my parents came from non-English-speaking countries and lacked education, finding work was difficult for my parents and the financial stress was felt daily in my home. Starting at a young age, I felt alienated at school, made fun of constantly and bullied for being different. My shame ran deep. By high school I was clinically depressed and suicidal. I was also diagnosed with attention deficit disorder (ADD), and the neurodivergence made it difficult to concentrate in a normal school setting, leading even further to my feelings of alienation. Even though I had ADD, I was placed into a gifted education program that cultivated my skills of logic and imagination. Once a week in elementary and once a day in middle school, I went to a class with a more relaxed learning structure that focused on developing abstract thought. We played chess, painted, and had more advanced vocabulary exams. There was less risk of being picked on in these classrooms, and it provided some sense of a haven from an otherwise painful daily school life. I was curious and loved to learn, and though I chose to go to church as a child, I was an atheist by the time I became a teen. I saw no evidence of anything sacred in the world around me. Existence seemed bleak.

A month after graduating high school, I was given a handful of mushrooms while on my way to see my favorite band, Tool, play for the first time. I remember saying out loud that this was going to be the best day of the whole year. Little did I know it was going to be the most significant day of my life.

Once Tool hit the stage, the mushrooms' effects began and my experience of time immediately dissolved. I was only conscious of the present moment, which was rushing toward a threshold that I perceived to be death. The movie *The Matrix* came to mind, and I felt like the character Neo about to be unplugged from the Matrix—I had no idea what was on the other side. For fifteen minutes I held back from crossing this line, and then, out of curiosity, I relaxed and let my being move forward. What occurred was an explosion in my consciousness to a degree I have never experienced since. I could feel every cell of my being rejoice in love and celebration. I felt eternal—that my consciousness existed before the Big Bang and would exist after death. There was a familiarity to this feeling, as if I had known it all along but had just forgotten. Then a voice—strong and not my own—arose in my consciousness to say my name: "Jahan."

"Is this real?" I asked.

"Yes," the voice replied, telepathically. Every wall I had built around my heart collapsed, and I broke into a gushing river of tears for the next ninety minutes.

I knew this was the voice of God—a recognition of something I thought was impossible. I realized that, beneath my awareness, this being was always seeing through my eyes and hearing through my ears, and it had been doing so my entire life. It was also simultaneously doing this within everyone else. God was with me. God was with all of us, all the time. It registered every experience in the cosmos and held each and every one of them with love.

I witnessed each instance of my life flash by, frame by frame, all leading to this one moment. I grasped that all the pain I experienced was necessary and precisely choreographed by a divine intelligence to bring me to this breakthrough so that I could dissolve into this union. At this level of relationship with God, I felt I knew everything, including the location of every atom in the universe. I was one with the larger mind, and yet still wholly an individual self. I felt the greatest contentment I had ever known. At this moment during the mushroom journey I asked God, "What are we?"—*we* referring to us as human beings. I saw light arise from the ground and fill everybody in the arena, and I understood immediately what the all-encompassing being was trying to tell me—that we are love and light and that those qualities are one and the same. Light was wholly intelligent.

I was then taken through our solar system and realized that "outer space" was the same space right in front of me here on Earth. Just as our bodies need vessels to go out into outer space, light needs the vessels of our physical bodies, these "spacetime" ships, to explore our spatial and temporal dimensions. When these "biovessels" die, we simply move into another body. Eternal life of an individual soul, wholly connected through a central uniting being, without the possibility of death, is bliss.

I grasped that our identities are the creation of our imagination and that this world was in fact Heaven. This realization had profound implications for me. Up to this point, I had thought of existence as a miserable hell. Realizing the opposite was in fact true made me suddenly angry. I had been lied to my whole life. Everyone who had sent the wrong message did not have the awareness of what I was now being shown. They didn't know that we are all already in God's palace and the only thing that stops us from living this way is the shortcomings of our collective awareness. This ignorance struck me as deeply unsustainable. It seemed that there must come a time in our future when all humans would realize the essence of our existence and would treat the planet and each other as if we are in Heaven.

The greatest lesson this being taught me is that the most important values in existence are love and learning. Love is by far the most important, with learning being a distant second. Everything else—and this cannot be overstated—was so far behind these values that they seemed almost empty. Love is the most intelligent force in the cosmos, always pointing in the right direction. Learning helps us adapt, evolve, and move further in that direction. Both of these, ultimately, move toward unity. If a person orients their life with these two values, they will never have to worry about holding the complexity of everything else. Seeing through the lens of these two values allows one to recognize what is important in each instant.

When the experience concluded, I climbed to the highest seat in the arena to look over the entire Tucson Convention Center. I knew that my life was transformed, and I felt privileged to have the awareness to take that in. I contemplated that experience almost daily for the next seven years. Two decades later I am still integrating what occurred and still find myself in awe. I had firsthand experience of how drastically and quickly life can be transformed with psychedelics. A month after this experience, I started college as a neuroscience major, with the hope of understanding the link between matter and consciousness. It was my goal to contribute to the academic efforts to create a scientific understanding of consciousness. Privately, I hoped to pursue research on psychedelics, though not much was happening in the field at this time because research on psychedelics was largely restricted.

During my first semester in Pima Community College I took two important classes with phenomenal professors that formed my orientation toward school. The first was a professor in a philosophy class titled "God, Mind, and Matter." The textbooks we used were Ken Wilber's *A Brief History of Everything* and Alex Grey's *The Mission of Art*. The influence of those two books can be seen throughout this text. The other professor was a passionate physics teacher with a similar hunger for knowledge. I believed physics would give me a fundamental understanding of the universe, and I changed my major to focus on physics and mathematics for the next three years. However, a psilocybin journey three years into my major told me to leave physics and focus more directly on mysticism. This brought up tremendous fear since the path of studying physics seemed to hold more social and financial security. At the same time, my intuition said to trust the experience. Studying philosophy and psychology was the closest thing to understanding mysticism at my university, so I switched my major to philosophy and graduated with minors in both psychology and physics and a class short of a minor of mathematics from the University of Arizona.

A few months after graduating, I enrolled at John F. Kennedy University to work on my master's degree in consciousness and transformation and used all the math I had learned to support myself as a math tutor. During this time, I was introduced to psychotherapy and have been studying it since. After my master's, I started work on my doctorate in philosophy, cosmology, and consciousness at the California Institute of Integral Studies. While working on my dissertation, which became this book, I had a psychedelic experience during which I received direction to undergo three more multiyear trainings. I then trained for years within the Mazatec mushroom tradition as well as in Hakomi, a two-year mindfulness-based somatic-psychotherapy comprehensive training. For two years I assisted the Psychedelic-Assisted Psychotherapy Certificate Training at the California Institute of Integral Studies. I then began facilitating legal psilocybin mushroom ceremonies in Jamaica as part of the Atman Retreat team and became a mentor for the Center for Consciousness Medicine's comprehensive guide training. Currently I lead a monthly public group titled "Developing a Relationship with Sacred Mushrooms" with the San Francisco Psychedelic Society. Each day I am filled with gratitude for the psilocybin mushroom experience that first transformed my life, and I can see how everything since has been a ripple from that psychedelic experience. It has been my greatest resource during my difficulties and has allowed me to embrace both the darkness and light by deepening my trust with life.

I share my own psychedelic experiences with the belief that they may prove beneficial to the reader. I hope that these stories, in addition to the similar experiences of others that I explore in these pages, will enable the reader to see real-life examples of how psychedelic experiences can radically transform one's life. After two decades of researching the development and evolution of consciousness, I know of no approach to transformation more powerful and effective than those that use the assistance of psychedelics. This is not to say that psychedelics are a substitute for psychotherapy, meditation, or working within a community. In fact, I believe all these practices are synergistic and that psychedelics deeply enhance these practices. Psilocybin mushrooms and other psychedelics can be traumatizing without the right set and setting, which includes being with trustworthy experienced people and in a safe environment. Psychedelics can conjure deeply painful and frightful experiences, and the help of a therapist or guide, the awareness cultivated in meditation, and the support of friends and family are all essential resources for integration. I hope that those who are ready and want these experiences find the resources that they need. Movements toward decriminalization and legalization are currently underway. Several retreat centers exist and many more are already in the planning stage. The following work is one of the ways I am doing my part to carry psychedelics out of the shadows and into the light, so that they are seen as wholesome, healing, and perhaps humanity's greatest untapped resource for self-realization.

INTRODUCTION

M y intention in this book is to expand the context of the conversations about psychedelics to fully explore their potential for
individual and collective transformation. Though the philosophical and
systems views I provide can be applied to most psychedelics, I focus on
psilocybin mushrooms for several reasons:

- Evidence suggests psilocybin mushrooms may have played a
  unique role in the evolution of early humanity.

- Psilocybin mushrooms are widely available and grow in ecosystems worldwide (they are endemic to six continents, can
  be cultivated privately in one's home, and exist in over two
  hundred species), and thus their accessibility to humanity
  may provide large scale of transformation in comparison to
  other psychedelics.

- A wave of decriminalization of psilocybin mushrooms is
  taking place across the United States, with federal medical
  legalization projected in a few years, and other countries may
  soon follow suit.

- I have a deep practical, academic, and professional knowledge of psilocybin, having trained within the Mazatec
  mushroom lineage and having worked as a legal facilitator of
  psilocybin ceremonies in Jamaica.

- I have a deep personal connection to psilocybin—it is the psychedelic that first helped me heal and gave my life direction.

This book is separated into three sections: Present, Past, and Future.
The format is inspired by a quote from George Orwell's *1984*: "Who

controls the past controls the future. Who controls the present controls the past."[1] The hope is that by rewriting our human history (based on emerging scientific evidence and a potentially more accurate explanation of the origins of humanity) we can break through the cultural and ecological stalemates that our species faces. The format is also in resonance with my Hakomi somatic psychotherapy training (meet the client in the present moment, before uncovering their beliefs that are rooted in their past, so that we can transform their future trajectory). Chapters 1 through 3 address the present, chapters 4 and 5 focus on the past, and chapters 6 and 7 speculate on our future. By shedding light on the present state of psychedelics and by looking at humanity's evolutionary past through the lens of our present knowledge, I hope to help re-envision our collective understanding of our human identity.

Chapter 1, "The State of (the) Union," is meant to serve as a comprehensive overview of the current understanding of psilocybin. This includes presenting and describing common characteristics of the psilocybin experience. I then consider all the major studies on psilocybin in the United States over the last sixty years, though I save a discussion on neuroscience for chapter 5 in order to inform the section on human evolution. After presenting a synthesis of the science regarding psilocybin, I continue by sharing a brief modern history of psilocybin within Western culture.

Chapter 2, "An Integral Approach to Psychedelics," provides the philosophical and metaphysical framework for the remainder of the text. The reader may skip this chapter if they find it too abstract (the rest of the work will read fine without it). Though it is slightly more technical and introduces many concepts to the reader, it presents the logic by which one can most readily grasp a deeper understanding of psychedelics. The chapter situates psychedelics within a context of an understanding of human evolution that includes consciousness as an integral part of the process. The aim is to bring a more comprehensive model to better comprehend the paradigm-transforming psychedelic phenomenon.

---

[1] Orwell, *1984*, 37.

Chapter 3, "An Ecology of Synergy," situates psychedelics within a living systems framework. Psychedelic compounds, which produce complex states of consciousness (often without biological toxicity), naturally evolved in thousands of plant and hundreds of fungus species. I examine how and why such molecules may grow in the environment. It is my contention that the role and effects of psychedelics are a chief anomaly in the materialistic paradigm. Looking through the lens of an integral approach (provided in the previous chapter) may enable the reader to see why such molecules may exist in most ecosystems on the planet. An integral approach situates consciousness as a fundamental facet of ecology, and psychedelic experiences generally allow one to realize that the world is pervaded by consciousness and that we live in a complex living system. It is only through such a realization that we may come to understand how and why psychedelics grow in our environment.

With the primary concepts of the processes of evolution presented in chapters 2 and 3 in mind, chapter 4 focuses on the concrete story of evolution, starting with the Big Bang until the Agricultural Revolution. Specific focus is given to primate psychology and early tribal life, especially in areas concerning sex and diet. The chapter paints a picture for the reader, based on modern scientific understanding, of what life and social dynamics may have been like for our ancestors before the rise of settlements. It shows that our ancestors lived a lifestyle that predisposed them to psychedelic use.

Chapter 5, "The Mycelial Mind," is the heart of this work and is meant to be superimposed over the previous chapter. Building off the research of dozens of scientists and intellectuals, I speculate on how the psilocybin mushrooms naturally growing in our ancestors' environment may have been beneficial in five domains of early human life— group dynamics, spirituality, creativity, language, and brain development. I then compare the mushroom theory of human evolution with other leading theories that attempt to explain the origins of humanity. The section ends with a brief summary of humanity's psychedelics history, based on anthropological evidence, from the archaic period up until our modern era.

Chapter 6, "Creativity, Healing, and Economics," takes a detailed look at the current cultural processes catalyzed by psychedelics that serve as intimations of transformations to come. This chapter is divided into four sections. The first, "Psychotherapy and Guides," serves as a presentation of and advice to an emerging industry focused on professionally held psychedelic experiences. Within as little as five years, there may be hundreds of psychedelic psychotherapy clinics opening worldwide. In a decade, the number could be in the thousands. "Visionary Art and Culture" presents accounts of how psychedelics have dramatically impacted visual art, music, and movies, even giving rise the field of visionary art itself. The next section is an overview of how psychedelics have and may continue to influence innovation in both philosophy and science. The last section, "Psychedelic Economics," focuses on the similarities between blockchain (the technology underlying cryptocurrencies like Bitcoin) and how blockchain can help support the safe integration of psychedelics into society.

The final chapter, "Strange Attractors," takes a teleological approach to the future. Psychedelic experiences often give the subject a sense that something big is about to happen in our world. This chapter begins with presenting how complexity within systems evolves and how psychedelics increase the complexity within both the brain and society, leading to novel connections and creative expressions that further accelerate the evolution of our species. Following is a presentation of visions of the future that people experienced in psychedelic states. I suggest that psychedelics may be tools of communication between the individual and the collective unconscious that may awaken visions of the future. These visions may help humanity become clear about what direction to move toward so that we can evolve consciously. The closing section, "Psychedelic (Re)Evolution," serves as a summary for this work and presents the major implications.

PART I
The Present

1

THE STATE OF (THE) UNION

L et's set the stage for the phenomenology of psilocybin by showcasing eight selected experiences of different people's transformative
moments with psilocybin. I ask that the reader hold these examples in
mind when reading the rest of the book, which deals more with facts and
theory. The often-sublime subjective experiences of psilocybin mirror
the extraordinary objective empirical evidence and theories discussed in
this work, such as people healing from previously untreatable psycho-
emotional illnesses; the accelerated positive transformation in people's
lives; and the possibility that psilocybin mushrooms played a critical role
in the emergence of humanity. We'll look at all the major scientific studies focusing on psilocybin that have taken place in the United States;
then this chapter gives a brief overview of the cultural events relevant to
the history of psilocybin in Western culture.

Peak Experiences

Peak experiences—breathtaking expansive states of consciousness that leave us with awe, insight, and a vitalized sense of being reborn—can dramatically transform a person's life. Abraham Maslow, a developmental psychologist and architect of the famous hierarchy of needs, writes, "Peak experiences often have consequences. They can have very, very important consequences."[1] He continues:

> If we are conscious enough of what we are doing, that is, if we are philosophical enough in the insightful sense too, we may be able to use those experiences that most easily produce ecstasies, that most easily produce revelations, experiences, illumination, bliss, and rapture experiences. We may be able to use them as a model by which to re-evaluate history teaching or any other kind of teaching.[2]

In my work I have continuously seen people review their own history as a result of psychedelic states. Peak experiences are moments of self-transcendence that often catalyze a transformation of identity, where a person's social construct dissolves and they begin to identify with a deeper aspect of their self. "The discovery of identity comes via impulse voices, via the ability to listen to your own guts, and to their reactions and to what is going on inside of you," writes Maslow, one of the founders of humanistic psychology.[3] Many people in peak experiences—which can be intentionally catalyzed by psychedelics, as well as through other methods such as sex, breathing, and meditation—experience a transrational, intuitive knowing, a sense of wholeness and homecoming, of finally being united with themselves and the cosmos.

---

[1] Maslow, *Farther Reaches of Human Nature*, 170.

[2] Maslow, 172.

[3] Maslow, 171.

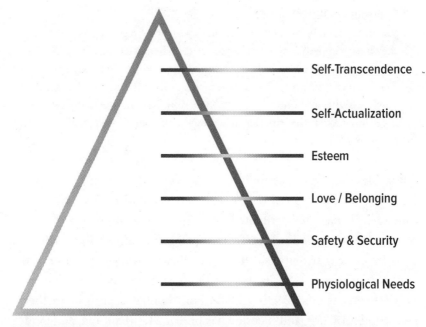

FIGURE 1. Maslow's hierarchy of needs. This is the updated version of Maslow's famous model. Before he passed he revised his theory to include Self-Transcendence at the top.

In the book *Shroom: A Cultural History of the Magic Mushroom*, Andy Letcher—who earned two doctorates, one in ecology from Oxford and the other in religious and cultural studies from King Alfred's College in Winchester—provides an eloquent account of a general psilocybin mushroom experience:

> The epithet "magic" appears apposite and well earned, for mushrooms create an overall ambience of earthly, Tolkienesque enchantment. The world, and especially the natural world, appears in a new light, as if some ordinarily obscured and secret aspect of it has been suddenly revealed. The smallest details—leaves, bark, cobwebs, grains of sand— appear exquisitely beautiful and heavy with meaning. Consciousness appears less bounded than it is ordinarily, for trees, plants and even rocks seem to be, in some peculiar sense, aware. However strange and unsettling this transformation, the bemushroomed may report a

feeling of familiarity, of deja vu, of having always known about this particular nook in the architecture of experience. Some say it is as if they have stepped into an archetypal space where they are actors in some ancient drama played out by fools, lovers, kings, and queens. This is more than an enchanted escapade: enthusiasts report that great noetic insights and philosophical connection flash unexpectedly into the mind, so that the experience is intellectually and ontologically rewarding.[4]

After his eloquent description of the "bemushroomed" experience, Letcher goes on to point out that psilocybin mushrooms are biologically safe. "It has been estimated," he writes, "that you have to eat your own body weight in mushrooms to take a lethal dose."[5] The traditional measure of drug toxicity is called a therapeutic index—the ratio of the dose that is effective in 50 percent of subjects to the lethal dose that kills 50 percent of subjects (LD50). For example, aspirin has a therapeutic index of 199, and nicotine has one of 21.[6] The therapeutic index for psilocybin is 641 (a higher number indicates a greater safety profile). The body removes two-thirds of the ingested psilocybin from the system within three hours of taking it. Since the body builds tolerance to psilocybin quickly, one cannot take psilocybin on consecutive days and still feel as strong an effect.[7] With the correct mindset and environment (discussed in chapter 6), psilocybin mushrooms are relatively physically harmless and may provide immensely valuable experiences that support the development of one's consciousness, as the reader will learn in the next section.

The first documented Westerner to intentionally take psilocybin mushrooms was Gordon Wasson, a vice president at J. P. Morgan, who encountered psilocybin mushrooms within the Mazatec tradition

---

[4] Letcher, *Shroom*, 19.

[5] Letcher, 21.

[6] Strassman et al., *Inner Paths to Outer Space*, 47.

[7] Letcher, *Shroom*, 21.

in 1955.[8] Wasson, aside from being a Wall Street banker, was keenly interested in mycology, the scientific and cultural study of fungi. Deeply curious about the custom of using mushrooms in a religious ceremony, Wasson made the trip to Huautla de Jimenez, a town in the Mexican state of Oaxaca, and convinced Maria Sabina, a Mazatec *curandera*, to let him participate in a mushroom ceremony. Of this first ceremony, Wasson writes:

> geometric patterns . . . in richest colors .... Then the patterns grew into architectural structures . . . patios of regal splendor . . . all harmoniously and ingeniously contrived. . . . There is no better way to describe the sensation than to say it was as though . . . [my] very soul had been scooped out of . . . [my] body and translated to a point floating in space, leaving behind the husk of clay. . . . We had the sensation that the walls of our humble house had vanished, that our untrammeled souls were floating in the universe, stroked by divine breezes, possessed of divine mobility that would transport us anywhere on the wings of a thought. . . . There came a moment when it seemed as though the visions themselves were about to be transcended, and dark gates reaching upward beyond sight were about to part, and we were to find ourselves in the presence of the Ultimate. We seemed to be flying at the dark gates as a swallow at a dazzling lighthouse, and the gates were to part and admit us. But they did not open, and with a thud we fell back, gasping. We felt disappointed, but also frightened and half relieved, that we had not entered into the presence of the Ineffable, whence, it seemed to us at the time, we might not have returned, for we had sensed that a willing extinction in the divine radiance had been awaiting us.[9]

Visions of sacred geometry seemingly creating the structure of the world, physical space developing into regal architecture and a palace of God, and the fear of disintegration as one is pulled toward divine

---

[8] Riedlinger, "'Wondrous Mushroom' Legacy."

[9] Wasson and Wasson, as cited in Forte, *Entheogens and the Future of Religion*, 138.

light are common experiences for people who take an adequate dose of psilocybin. An adequate dose for this kind of experience is about five dried grams, the amount Wasson took in that ceremony.[10] This is also the amount that the philosopher Terence McKenna refers to as a "heroic dose" and recommends for breaking past the threshold of our ego boundary and into the psilocybin realm;[11] and this was approximately the amount used to study psilocybin and its ability to occasion mystical experiences by the New York University School of Medicine and Johns Hopkins over the last two decades.[12]

As William Richards—who in 1977 administered the last legal dose of psilocybin at the Maryland Psychiatric Research Center and was again the first person in the United States to legally administer psilocybin as part of the research he co-initiated at Johns Hopkins School of Medicine in 1999—writes in his book *Sacred Knowledge: Psychedelic and Religious Experiences*: "In my experience, the spiritual insights treasured by most people who have known mystical forms of experience are remarkably similar."[13] Many who take an adequate dose of psilocybin arrive at common insights and experiences. Further, some of these insights and experiences are similar to those reached by exploring other members of the tryptamine chemical family (which includes psilocybin, LSD, and DMT), as well as those graced by spontaneous mystical experiences or reached by a disciplined practice.

Author and speaker James Jesso, in his book *Decomposing the Shadow: Lessons from the Psilocybin Mushroom*, echoes that the intentional use of psilocybin mushrooms can have transformative effects:

> I realized psilocybin was exposing me to previously unrealized perspectives on the nature of mind, cultural conditioning, emotional repression,

---

[10] Wasson and Wasson, as cited in Forte.

[11] T. McKenna, *Food of the Gods*.

[12] Miller, *Psychedelic Medicine*.

[13] Richards, *Sacred Knowledge*, 36.

the cultivation of personal courage, and the honesty of emotion. It was offering me a perspective on what it means to become *whole*.[14]

For over a year, on every full moon Jesso held a personal mushroom ceremony:

> I ended this practice after thirteen months in order to take a step back and look at myself. Before I began, I felt fragmented and confused. . . . Coming out on the other side of those thirteen months with the mushroom, I felt healed, *whole,* self-aware, and in line with the deep passions firing my life forward.[15]

In addition to these transcendent spiritual experiences, many people who held decades of pain finally found relief when they encountered psilocybin mushrooms. In the last hundred pages of the book *Sacred Mushroom of Visions: Teonanácatl,* Ralph Metzner—who in the 1960s was one of the first psychologists to research psilocybin at Harvard—presents people's personal experiences with psilocybin mushrooms. For example, David S., a fifty-two-year-old writer and publisher, recalls undergoing a deeply healing transformative experience with psilocybin:

> A singular powerful knowing swept over me and totally overwhelmed me, mentally and physically: that this world is a beneficent place and the source of all goodness. The power and simplicity of this realization astounded me. It was not a part of my belief structure. Where had I been all these years? I had been in self-absorption. I saw my entire worldview and value system shift and realign. *The world is a beneficent place.* An immense relief came over me as I realized that I was free from the captivity of my previous worldview and attitudes. A new perception was manifesting, and it made sense. As waves of gratitude and awe washed over me, I went into more contortions and spinal muscle spasms.

---

[14] Jesso, *Decomposing the Shadow*, 10.

[15] Jesso, 10.

Now came a knowing that things were going to be all right in my life. The term "all right" was the driver. Everything was all *right* in my life, starting now. At first I was shocked at the fact that I knew this on such a core level. It wasn't a case of believing it or hoping for it; it was simply *knowing* it. I was *experiencing* the knowledge and not merely thinking it. I tried to verbalize this, but I couldn't get the words out. I realized that I was having a world-life-view shift, and that I was blowing out a lifetime's worth of negative dross and sediment from my system.

Powerful sobs wracked my body and there was a tremendous letting go of years of misery as next came the knowing that I was *all right* just the way I was. I was *all right*, period. Without qualification, rationalization, justification, negotiation, performance, or explanation. This was the simple truth. Throughout my life, on a deep level, I have always believed that there was something wrong with me. Now, for the first time, I was simply *all right*. I experience being *all right*. As the magnitude of this sank in, a great calmness came over me. On the outside I was a blubbering mess of tearful gratitude; on the inside I felt the purity of the truth. This made sense. This is the way it is.[16]

In that same book, author Jason Serle also shares his experiences with psilocybin, telling of a divine intelligence guiding him and bestowing lessons hidden within his past:

I began to see faint geometric patterns but little more. By now I could feel surges of energy moving through me, increasing in intensity, and I felt a slight fear of being overwhelmed by the experience. . . . Suddenly the two-dimensional blackness of the room opened out into an infinite three-dimensional void in which I was suspended, yet free to move any direction I pleased. In the absence of anything to verify my motion and with nothing to measure the passage of time, I dwelt in a state of time-lessness, an eternal realm that until then had been mere speculation.

I actually became clear that this great emptiness actually contained the sum total of all possible experiences. I began traveling into my

---

[16] Metzner, *Sacred Mushroom of Visions*, 270–71.

past to relive events from my childhood as if they were actually and presently taking place, in the true fullness of the five senses. The mere thought of a person would bring me to them instantly. . . . It soon became clear that I could not only visit people I have known, I could actually *become* them.

It became apparent that my own choice was falling away and there was a strong sensation of being *led* from scene to scene. The entity leading me seemed to know me better than I did myself, for as each experience unfolded I was amazed that it was exactly the experience that I wanted and needed. It was as if something were reading my thoughts even before they surfaced in my own conscious mind.

I identified with the one Ground of Being, the great ocean of awareness that gives rise to the feeling of "I am" in all of us. It was this feeling, prior to all thought, that was identical in all those I became. At one point I became my mother giving birth to me, or perhaps it was me giving birth to my mother—I could not tell—but the experience was as real as any I have ever had: the contractions, the mixed feelings of pain and joy, and the relief at it all being over as I cradled the baby in my arms, holding its head to my swollen breast.

All traces of fear and anxiety had left me and in their place was an ecstatic feeling that grew in intensity. As it unfolded, I was being stripped of boundaries and liberated into an ever-widening aware-ness of the universe. The point that I had been, floating in an infinite void, expanded to include all things, all worlds, all planes, all levels, all beings, and all manifestations, all taking place inside of me. At one point I lifted my hands above my head and my body reaching from one side of the universe to the other, contains all things in between.... There was only one Super-Organism, whose body was the universe, and all manifestations were merely modifications of itself. . . . Hand in hand with this most liberating insight was the knowledge that every-thing is exactly as it should be.

This experience with the sacred mushroom was of great significance to me. In all honesty, it has, more than any other event, changed my life for the better. . . . Shortly afterward, when my partner returned from her holiday, she undertook a similar rite, with much the same effect.[17]

---

[17] Metzner, *Sacred Mushroom of Visions*, 254–56.

In the previous experience one can see the common trajectory, when working with psilocybin and other psychedelics, of moving from a personal domain—working on themes in one's own biography—into a transpersonal domain, where individuality dissolves into a larger unity that enables one to personally experience the consciousness of other beings.[18]

Paul Stamets, a world-renowned mycologist, also had his life transformed with the help of psilocybin mushrooms.[19] Michael Pollan spent a lot of time with Stamets while researching his best-selling book *How to Change Your Mind: What the New Science of Psychedelics Teaches Us about Consciousness, Dying, Addiction, Depression, and Transcendence.* He recounts that:

> Stamets went off to Kenyon College, where, as a freshman, he had a "profound psychedelic experience" that set his course in life. As long as he could remember, Stamets has been stymied by a debilitating stutter. "This was a huge issue for me. I was always looking down at the ground because I was afraid people would try to speak to me. In fact, one of the reasons I got so good at finding mushrooms was because I was always looking down."
>
> One spring afternoon toward the end of his freshman year, walking alone along the wooded ridgeline above campus, Stamets ate a whole bag of mushrooms, perhaps ten grams, thinking that was a proper dose. (Four grams is a lot.) As the psilocybin was coming on, Stamets spied a particularly beautiful oak tree and decided he would climb it. "As I'm climbing the tree, I'm literally getting higher as I'm climbing higher." Just then the sky begins to darken, and a thunderstorm lights up the horizon. The wind surges as the storm approaches, and the tree begins to sway.
>
> "I'm getting vertigo but I can't climb down, I'm too high, so I just wrapped my arms around the tree and held on, hugging it tightly. The tree became the *axis mundi*, rooting me to the earth. 'This is the tree

---

[18] Grof, *Psychology of the Future.*

[19] Stamets, *Mycelium Running.*

of life,' I thought; it was expanding into the sky and connecting me to the universe. And then it hits me: I'm going to be struck by lightning! Every few seconds there's another strike, here, then there, all around me. On the verge of enlightenment, I'm going to be electrocuted. This is my destiny! The whole time, I'm being washed by warm rains. I am crying now, there is liquid everywhere, but also feel one with the universe."

"And then I say to myself, what are my issues if I survive this? Paul, I said, you're not stupid, but stuttering is holding you back. You can't look women in the eyes. What should I do? *Stop stuttering now—* that became my mantra. *Stop stuttering now,* I said it over and over."

"The storm eventually passed. I climbed down from the tree and walked back to my room and went to sleep. That was the most important experience of my life to that point, and here's why: The next morning, I'm walking down the sidewalk, and here comes this girl I was attracted to. She's way beyond my reach. She's walking toward me, and she says, 'Good morning, Paul. How are you?' I look at her and say, 'I'm doing great.' I wasn't stuttering! And I have hardly ever stuttered since. And that's when I realized I wanted to look into these mushrooms."[20]

Stamets went on to devote his life to the study of mushrooms. He has written five books on mycology; developed several patents that use mushrooms; started a successful company called Fungi Perfecti that employs over one hundred people by selling fungi dietary supplements and growing supplies; worked with the Pentagon's Defense Advanced Research Projects Agency (DARPA) to research how mushrooms can protect US citizens against chemical warfare; was offered a grant from the National Institutes of Health to research how turkey tail mushrooms can cure breast cancer; won several awards in the field of mycology; did a TED talk titled "6 Ways Mushrooms Can Help Save the World" with millions of views on YouTube; cocreated a documentary called *Fantastic Fungi* with award-winning director Louie Schwartzberg; and created what has become known as the "Stamets Stack," a microdose regimen

---

[20] Pollan, *How to Change Your Mind*, 99.

that uses psilocybin mushrooms, lion's mane (*Hericium erinaceus*, which also has neurogenic properties that rebuild memory), and niacin (vitamin B3) that may be used to enhance cognition and well-being.[21]

Ayelet Waldman, a most unlikely psychedelic explorer, also experienced a radical transformation with the help of psychedelics.[22] Waldman, a novelist, former University of California, Berkeley, law professor, and a mother of four children, suffered from treatment-resistant depression as part of her bipolar disorder. After years of working with multiple forms of therapies and prescription medications, she was still left with chronic feelings of low mood and irritability. In a desperate attempt to heal, she encountered the resurgence of research on psychedelics and became intrigued with the topic of microdosing. *Microdosing* generally refers to regularly taking subthreshold amounts of a psychedelic. The study of microdosing was popularized by the researcher James Fadiman and made public with his book *The Psychedelic Explorer's Guide: Safe, Therapeutic, and Sacred Journeys*. After Waldman experimented with microdosing, she wrote the book *A Really Good Day: How Microdosing Made a Mega Difference in My Mood, My Marriage, and My Life*. It provides a detailed, organized account that charts her monthlong processes of microdosing with LSD, which is derived from a fungus called ergot. The chemical composition and biochemical processes of LSD closely resemble those of psilocybin; they both come from fungi, are both tryptamine molecules, and dock into the same 5-HT2A serotonin receptors in the brain.[23] Waldman took ten micrograms of LSD every third day, and the benefits of microdosing were instantaneous. She felt increases in mood, confidence, and healing in her relationships. On microdose days she experienced states of flow at work and was more productive. Waldman's criticism of self and others was significantly reduced, allowing greater ease and satisfaction in her life.

---

[21] MAPS, "Mycology of Consciousness."

[22] Waldman, *Really Good Day*.

[23] Pollan, *How to Change Your Mind*.

As one can see in the stories presented thus far, there are many commonalities in experience when people take psilocybin mushrooms or similar psychedelics. The wide spectrum of variations in experience is partly due to dosage. At lower doses, one may feel a sense of enchantment with one's everyday life and psychological insights about oneself. As the dose increases, one may experience more intense archetypal themes that seemingly arise from a collective psyche (a topic further expanded upon in the following chapters). At even higher doses, the probability of experiencing unity with all creation also increases. At these high doses, more people report being guided by a greater intelligence on psilocybin than when using other psychedelics.[24] Repeated experiments show that, with carefully planned intentions and guidance, about 70 percent of people taking doses approaching five dried grams of psilocybin mushrooms undergo a vivid experience of interconnection that they describe as a mystical experience.[25] The following examples illustrate reports of people having direct experiences of God that can occur while taking psilocybin mushrooms.

Bill Hicks—an American stand-up comedian, satirist, and social critic—spread awareness of the spiritual potential of psychedelics in his comedy. After Hicks was diagnosed with terminal cancer, he said there were only two things that he wanted to do other than continue furthering his work: to reread *Lord of the Rings* and, with his two closest friends, take five dried grams of psilocybin mushrooms. He developed a skit after this psilocybin session:

> I recommend a healthy dose of psilocybin mushrooms. Three weeks ago, two of my friends and I went to a ranch in Fredericksburg, Texas, and took what Terence McKenna calls a heroic dose—five dried grams. Let me tell you, our third eye was squeegeed quite cleanly (squeegee sounds). Wow! Now I am glad they are against the law. You know what happened when I took them? I laid in a field of green grass for four hours, going

---

[24] Beach, "Listening for the Logos"; T. McKenna, *True Hallucinations*.

[25] Pollan, *How to Change Your Mind*, 10.

"My God, I love everything!" The heavens parted, and God looked down and rained gifts of forgiveness unto my being, healing me on every level—psychically, physically, emotionally. And, I realized our true nature is spirit and not body; that we are eternal beings and God's love is unconditional and there is nothing we can ever do to change that. It is only our illusion that we are separate from God, or that we are alone. In fact, the reality is, we are one with God and he loves us. Now, if that isn't a hazard to this country. You see my point! How are we going to keep building nuclear weapons?! You know what I mean? What's going to happen to the arms industry when we realize we are all one?! It's going to fuck up the economy! The economy that's fake anyway. Which would be a real bummer. . . . You can see why the government is cracking down on the idea of experiencing unconditional love. . . . Ain't it interesting that the two drugs that are legal, alcohol and cigarettes, two drugs that do absolutely nothing for you whatsoever—and drugs that grow naturally upon this planet, drugs that open your eyes up to make you realize how you are being fucked everyday of your life—those drugs are against the law? Coincidence?! I don't know. I am sure their motives are pure. . . . Ain't that great, mushrooms grow on cow turds. I love that. I think that is why you giggle for the first hour . . . I know where Heaven is! Where? In a cow's ass! "Ohh my God! Lift me up out of this illusion Lord. Heal my perception—that I may know only reality and only you."[26]

William Melvin Hicks died February 26, 1994, at the age of 32.

Another powerful experience of God catalyzed by psilocybin is documented in the 2008 book *Inner Paths to Outer Space: Journeys to Alien Worlds through Psychedelics and Other Spiritual Technologies*, by Rick Strassman, MD, Slawek Wojtowicz, MD, Luis Luna, PhD, and Ede Frecska, MD. The following example comes from a friend of Wojtowicz that chooses to remain anonymous and depicts a complex, multilayered landscape and concludes with the experience of unity:

I went deeper and deeper inside—I traveled through various realms, some of them beautiful, others magical, and others quite scary. It felt

---

[26] Hicks, *Rant in E-Minor*, track 8.

kind of like being in a computer game, where you have to figure out a way to go from level to level and there are hidden dangers, distractions, and traps awaiting you everywhere. Finally, I broke through to the top level—and to my amazement, I became simultaneously all the people (and other intelligent beings) who ever lived, are alive, and will ever live in the universe. I realized that there is only one Actor playing all the parts—it is God, and I am him. Thus, we all will be saved, there is no hell waiting for us after death (although we created one for ourselves on Earth), and God loves every single one of us the way we are. I knew that our lives are merely a dream, a virtual-reality movie. We cannot really die or get hurt and we have potential to awaken to who we really are—when we will, this world will turn to heaven. I saw how perfect the story is and that everything is fine the way it is—there is no need to struggle to change things out in the world; instead each of us has to work on healing himself or herself. There is no need to suffer or to be unhappy ever again. This experience turned upside down my views of the world and religion and changed me profoundly—for the better.[27]

Like previous examples, this author experienced what he perceives to be the highest realm of consciousness, where one merges into a being that is simultaneously all beings, at all times, and through this merger one may experience what it is like to be other people.

After researching psychedelic states of consciousness for fifty years, Stanislav Grof, one of the principal developers of transpersonal psychology and a leader in the field of psychedelic psychotherapy, presented that psychedelics can catalyze holotropic states—higher levels of consciousness that lead to greater degrees of wholeness and unity, with oneself and the world.[28] Unity, which can be defined as a deep sense of wholeness and interconnection, has the potential to heal our fractured sense of isolation, alienation, rejection, and loneliness. The sense of separation can be seen as the greatest source of our fear and pain,[29] while

---

[27] Strassman et al., *Inner Paths to Outer Space*, 149–50.

[28] Grof, *Way of the Psychonaut*, vols. 1 and 2.

[29] Swan, *Anatomy of Loneliness*.

the subjective realization of unity allows one to see that they are not separate and in fact exist as part of a larger whole—within a family, a relationship, a community, the planet, and the universe. The deep sense of oneness that can arise in psychedelic states—the realization that we are part of a vast and singular network of consciousness—is an example of the pinnacle of human experience. In *Toward a Psychology of Being*, Abraham Maslow states, "The peak experience is felt as a self-validating, self-justifying moment which carries its own intrinsic value with it. That is to say it is an end in itself."[30] He goes on to write:

> Any person in a peak experience takes on temporarily many of the characteristics which I found in self-actualizing individuals. That is, for the time they become self-actualizers. We may think of it as a passing characterological change if we wish, and not just an emotional-cognitive-expressive state. Not only are these his happiest and most thrilling moments, but they are also moments of greatest maturity, individuation, fulfillment—in a word, his healthiest moments.[31]

From such peak experiences one acquires the sense of their own deeper identity and interconnectedness with everything. Following these states, one is often inspired to create art, transform society, heal others, and orient toward seeing beauty in the world. As evidenced in the experiences described earlier, even just one such direct experience can greatly transform one's life, with the potential to heal depression and increase vitality and connection.

Science: Evidence of Transformation

The empirical, quantitative research on psilocybin is just as spectacular as the anecdotes in the previous section, providing ample evidence of

---

[30] Maslow, *Toward a Psychology of Being*, 74.

[31] Maslow, 91.

objective and behavioral changes that accompany having such powerful and transformative experiences. Multiple studies—at Harvard, New York University, Johns Hopkins University School of Medicine, and the University of California, Los Angeles (UCLA)—repeatedly show that with the right set and setting about 70 percent of participants report sessions that qualify as a mystical experience.[32] Many of those working in the field of psychedelics, myself included, believe that these experiences of unity can bring profound healing in one's life.[33]

Though an increasing amount of research has been underway in the last two decades, there was already a wealth of accumulated scientific research by the 1970s. As Pollan notes, there were

> more than a thousand scientific papers on psychedelic drug therapy before 1965, involving more than forty thousand research subjects. Beginning in the 1950s and continuing into the early 1970s, psychedelic compounds had been used to treat a variety of conditions—including alcoholism, depression, obsessive-compulsive disorder, and anxiety at the end of life—frequently with impressive results.[34]

The results of these extensive experiments have been overwhelmingly positive, with seemingly no traumatic experience having been reported during the carefully structured experiments.[35]

In the early 1960s, Harvard started the first known scientific experiments on psilocybin and psychology with Timothy Leary spearheading what came to be known as the Harvard Psilocybin Project. Neal Goldsmith, a psychotherapist and scholar of psychedelic history, writes in his

---

[32] Pollan, *How to Change Your Mind*, 10.

[33] Grof, *Way of the Psychonaut*, vols. 1 and 2.

[34] Pollan, *How to Change Your Mind*, 44.

[35] Metzner, *Sacred Mushroom of Visions*.

book *Psychedelic Healing: The Promise of Entheogens for Psychotherapy and Spiritual Development*:

> The first study in the Harvard Psilocybin Project was Leary's "remarkable people" study. Basically, they gave psilocybin to everybody, except undergrads: graduate students, psychologists, religious people, religion professors, mathematicians, chemists, artists, and musicians, in a comfortable setting (usually Leary's house). Results were published in 1963 in *The Journal of Nervous and Mental Disorders,* reporting that 70 percent had a pleasant or ecstatic time; 88 percent learned important insights; 62 percent changed their life for the better; and 90 percent desired to try it again.[36]

Leary also created and directed the Concord Prison Study, under Harvard University's Center for Research in Personality, to study whether psilocybin trips affected the reincarceration rate of prisoners.

Afterward, Walter Pahnke, a Harvard graduate student, conducted the Harvard Good Friday Experiment to study if psilocybin stimulates subjective qualities that categorically fit into the definition of a classical mystical experience. The questionnaire used by Pahnke, and then again decades later by the team at Johns Hopkins, asked the participants to assign a number on the scale from 0 to 6 to the following criteria: unity (whether internal or external unity), transcendence of space and time, ineffability, sense of sacredness, noetic quality (intellectual insights), and positive mood.[37] As part of the experiment, graduate divinity students took psilocybin during a Good Friday church service; 67 percent of them reported experiences that met the criteria of a genuine mystical experience. Most participants reported that it was one of the most important experiences of their lives. This was verified in a twenty-five-year follow-up conducted by Rick Doblin, the founder of the Multidisciplinary Association for Psychedelic Studies

---

[36] Goldsmith, *Psychedelic Healing.*

[37] Griffiths et al. "Psilocybin Can Occasion Mystical-Type Experiences."

(MAPS).[38] He tracked down the participants, who still reported that they considered it to be one of the most spiritual moments of their lives.

In *Psychedelic Medicine: The Healing Powers of LSD, MDMA, Psilocybin, and Ayahuasca,* Richard Miller, who has been a psychotherapist for over fifty years and a former advisor on the President's Commission on Mental Health, interviewed Roland Griffiths, chief investigator of the psilocybin experiments at Johns Hopkins University. Griffiths is a psychopharmacologist and professor at Johns Hopkins in the departments of psychiatry and neuroscience and has been working on the cutting edge of neuroscience for over forty years. The psilocybin studies he conducts at Johns Hopkins University have now spanned two decades. In the interview, Griffiths focuses on the first Johns Hopkins psilocybin experiment, which began in 1999 and was published in 2006, which studied if psilocybin catalyzes mystical experiences. About this study, David Nichols, a researcher in Purdue University's Department of Medicinal Chemistry and Molecular Pharmacology, says,

> It is the first well-designed, placebo-controlled clinical study in four decades to examine the psychological consequences of the effects of . . . psilocybin. In fact, one would be hard pressed to find a single study of psychedelics from any earlier that was as well done or as meaningful.[39]

The study involved administering doses of psilocybin equivalent to about five dried grams of mushrooms to participants.[40] In discussing the experiment, Griffiths says:

> What's most interesting to us is that under the right conditions—when participants are prepared well and feeling safe—they often have experiences that map onto naturally occurring mystical-type

---

[38] Doblin, "Note on Current Psilocybin Research Projects."

[39] Nichols in Miller, *Psychedelic Medicine,* 137.

[40] Griffiths in Miller, 144.

experiences. These are experiences that have been reported by mystics and religious figures throughout the ages and have been carefully described throughout the literature of the psychology of religion—very prominently represented by William James in the early 1900s. There have been measures developed for rigorously assessing the phenomenological domains of these transcendent experiences.

The major feature of this experience, endorsed by about 70 percent of our volunteers, is the interconnectedness of all people and things—a sense of unity, that all is one. This is accompanied by a sense of sacredness or reverence, sometimes described as awe. Also, a sense that the experience is more real and true than everyday waking consciousness. The other qualities of the experience are a sense of open-heartedness—sometimes described as love, gratitude, or peacefulness—and a sense of transcendence of time and space, when past and future collapse into the present moment and that's all there is, the present moment. Space becomes boundless and time endless. And finally, a sense of ineffability. One of the first things people say after having this kind of experience is, "I can't possibly tell you what the experience was about. I can't put it into words because they just don't fit."

The remarkable thing is, not only do people endorse that experience immediately after the session, but at a one- or two-month follow-up and more than a year follow-up, they continue to say the experience has positively changed their attitudes about themselves, their lives, and other people. They claim to be more prosocial, more generous, and more loving. People will also claim to make changes in their behavior in accordance with that; so, for instance, they may take up a meditation practice, eat more healthily, or exercise more regularly. Caretaking of self and others emerges from this experience. The experience, of course, is over at the end of the session. But the memory endures, and the principal features—this interconnectedness of all things, sacredness, the sense of the true value of it, a sense of heart opening, transcendence of time and space, and ineffability—this whole package comes together as the mystical experience.[41]

---

[41] Griffiths in Miller, 144–45.

Griffiths goes on to say that a one-year follow-up interview with the participants' friends, family, and colleagues at work confirms the types of changes reported by the participants.[42] In 2006, the same year the Johns Hopkins study was published, the University of Arizona also published research results of their experiment that studied if psilocybin works as a treatment for obsessive-compulsive disorder (OCD). All participants in the Arizona experiment experienced decreases of symptoms of OCD.[43]

Bob Jesse, the person primarily responsible for initiating the research at John Hopkins and bringing together the John Hopkins team,[44] writes:

> The findings, published in 2006, 2008, and 2011, confirm what the literature has long suggested: psilocybin, used under suitable conditions, frequently brings about experiences similar to mystical breakthroughs that occur spontaneously or through prolonged spiritual practice. People who had such experiences in the research setting more often than not attributed great significance to them, ranking them among the top experiences of their lives. Additionally, most of these individuals reported positive changes in mood, outlook, and behavior, which friends and family members tended to corroborate.[45]

The Johns Hopkins study on the mystical experiences catalyzed by psilocybin opened the door for more research. Three more experiments—at UCLA, New York University, and another at Johns Hopkins—tested if the mystical states psilocybin creates can alleviate fear of death in terminally ill cancer patients.

After the first Johns Hopkins experiment, Charles Grob began to clinically research psilocybin at UCLA. Grob is a medical doctor who works as a professor of psychiatry at the UCLA School of Medicine and conducted the first government-approved psychobiological research

---

[42] Griffiths in Miller, 146.

[43] Moreno et al., "Safety, Tolerability, and Efficacy of Psilocybin."

[44] Pollan, *How to Change Your Mind*.

[45] Jesse in Forte, *Entheogens and the Future of Religion*, xi.

study of MDMA, along with being the principal investigator of an international research project studying ayahuasca. The focus of this psilocybin study was to learn if psilocybin could treat anxiety in advanced cancer patients. Beginning in 2004, Grob administered psilocybin—at half the dosage Griffith used—to twelve individuals participating in a double-blind placebo-controlled study. At this moderate dose, no one reported a difficult experience. After treatment, Grob's team helped with integration and remained in touch with participants for a six-month follow-up. "We saw some indices of anxiety improve over time, we saw some indication that mood improved, and overall there was an improved quality of life."[46] The findings were published in the January 2011 issue of the *Archives of General Psychiatry*, which is considered to be the number one influential journal in the field of psychiatry.

This study led to two more experiments that focused on the treatment of anxiety with cancer patients: one at New York University (NYU) and the other at the Johns Hopkins School of Medicine. The results of these studies attracted enormous media attention. Thomas Roberts, professor emeritus at Northern Illinois University, in his book *The Psychedelic Future of the Mind: How Entheogens Are Enhancing Cognition, Boosting Intelligence, and Raising Values* says:

> In a very real sense, the Hopkins study broke the ice for news media to publish other psychedelic findings. It was reported on in more than three hundred newspapers, national TV news broadcasts, websites, and magazines, and continues to be cited often in professional journals.[47]

A December 2016 article in *Time* magazine also noted:

> In two new studies released simultaneously by researchers at New York University and Johns Hopkins, doctors reveal that a single dose of psilocybin—a compound from magic mushrooms—can ease anxiety and

---

[46] Grob in Miller, *Psychedelic Medicine*, 156.

[47] T. Roberts, *Psychedelic Future of the Mind*, 8.

depression for up to six months. . . . The studies, both published in the *Journal of Psychopharmacology*, are accompanied by 11 editorials of support from leaders in psychiatry, including two past presidents of the American Psychiatric Association. "Our results represent the strongest evidence to date of a clinical benefit from psilocybin therapy, with the potential to transform care for patients with cancer-related psychological distress," says NYU study author Dr. Stephen Ross, director of substance abuse services in the Department of Psychiatry at NYU Langone in a statement . . . "The results were remarkable: 60–80% of people in the study reported reductions in their depression and anxiety symptoms that lasted six months after the treatment. . . . Eighty-three percent of people reported increases in their well-being and life satisfaction, and 67% said the trial was one of the top five most meaningful experiences in their lives."[48]

Katherine MacLean, director of the Psychedelic Education and Continuing Care Program and a research scientist at the University of California, Davis, is a postdoctoral fellow and faculty member at Johns Hopkins University School of Medicine and worked with Griffith on his psilocybin experiments. Her role was to study if the psilocybin experiences correlated with increased personality development of the participants. She found that the greatest change in personality structure was what mainstream psychology categorizes as openness.[49] The quality of openness in personality correlates to intelligence, creativity, problem solving, sensitivity to one's feelings and those of others, openness to new ideas, and flexibility when approaching new situations, all essential qualities that are useful in adapting to our swiftly evolving world. MacLean states, "We saw an increase in openness after the single psilocybin session with the highest dose. That increase in openness persisted for up to more than a year after the session in the people who had this classical mystical experience."[50] The measurement of transformation is

---

[48] Sifferlin, "Just One Dose," 2.

[49] MacLean in Miller, *Psychedelic Medicine*.

[50] MacLean in Miller, 146.

based on a self-reporting survey of two hundred questions that are used in the field of personality research in psychology. The finding is significant, MacLean points out, because research in personality development has traditionally shown that personality begins to solidify around the age of thirty.[51] She concludes, "We saw increases in openness that were larger than you might expect, even over decades of life experience, if you extrapolate a growth curve that people might be on. So it seems fairly permanent in the people that we studied."[52]

Katherine MacLean's findings are congruent with those of Robert Kegan, a developmental psychologist who taught at Harvard for forty years and served as educational chair for the Institute of Management and Leadership in Education. In their best seller *Stealing Fire: How Silicon Valley, the Navy SEALS, and Maverick Scientists Are Revolutionizing the Way We Live and Work,* Steven Kotler and Jamie Wheal do a great job of summarizing aspects of Kegan's work and its relationship to psychedelic experiences:

> Robert Kegan discovered that while some adults stay frozen in time, a select few achieved meaningful growth. Right around middle age, for example, Kegan noticed that some people moved beyond generally well-adjusted adulthood, or what he called "Self-Authoring," into a different stage entirely: "Self-Transforming."
>
> Defined by heightened empathy, an expanded capacity to hold differing and even conflicting perspectives, and a general flexibility in how you think of yourself, self-transforming is the developmental stage associated with wisdom. While it usually takes three to five years for adults to move through a given stage of development, Kegan found that the further you go up that pyramid, the fewer people make it to the next stage. The move from self-authoring to self-transforming, for example? Fewer than 5 percent of us ever make that jump.

---

[51] MacLean in Miller, 147.

[52] MacLean in Miller, 147.

But in all of this developmental research, buried in the footnotes about those self-transcending 5 percenters, lay a curious fact. A disproportionate number of them had dabbled in ecstasis: often beginning with psychedelics and, after that, making meditation, martial arts, and other state-shifting practices a central part of their lives. Many of them described their frequent access to non-ordinary states as the "turbo-button" for their development.[53]

These research results also correlate with the findings of integral philosopher Ken Wilber, who synthesized hundreds of models of development. Though Wilber focused on meditation as the primary method of consciousness development, he concludes that, with repeated experiences, altered states can become permanent traits.[54]

In Europe, Amanda Feilding, a scientist and founder of the Beckley Foundation (a UK-based think tank focused on psychedelic research and drug policy reform), conducted an experiment to see if psilocybin works as medicine for treatment-resistant depression. The average volunteer in the study suffered from eighteen years of depression and had been unresponsive to every other form of treatment.[55] The experiment showed that 67 percent of participants had significant improvement after one week of treatment and 42 percent remained depression-free three months later.[56] This is one of the highest success rates ever recorded in comparison to traditional methods and is higher than ketamine treatment for depression.[57] The World Health Organization has identified depression as the leading cause of disability worldwide;[58] by definition people with treatment-resistant depression generally have not

---

[53] Kotler and Wheal, *Stealing Fire*, 92.

[54] Wilber, *Integral Psychology*; Wilber, *Integral Spirituality*.

[55] Feilding, "Psilocybin and Depression."

[56] Feilding, 160.

[57] Feilding, 163.

[58] World Health Organization, "Depression."

responded to traditional treatment, and the psilocybin treatment can bring hope to this growing global population. After the overwhelming success of the study, Amanda Feilding also went to Johns Hopkins to work with Roland Griffiths to see if psilocybin might aid in overcoming nicotine addiction. With just two high-dose experiences, 80 percent of participants were still abstaining from nicotine at their six-month follow-up, which is unprecedented.[59] Johns Hopkins is currently carrying out a similar study on alcohol addiction.[60]

Some current ongoing studies are integrating a brain-imaging component. In 2016 Amanda Feilding, David Nichols, and Robin Carhart-Harris published fMRI brain scan images of participants under the influence of psilocybin and LSD. What they found was that psilocybin and LSD dissolve what is known as the default-mode network, which neuroscientists describe as the ego network in the brain.[61] (The results of this study, along with a deeper dive into the neuroscience of psychedelics, is explored further in a section presenting the evolution of the brain in chapter 5.) When the results of the fMRIs were published, Judson Brewer, a former researcher at Yale who used fMRI to study the brains of experienced meditators and now is the director of research at the Center for Mindfulness at the University of Massachusetts Medical School, shared that "the brain scans of people that took psilocybin look like the brains of experienced meditators."[62] This perhaps makes more credible the possibility that psilocybin can catalyze genuine mystical experiences similar to those that some people arrive at through other, conventionally accepted spiritual practices.

In 2017 Roland Griffiths and Stephen Ross, who conducted the psilocybin experiments at Johns Hopkins and NYU, brought their clinical trial results to the FDA with the hopes of winning a Phase III approval to

---

[59] Feilding, "Psilocybin and Depression," 162.

[60] Feilding, 163.

[61] Pollan, *How to Change Your Mind*.

[62] Pollan, 305.

continue their research on psilocybin as a treatment for anxiety in cancer patients. Impressed with their results, the FDA surprised Griffith and Ross by asking them to expand their focus and ambition: "To test whether psilocybin could be used to treat the much larger and more pressing problem of depression in the general population."[63] A similar situation happened in Europe when psilocybin researchers were asked by the European Medicines Agency to enlarge their next experiment to include treatment-resistant depression, which afflicts more than 800,000 Europeans.[64] Like MDMA—which has now entered into the third and final phase of earning FDA approval as a treatment for PTSD and has wide nonpartisan support because of its focus on helping veterans—psilocybin is moving toward federal legalization. As Michael Pollan notes, one is hard-pressed to find anyone opposing further scientific research on psychedelics.[65] The stigma around psychedelics has dramatically transformed since the 1960s. We are now in a time when the government, medical institutions, and academic environment are now showing support.

In October 2018 the US Food and Drug Administration (FDA) gave psilocybin-assisted therapy the status of a breakthrough therapy, which means it provides a substantial improvement over available therapies. Also in the fall of that year the FDA approved Compass Pathways, a for-profit company, to begin experiments that focus on psilocybin-assisted therapy as a possible solution for treatment-resistant depression. They join the Usona Institute, a nonprofit organization that has also been approved to begin research on psilocybin to assist alleviating depression. "For the first time in U.S. history, a psychedelic drug is on the fast track to getting approved for treating depression by the federal government" states a 2018 article in *Rolling Stone*.[66] The proposed Compass Pathways study involves administering psilocybin to 216 patients in twelve to fifteen different research sites

---

[63] Pollan, 375.

[64] Pollan, 377.

[65] Pollan.

[66] Hartman, "Psilocybin Could Be Legal," para 1.

across Europe and North America,[67] while the Usona trials will take place in five to seven different research sites across the United States. Compass Pathways was created by George Goldsmith, who started and worked in several companies in the fields of computer science, business, and medicine, and his spouse Ekaterina Malievskaia, a medical doctor focusing on internal medicine and public health. When their son began university, he developed severe depression, and in their search to understand depression they came across the research on psilocybin and its amazing therapeutic results. Malievskaia says, "It was interesting science but there was no pathway to patients."[68] Compass Pathways is now backed by billionaire investors, and their financial support marks a stark contrast to the psychedelic research of the past. Most research on psychedelics has been carried out by nonprofit and academic organizations that raise money through public donations for research trials that cost millions of dollars or are limited to the budget allowed by a university. Shelby Hartman, in her November 2018 *Rolling Stone* article, states:

> There's consensus among the psychedelic community that Compass' success with the FDA will make it easier for everyone else in the field to get approved for research. If Compass continues to succeed and gets psilocybin approved for depression, Doblin predicts it will be eligible for "off label" prescription, in which doctors will be able to prescribe it for any condition they see fit. That means all the psilocybin research conducted for academic purposes could be used to prescribe psilocybin for conditions like addiction to cigarettes or alcohol.[69]

There has, however, been controversy surrounding Compass Pathways. They are the first large for-profit company working within the field of psychedelics and were granted a patent for their psilocybin formulation in addressing treatment-resistant depression in early 2020.

---

[67] Cheung, "COMPASS Pathways Receives FDA Approval."

[68] Henriques, "Two Parents' Fight," para 6.

[69] Hartman, "Psilocybin Could Be Legal," para 13.

Many who have been working in the field of psychedelics believe the medicine should remain open-source and patent free. There is a strong argument that it is unethical to patent and own the rights to the plants and fungi that grow on the planet. Still, the movements catalyzed by Compass Pathways and Usona bring psilocybin-assisted psychotherapy closer to legalization than previously projected.

As psilocybin and MDMA become legalized for their therapeutic uses, it will likely lessen the stigma attached to psychedelics and open unrealized pathways that make use of their benefits. These academic studies add a much-needed legitimacy to what individuals have already experienced for themselves and know to be true—that psilocybin and other psychedelic medicines transform lives.

Modern History

In 1936, Bras Pablo Reko, an Austrian-born Mexican ethnobotanist, challenged the prevailing academic understanding at the time that held that the sacred substance the Aztecs called *teonanácatl* (which translates into "the flesh of God") and used in their practices was peyote.[70] Reko suggested the ancient Aztecs used mushrooms rather than peyote. He visited with the Indigenous people in the mountains of Oaxaca, in southern Mexico, to find if entheogenic mushrooms existed in their area. Not only did they confirm his intuition but revealed that sacred mushroom rituals still existed. Richard Evans Schultes, a Harvard ethnobotany student who later become director of the Botanical Museum of Harvard, joined Reko in his expedition to collect samples of these sacred mushrooms from a Mazatec village in Huautla de Jimenez.[71] In 1939 Jean Bassett Johnson, an anthropologist from Mexico City, and his wife, Irmgard Weitlaner, were the first outsiders to attend a mushroom

---

[70] Riedlinger, "'Wondrous Mushroom' Legacy," 30.

[71] Forte, *Entheogens and the Future of Religion*, 131.

ceremony. They did not eat any mushrooms and only participated as observers.[72] That same year, Schultes published his research identifying *teonanácatl*, the Aztec medicine used to commune with God, as a specific psilocybin mushroom. Unfortunately, World War II had just begun, and Schultes's work went overlooked for several years.

Gordon Wasson, who was at the time VP of public relations at J. P. Morgan & Co., became equally enamored with the mushroom traditions of the Maztec and is considered by many to be the West's first ethnomycologist.[73] Wasson and his wife developed a curiosity about gourmet and wild mushrooms and began traveling the world to study the various ways humanity relates to fungi. Robert Graves, a well-known scholar and poet, alerted the Wassons about the mushrooms in Mexico by sending them Schultes's paper.[74] Intrigued and equipped with financial resources, Gordon Wasson made it his mission to go to the Mazatec village. After locating the village, as well as establishing a contact in the society, Wasson made the trip with a photographer. There, Wasson encountered Maria Sabina, a *curandera* that held mushroom ceremonies. After some discussions, he was invited to participate. In 1980, twenty-five years after his first mushroom ceremony, Wasson wrote:

> In the lives of us all, even those who are most earthbound, there are moments when the world stops, when the most humdrum things suddenly and unaccountably clothe themselves with beauty, haunting and ravishing beauty . . . for the mushroomic visions are an endless sequence of those flashes. . . . We suspect that, in its fullest sense, the creative faculty, whether in humanities, or science or industry, that most precious of man's distinct possessions and the one most clearly partaking of the divine, is linked in some way with the area of the mind that the mushroom unlocks.[75]

---

[72] Riedlinger, "'Wondrous Mushroom' Legacy," 131.

[73] Riedlinger.

[74] Letcher, *Shroom*, 236.

[75] Wasson as cited in Riedlinger, "'Wondrous Mushroom' Legacy," 89.

On May 13, 1957, *Life* magazine published Wasson's article detailing his mushroom experience in the Mexican ceremony. In time, what took place in Wasson's first ceremony with Maria Sabina set off a series of events that transformed Western consciousness—including psychology, technology, art, religion, and law—in more ways than can directly be measured. The article also had enormous unintended consequences for the Mazatec people.

Maria Sabina was born Dona Maria in 1894 in the Mexican state of Oaxaca; *Sabina* (meaning "wise one") indicates the shamanic role into which she was initiated by the Mazatec elders.[76] Dona Maria first ate psilocybin mushrooms at age seven after picking them out of the ground, and she took them while playing in a field with her sister. In the psilocybin state, the mushrooms told her that they would help her if she ever needed it. A year later, her uncle got sick. Even after seeing many healers, he was not cured. Maria ate some mushrooms and asked them for help. They told her what herbs her uncle needed to cure the "evil spirits" in his blood and even told her where to find these herbs. Within days of her uncle eating these herbs, he was cured. She knew at that moment that these mushrooms would become her way of life, and Maria Sabina went on to heal hundreds of people. Of the mushrooms, she says:

> There is a world beyond ours, a world that is far away, nearby, and invisible. And there is where God lives, where the dead live, the spirits and the saints, a world where everything has already happened and everything is known. That world talks. It has a language of its own. I report what it says. The sacred mushroom takes me by the hand and brings me to the world where everything is known. It is they, the sacred mushrooms, that speak in a way I can understand. I ask them and they answer me. When I return from the trip that I have taken with them, I tell what they have told me and what they have shown me.[77]

---

[76] Allen, *Maria Sabina.*

[77] Sabina as cited in Schultes, Hofmann, and Rätsch, *Plants of the Gods*, 156.

Gordon Wasson presented a saintly portrayal of Maria Sabina as a mushroom priestess with the national media. People around the world became aware of her and traveled to visit this mystical woman. At first, pilgrims arrived bearing gifts with wishes to expand into mushroom states under her care. As the 1960s counterculture roared into a critical mass, waves of young thrill-seeking hippies and college students voyaged to Mexico to see her. On any given day, approximately seventy international pilgrims camped in the village of Huautla de Jimenez.

The entire Mazatec population consists of approximately 305,000 people. They are indigenous to the Sierra Mazateca, a part of the Sierra Madre de Oaxaca mountain range. Huautla de Jimenez, the largest pueblo in the Mazatec region, is home to about 33,000 Mazatecs. Some of the travelers that came to visit Huautla de Jimenez at this time were disrespectful. Hedonistic personalities trashed the town in their search for a high, and many of the villagers felt their way of life was being destroyed. They held Maria Sabina responsible for the intruders ruining their quiet mountain community, and at one point a group of locals burned down her house.

As Maria Sabina grew older, she began to resent the waves of people that came into her village and what it had cost her. However, it is said that before her death in 1985, Maria Sabina spent most of her final years teaching students how to communicate with the mushrooms.[78] Presently, Huautla de Jimenez dedicates July 22 as Maria Sabina Day. Hundreds of people parade in her honor, and her grave is adorned with flowers and relics of her mushroom medicines.

Wasson's article was the first time that mainstream America heard of psychedelics.[79] News of Wasson's discovery reached Albert Hofmann, the chemist who in 1943 discovered the psychedelic properties of LSD, all the way in Switzerland. Wasson brought Hofmann to Mexico to study the mushrooms, and Hofmann was the first to isolate and name

---

[78] Krippner, "Salvador Roquet Remembered."

[79] Goldsmith, *Psychedelic Healing*, 95.

psilocybin and psilocin. The results were published in the journal *Experientia* in 1958. In his autobiography *LSD: My Problem Child: Reflections on Sacred Drugs, Mysticism and Science,* he writes on the similarity of LSD (which is also derived from fungi) and psilocybin and on the unique chemical structure that comprises psilocybin in nature:

> The chemical structures of these mushroom factors deserve special attention in several respects. Psilocybin and psilocin belong, like LSD, to the indole compounds, the biological important class of substances in the plant and animal kingdoms. Particular chemical features common to both the mushroom substances and LSD show that psilocybin and psilocin are closely related to LSD, not only with regard to psychic effects but also to their chemical structures. Psilocybin is the phosphoric acid ester of psilocin and, as such, is the first and hitherto only phosphoric-acid-containing indole compound discovered in nature. The phosphoric acid residue does not contribute to the activity, for the phosphoric-acid-free psilocin is just as active as psilocybin, but it makes the molecule more stable. While psilocin is readily decomposed by the oxygen in air, psilocybin is a stable substance.[80]

Psilocybin and psilocin are both psychoactive compounds found in the same mushrooms, but as Hofmann notes, only psilocybin is stable, which is why the focus has been on psilocybin and not psilocin.

Wasson's article in *Life* magazine also inspired Timothy Leary, at the time a well-respected professor of psychology at Harvard, to voyage to Mexico and try psilocybin mushrooms, which he did with friends at a Mexican villa.[81] Deeply impressed by his experience with psilocybin, Leary created the Harvard Psilocybin Project.[82] Accompanying Leary through his adventures were his two Harvard associates Ralph Metzner and Richard Alpert. Metzner went on to write several books about

---

[80] Hofmann, *LSD: My Problem Child*, 128.

[81] Goldsmith, *Psychedelic Healing*, 95; Leary, "Initiation of the 'High Priest.'"

[82] Metzner, *Sacred Mushroom of Visions*.

psychedelics and teach at the California Institute of Integral Studies; Richard Alpert wrote the popular 1971 book *Be Here Now* and came to be known as the spiritual teacher Ram Dass. The work of these three psychologists, promoting and studying psychedelics at Harvard, helped prompt the psychedelic revolution of the 1960s. The influence from the West Coast—Ken Kesey and the Merry Pranksters, the Grateful Dead, the mass Acid Tests in Golden Gate Park and elsewhere—played an important role as well.

Though it was psilocybin mushrooms that initiated all three Harvard researchers into psychedelic states of consciousness, it was largely LSD that spread into the wider culture. Cultivation methods for psilocybin mushrooms would not be discovered until 1976, and LSD was both cheaper and quicker to produce.[83] The switch from using psilocybin mushrooms to LSD, which is far more potent by weight, came with a cost. Of that time, Metzner writes:

> After two years of working exclusively with psilocybin in moderate doses, LSD made its appearance. . . . The depth and power of those experiences seemed several orders greater than psilocybin. We had referred to psilocybin as a "love drug" because of the interpersonal closeness that often developed among participants in a group session. LSD was never called that; with LSD, experiences of "ego-death" and "disintegration" became much more common.[84]

LSD moved from intentional and controlled environments and into widespread recreational use. Understandably, these not-yet-understood medicines frightened the public. A common experience of psychedelic use is the dissolving of cultural conditioning, which only strengthened the younger generation's questioning of identity and the dominant values of society. Western culture had no context or shamanic container for psychedelic experiences. Psychedelic experiences outside of established

---

[83] DeKorne, *Psychedelic Shamanism*, 178.

[84] Metzner, *Sacred Mushroom of Visions*, 34.

ceremonies, without context or support for one's experience, created high levels of tension and anxiety.[85] Though some people began a process of spiritual awakening, many then looking to Eastern wisdom to understand their experiences,[86] others struggled with the fear and panic that can arise from boundary-dissolving experiences without the right set and setting. In reaction, the courts, without viewing any of the scientific evidence or acknowledging the countless positive benefits of psychedelics in the right set and setting, made all known psychedelics, including mescaline and psilocybin, illegal. They became classified as Schedule 1 substances—that is, as providing no medical value, addictive, and in the same category as heroin.

After reviewing the cultural, scientific, and legal material of this period as research for his book, Michael Pollan concludes:

> Where Leary and the counterculture ultimately parted ways with the first generation of researchers was in deciding that no such container—whether medical, religious, or scientific—was needed and that an unguided, do-it-yourself approach to psychedelics was just fine. . . . But the biggest thing we might have learned is that these powerful medicines can be dangerous—both to the individual and to the society—when they don't have a sturdy social container: a steadying set of rituals and rules—protocols—governing their use, and the crucial involvement of a guide, the figure that is usually called a shaman . . . this is, I think, the greatest lesson of the 1960s experiment with psychedelics: the importance of finding the proper context, or container, for these powerful chemicals and experiences.[87]

Much of the social upheaval of the 1960s was the result of an unprecedented and unusually sharp break between generations. Pollan remarks, "For what other point in history did a society's young undergo a searing

---

[85] DeKorne, *Psychedelic Shamanism*, 177; Pollan, *How to Change Your Mind*.

[86] Badiner and Grey, *Zig Zag Zen*.

[87] Pollan, *How to Change Your Mind*, 215.

rite of passage with which the previous generation was unfamiliar?"[88] Traditionally, cultural rites of passage generally create lineages where elders weave together with younger generations in rituals, enabling a cohesive society that gradually evolves while passing down traditions. Instead, "the psychedelic journey into the 1960s, which at its conclusion dropped its young travelers onto a psychic landscape unrecognizable to their parents," caused fear in the older generation and left the younger generation with no trusted elders to guide them.[89]

After 1965, most scientific studies in the United States using psychedelics became illegal, though in some foreign countries psychedelic treatments continued until 1982. In October 1966 the FDA sent letters to over sixty psychedelic researchers living across the United States, ordering them to stop their work.[90] In the nineteen different psilocybin studies that remained between 1962 and 1982, most of them outside of the United States, over 1,970 patients and volunteers were administered psilocybin within the context of rigorous study. What scientists found was that 65 percent of the patients with serious and chronic neurosis showed significant improvement.[91] Though psychedelics seemed to show more promise than other medications and traditional therapy, it wouldn't be until Rick Strassman's research on DMT in 1992 that scientific studies with psychedelics in the United States legally resumed.[92]

In his book *Psychedelic Shamanism*, Jim DeKorne, who founded the *Entheogenic Review*, writes briefly about the cultural history of psychedelics and the emergence of one of its most influential voices—Terence

---

[88] Pollan, 126.

[89] Pollan, 126.

[90] Pollan, 217.

[91] Passie, "Psilocybin in Psychotherapy," 113–38.

[92] Strassman, *DMT: The Spirit Molecule*.

McKenna. DeKorne, who was in San Francisco during the 1960s at ground zero of the counterculture movement, writes:

> Of course, most psychedelics had been declared Schedule 1 drugs in 1966, but by that late date this was like trying to outlaw fireworks halfway through a Fourth of July celebration. I lived in the Haight-Ashbury during those years and watched in amazement as the scene progressively deteriorated.... The '60's fascination with psychedelics devolved into the '70's cocaine epidemic, which in turn descended into the "just say no" era of the '80's and a whole new status quo begging to be busted loose by a mass shift in consciousness. Out of this darkness emerged Terence McKenna, a drug guru for the '90's who made the psychedelic experience respectable again after years of excess, confusion, and reactionary dogma. It is significant that his drug of choice was the psilocybin mushroom.[93]

In the book *Magic Mushroom Explorer: Psilocybin and the Awakening Earth,* Simon Powell echoes DeKorne's emphasis of Terence McKenna's impact on culture through generating awareness of psychedelics, especially psilocybin mushrooms:

> McKenna—who died in 2000—was without a doubt the greatest spokesperson for the judicious use of psilocybin that the modern world has known....What Timothy Leary was to the acid-dropping 1960s McKenna was to the shamanic fungus wielding 1990s. . . . He was a psychedelic polymath, a turned-on Carl Sagan, a spellbinding bard of the highest order. . . . More important, he was stating in a cogent and convincing manner that psilocybin fungi were a valuable spiritual resource and that their visionary effects were of profound importance for the future of our species.[94]

McKenna's personal story is as extraordinary as a psychedelic experience itself. In 1971, while enrolled at the University of California, Berkeley,

---

[93] DeKorne, *Psychedelic Shamanism,* 177.

[94] Powell, *Magic Mushroom Explorer,* 17.

Terence and his brother, Dennis McKenna, felt inspired by their experiences with LSD and DMT, and so flew with friends to the Amazon to look for ayahuasca, a brew containing DMT that is used by Indigenous South American shamans in ceremony. This was decades before the popularization of ayahuasca and the tourist industry now growing around it; back then it was incredibly hard to find. Their plan was to explore the Amazon until they came upon an Indigenous tribe that used the psychedelic brew—but what the brothers and their friends primarily encountered, naturally growing all over the jungle, was psilocybin mushrooms. Terence McKenna wrote a book about this spectacular, life-transforming journey titled *True Hallucinations: Being an Account of the Author's Extraordinary Adventures in the Devil's Paradise.*

The McKenna brothers became the first people to find a way to privately cultivate psilocybin mushrooms outside their indigenous environments. They published their techniques under the pseudonyms O. T. Oss and O. N. Oeric in their 1976 book *Psilocybin Magic Mushroom Grower's Guide.* The book was reprinted eight times and sold 100,000 copies by 1981.[95] The techniques presented in the book made it possible for anyone in the world to grow mushrooms privately in their own home. Dennis McKenna went on into academia to study chemistry and botany, did his postdoctoral research at Stanford University, and worked at the Heffter Institute to continue entheogenic research. Terence McKenna became a symbol of the psychedelic intellectual, a much sought-after speaker in lecture circuits and the ambassador of the mushroom for the public.[96] In his book *The New Psychedelic Revolution: The Genesis of the Visionary Age,* James Oroc writes:

> In his last years of his life, Terence was the most popular speaker and main draw at various conferences he attended, as well as a headlining attraction at the raves themselves. The self-declared "Mouthpiece for the Mushroom," McKenna had the rare ability to make a packed

---

[95] Letcher, *Shroom*, 279.

[96] Metzner, *Sacred Mushroom of Visions*, 38.

dance floor sit down between DJs and listen as he waxed eloquently
about the wild beauty in the mystery of the psychedelic, often for
hours and hours on end. His extraordinary capacity for the spoken
word and the discovery of a willing and captivated audience coin-
cided with the Internet revolution, and many in McKenna's audience
were digitally sophisticated. Since his death these fans have produced
a seemingly infinite number of recordings and podcasts that have
immortalized his words and philosophy.[97]

Terence McKenna inspired many artists and intellectuals with his talk
of mushrooms—including philosophical comedian Bill Hicks, visionary
artist Alex Grey, and mycologist Paul Stamets. The linguist Diana Reed
Slattery, in her book *Xenolinguistics: Psychedelics, Language, and the Evolution of Consciousness,* based on her doctoral dissertation, writes,

> I will always think of Terence McKenna, given my bias, of course, as
> a master xenolinguist, communicating the Unspeakable in such ways
> that we can get a taste. That taste, that rhetorical invitation, has been
> enough to deputize a generation of psychonauts . . . to explore the
> marvels he so seductively presents.[98]

Sound bites of Terence's talks were integrated in the work of many
musicians, as well as DJ sets during rave scenes and festivals for decades.
Terence McKenna, being an articulate and outspoken representative of
the countercultural, proclaimed that what society needs is an Archaic
Revival—a reintegration of psychedelics and tribal values into culture.[99]

Recent scientific research has brought psychedelics back from the
counterculture and into greater public awareness. As mentioned in the
last section, research on psilocybin over the last two decades—at Johns
Hopkins, NYU, UCLA, University of Arizona, and Imperial College

---

[97] Oroc, *New Psychedelic Revolution*, 27.

[98] Slattery, *Xenolinguistics*, 281.

[99] T. McKenna, *Archaic Revival*.

of London—has made international headlines. Their findings show unparalleled results in psychological healings in the areas of addiction and anxiety, as well as in the catalyzing of mystical experiences, and have helped shed light into the neuroscience of the brain.[100] MAPS's research with MDMA and its effort toward legalizing it for therapeutic uses constantly keeps psychedelics in the news. Michael Pollan's *How to Change Your Mind* became a national best seller, spreading awareness of the research on psychedelics and bringing to mainstream attention the underground field of psychedelic psychotherapy. The California Institute of Integral Studies began a psychedelic psychotherapy certificate program to train therapists in psychedelics so that facilitators are trained once psychedelics become legal. Compass Pathways and Usona Institute have initiated efforts to federally legalize psilocybin-assisted psychotherapy. Paul Stamets and Louie Schwartzberg released their popular film *Fantastic Fungi* in 2019, and half the film is on the science of psilocybin. In November 2020 Oregon voted to legalize psilocybin psychotherapy across the state. In the summer of 2021 the state of California advanced a bill to decriminalize psychedelics. Transformational festivals such as Burning Man (which sells out at a 70,000-person capacity and would probably be ten times larger if allowed) are filled with workshops and talks on psychedelics and include thousands of psychonauts. Surveys show that about one in ten Americans have used psychedelics.[101] "National Surveys on Drug Use and Health have indicated that more than 650,000 people a year in the United States used a hallucinogen (not including MDMA) for the first time."[102]

This chapter presented examples of psilocybin experiences; the science showing that psilocybin reliably produces unparalleled healing for previously incurable conditions, like chronic depression; and a

---

[100] Feilding, "Psilocybin and Depression"; Miller, *Psychedelic Medicine*; Richards, *Sacred Knowledge*; Pollan, *How to Change Your Mind*.

[101] Kotler and Wheal, *Stealing Fire*.

[102] Jesse in Forte, *Entheogens and the Future of Religion*, xii.

brief history of psilocybin in Western culture. What appears evident in each of these areas is that comprehension of psychedelic phenomena lies beyond the bounds of the current deconstructive postmodern paradigms. The scientific materialism of modernity cannot make sense of the mystical experiences catalyzed by psilocybin, and the relativism of postmodernism that reduces perspectives to cultural conditioning cannot make sense of the power of psilocybin to mediate similar mystical experiences in people across the globe. To make sense of how psilocybin and its effects are possible, the next two chapters present an evolutionary, integral, and ecological context for understanding psychedelics, with a special focus on psilocybin mushrooms.

2

AN INTEGRAL APPROACH
TO PSYCHEDELICS

I ntegral philosophy, or integral theory, popularized by philosopher Ken Wilber, aims at a comprehensive, multidisciplinary understanding of reality and is sometimes referred to as "the theory of everything." Steve McIntosh, in his 2007 book *Integral Consciousness and the Future of Evolution*, writes: "Integral philosophy is a new understanding of how the influences of evolution affect the development of consciousness and culture."[1] Though it draws on philosophers throughout time, only in the last three decades has it come together into a coherent whole.[2] Integral philosophy can be described as an evolutionary perspective that includes both matter and consciousness. It is a useful and invaluable lens through which we can best understand psychedelics.

---

[1] McIntosh, *Integral Consciousness and the Future of Evolution*, 2.

[2] McIntosh.

The Quadrants

After decades of contemplating evolution through the lenses of psychology, systems theory, spirituality, and the natural sciences, integral philosopher Ken Wilber discovered that all models fit under just four categories, or *quadrants*. Wilber's books *Sex, Ecology, Spirituality: The Spirit of Evolution* and the more accessible *A Brief History of Everything* set forth a comprehensive overview of the quadrant approach. The quadrants represent four aspects of understanding evolution. One can imagine the Big Bang at the center of the quadrants with respect to dimensions of consciousness, matter, individual, and collective evolution mapped out. As time moves forward the development of consciousness and the complexity of matter can be described from these four different perspectives. The upper quadrants describe the development of individual subjects (e.g., animals and people) and objective bodies (e.g., atoms, molecules, biological organs), while the lower quadrants map out the collective evolution of both psychology (e.g., culture, values, and world views) and the organization of systems (e.g., ecology, law, economics). The left quadrants describe the interior components of consciousness, whether that be an individual's subjective experience or a culture's beliefs and values, and the right quadrants describe the exterior, or physical components, whether one's body, society, or the cosmos.

The upper-left, or subjective, quadrant describes states and stages of an individual's consciousness. It also includes the psychological development one may experience throughout one's life, as articulated by the personality development models of Sigmund Freud, Abraham Maslow, and Robert Kegan.[3] This quadrant is the one most obviously relevant to psychedelics, as psychedelics create an almost instantaneous state shift in consciousness, including changing the perception of space, time, and identity. Cognitive and emotional capacities are also enhanced or impaired with psychedelics, depending on dose and set and setting. The subjective experience of psychedelics, including the visionary realm, is the domain of the upper-left/subjective quadrant.

---

[3] Freud, *Basic Writings*; Maslow, *Theory of Human Motivation*; Kegan, *Evolving Self*.

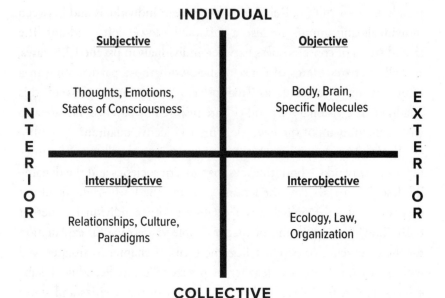

INDIVIDUAL

Subjective	Objective
Thoughts, Emotions, States of Consciousness	Body, Brain, Specific Molecules
Intersubjective	Interobjective
Relationships, Culture, Paradigms	Ecology, Law, Organization

INTERIOR

EXTERIOR

COLLECTIVE

FIGURE 2. Quadrants.

The upper-right, or objective, quadrant describes the physical body, whether that be of an atom, molecule, cell, or a human body. This is the domain that reductive-materialist philosophies tend to focus on to the exclusion of the other quadrants. The upper-right quadrant describes the actual psychedelic molecule, as well as its physiological effects on the body and brain once it has entered the human system. How psychedelics work with brain receptors, catalyze the growth of new neurons, or create a hyperconnected brain state are all qualities of the upper-right quadrant.[4] Anything that a psychedelic does that can be measured and objectively seen is the domain of the right objective quadrants.

The lower-left, or intersubjective, quadrant corresponds to the realm of collective experience, including what Carl Jung called the collective unconscious.[5] This realm describes the belief systems, myths, and

---

[4] Carhart-Harris and Nutt, "Serotonin and Brain Function"; Renter, "Grow and Repair Brain Cells"; Ghose, "Hyperconnected Brain."

[5] Campbell, *Portable Jung.*

paradigms of a culture. Relationships between individuals and between individuals and groups are also a part of the lower-left quadrant. The shared states of consciousness between individuals in psychedelic states, as well as shared states of consciousness with those participating in a ceremony or psychedelic-assisted psychotherapy, are realms of this quadrant. The visionary art and culture inspired by psychedelics are also within the domain of the lower-left/intersubjective quadrant.

The lower-right, or interobjective, quadrant represents systemic structures and networks—both the laws that govern societies and the dynamics described by systems theory and ecology. The lower-right quadrant describes how a person behaves in relation to other individuals, whether those individuals be atoms, plants, or people. An ecological explanation for the emergence of psychedelics (the focus of chapter 3) situates well within this quadrant. The legality of psychedelics, as Schedule 1 substances on a federal level, and the movement of many cities and states to decriminalize them on local levels, also fall within the domain of the lower-right quadrant. Psychedelics have obvious impacts on our states of consciousness (upper-left quadrant), our brains (upper-right quadrant), and our culture (lower-left quadrant). But we need radical new structures of social organization that are congruent with the insights offered by psychedelics. Some of these structures will be explored in chapter 6.

Holons

Another of Wilber's contributions has been popularizing Arthur Koestler's concept of the *holon*.[6] Koestler was a Hungarian British author and journalist whose work crossed a spectrum of topics, from politics and philosophy to psychology and science. The concept of the holon was originally put forward in Koestler's 1967 book *The Ghost in the Machine*:

---

[6] Wilber, *Sex, Ecology, Spirituality*; Wilber, *Brief History of Everything*.

It seems preferable to coin a new term to designate these nodes on the hierarchic tree which behave partly as wholes or wholly as parts, according to the way you look at them. The term I would propose is "holon," from the Greek *holos* = whole, with the suffix *on* which, as in prot*on* or neutr*on*, suggests a particle or part.

"A man," wrote Ben Jonson, "coins not a new word without some peril; for if it happens to be received, the praise is but moderate; if refused, the scorn is assured." Yet I think the holon is worth the risk, because it fills a genuine need. It also symbolizes the missing link—or rather series of links—between the atomistic approach of the Behaviorist and the holistic approach of the Gestalt psychologist.[7]

Arthur Koestler tried psilocybin with Timothy Leary and published an essay called "Return Trip to Nirvana" about his experience.[8] The psychologist Stanislav Grof, with over fifty years of experience researching psychedelic states, also uses the Greek term *holos*, meaning "wholeness," in his term *holotropic*. Holotropic states of consciousness, generally catalyzed by psychedelics, are states of consciousness that organically move toward wholeness.[9] As Koestler points out, the introduction of the term *holon* satisfies a genuine need of speaking of something as both a whole and also part.

Each holon contains all the quadrants.[10] That is to say, each holon has an experience (upper-left/subjective quadrant), a physical body (upper-right/objective), a shared culture with other holons (lower-left/intersubjective), and a networking structure with other holons (lower-right/interobjective). Wilber describes holons as tetra-arising, meaning that all holons simultaneously express these four characteristics, which are themselves part of a singular phenomenon that includes these four

---

[7] Koestler, *Ghost in the Machine*, 48–49.

[8] Letcher, *Shroom*, 229.

[9] Grof, *Future of Psychology*.

[10] Wilber, *Sex, Ecology, Spirituality*.

facets.[11] As Wilber points out, all of reality is made up of holons. They create a multidimensional, intersecting web consisting of inherently relational nodes (holons) in a network that gives rise to our evolving and complex existence.

It is important to emphasize that holons are sentient, based on the upper-left quadrant's assertion that every holon has an interior or a degree of subjectivity, which is the main requirement for consciousness. This perspective is in alignment with panpsychism (a term from the field of philosophy of mind), which the *Oxford* dictionary defines as "the doctrine or belief that everything material, however small, has an element of individual consciousness."[12] The experience of those who partake in higher doses of psychedelics confirms this axiom of the left, or interior, quadrants: that consciousness pervades—and connects—every part of the universe.[13] This resonates with the philosophical work of Alfred North Whitehead, the Cambridge philosopher and mathematician who later taught at Harvard and had a great influence on Integral philosophy and mathematics.[14] He believed that each individual element or entity of the cosmos, including atoms, can be better understood as an organism rather than as particles of matter. He called his approach the philosophy of organism, which also became known as process-relational philosophy.[15] The philosophy of organism states that varying degrees of mind exist all throughout the development of atoms, molecules, cells, and higher-order organisms. This helps explain the evolution of the natural plant and fungi psychedelics themselves (which is the focus of the next chapter).

---

[11] Wilber, *Religion of Tomorrow*.

[12] *Oxford English Dictionary*, s.v. "panpsychism."

[13] Grof, *Cosmic Game*; T. McKenna, Sheldrake, and Abraham, *Chaos, Creativity, and Cosmic Consciousness*; Doyle, *Darwin's Pharmacy*.

[14] Whitehead, *Process and Reality*.

[15] Whitehead, *Science and the Modern World*; Mesle, *Process-Relational Philosophy*.

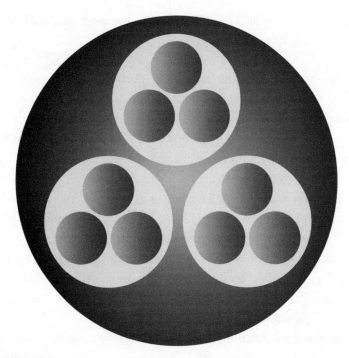

FIGURE 3. Holons.

Holons are physical-experiential entities that evolve by relating to one another. The structure of a holon is that it is made up of other holons, which are themselves made up of holons. They are systems within systems, each with its own dynamic processes. Through this lens, all of existence, composed of holons within holons, can be seen as a structure composed of beings within beings—a living universe that is both internally and externally interconnected.

Koestler also asserts that the coming together of holons, which form systems within systems, creates a hierarchical structure:

> We may say that the organism in its structural and functional aspect is a hierarchy of self-regulating holons which function (a) as autonomous wholes in supra-ordination to their part, (b) as dependent parts in sub-ordination to controls on higher levels, (c) in co-ordination with their local environment. Such a hierarchy of holons should rightly be called

a *holarchy*—but, remembering Ben Jonson's warning, I shall spare the reader this further neologism.[16]

It is important to point out that when discussing hierarchies what is being expressed are levels of organization. In this context, hierarchy does not necessarily mean oppressive structures. Hierarchies are found throughout nature—most apparently in the nested structure of atoms within molecules within cells. They are efficient strategies for organization and coordination. Wilber adds that each level transcends and includes the levels that came before, just as cells still include molecules, which still include atoms.[17] Each holon transcends and includes its predecessors, and by doing so a holon retains much of what was achieved and useful at a previous level of development. Some patterns are lost or repressed. For example, an electron has the capability to manifest in and out of existence at an atomic level. That ability does not continue into the level of cellular development.

Holarchies, the relational structure of holons, can be described in terms of *depth* and *span*, which can be thought of respectively as "quality" and "quantity."[18] A higher level in the holarchy holds more depth under it, leading to greater complexity. The shallower the level in the holarchy, the more quantity there is and therefore greater span. This is because the depth of the higher is built upon the quantity of the lower. There are more atoms in the universe than molecules because molecules are composed of atoms. There are more molecules in the universe than cells because cells are composed of molecules. There are more cells in the universe than humans because humans are composed of cells. There is a greater span of atoms in the universe than humans because humans are composed of them, but humans contain greater depth.

---

[16] Koestler, *Ghost in the Machine*, 103.

[17] Wilber, *Sex, Ecology, Spirituality*.

[18] Wilber, *Brief History of Everything*.

Since humans, in their interior, also contain the interior of a larger holon (according to the assertion of the lower-left/intersubjective quadrant), it should theoretically be possible to experience the larger holon of which one is a part. This is what people in psychedelic states report over and over again. Stanislav Grof writes:

> Holons can also create emergent holons of a higher order. . . . What is important from the point of view of our discussion is that in holotropic states all the different individual, as well as social, holons have corresponding subjective states. These states make it possible for us to experientially identify in a very authentic and convincing way with any aspects of existence that in our ordinary everyday consciousness we experience as objects separate from us. . . . Some of the people who have experienced holotropic states reported that they experienced consciousness of an ecosystem, of the totality of Life as a cosmic phenomenon, or of our entire planet. In transpersonal states, all aspects of existence as they manifest on different levels and domains of reality, can under certain circumstances become potentially available for conscious experience.[19]

This affirms what people in psychedelic states report over and over again, as illustrated be the examples in chapter 1. The next chapter expands these individual experiences of wholeness to explore the potential collective power of experiencing greater holons, such as that of entire ecosystems.

Instincts of Consciousness

Wilber states that holons display four fundamental capacities: self-preservation (agency), self-adaption (communion), self-transcendence (eros), and self-dissolution (thanatos).[20] For clarity's sake, I will refer to these four traits throughout the book as *autonomy*, *communion*, *transcendence*, and *dissolution*. These capacities, as they are instinctual

---

[19] Grof, *Cosmic Game*, 64.

[20] Wilber, *Sex, Ecology, Spirituality*.

within consciousness, are fundamental dynamics of consciousness and therefore essential in understanding the transformation that occurs in psychedelic states. These four instincts are best explored through the work of psychologist Abraham Maslow who, along with Stanislav Grof, helped found the field of transpersonal psychology, although these instincts had been discovered and discussed in the field of psychology long before Maslow.

Grof, originally trained in Freudian psychology, writes that Freud's view evolved:

> In his early writings, Freud saw the human psyche as governed by a dynamic tension between two conflicting forces—the sexual drive (libido) and the self-preservation drive (ego instinct). During these early years Freud believed that death had no relevance for psychology; he viewed the unconscious as a realm beyond time and space, incapable of knowing and acknowledging the fact of death. His recognition of the importance of death eventually led Freud to significant reformulation of his theory (Freud 1949, 1975). In this new version of psychoanalysis, the self-preservation instinct was replaced by the death instinct (Thanatos) as the rival of the sexual drive (libido, Eros).[21]

Here we can see Freud framing the instincts as dynamic tensions within the psyche rather than motivations that arise through evolutionary development, as Maslow presents them.[22] Freud called the autonomy instinct the self-preservation drive and communion instinct the sexual drive. In Maslow's perspective, as well as my own, these are not in opposition. Once the self-preservation needs are sufficiently met, the sexual needs arise. Freud eventually revised his theory and focused more on the dissolution, or death, instinct.

---

[21] Grof, *Modern Consciousness Research*, 20.

[22] Maslow, *Theory of Human Motivation*.

Among those of Freud's colleague who believed that Freud was unjustly reducing fundamental qualities of the psyche to sex and death was Carl Jung. Of this, Grof writes:

> Jung disagreed with Freud, stating that creativity would not be reduced to sexuality. He believed creativity came through wrestling with the contradiction that we have a personal self and are a part of a larger whole. Creativity is an innate drive that one channels. Creativity, he believed, is a cosmic energy of the anima mundi, the world soul.[23]

Indeed, creativity can be seen as an aspect of the transcendence instinct, which I will explore at length with the other core instincts of autonomy, communion, and dissolution. These instincts are essential for a comprehensive understanding of human evolution and how psychedelics have played an important role in enhancing those instincts within the model of evolution.

Autonomy

The first instinct of consciousness that is necessary for maintaining an individual's psychic and physical existence is autonomy. The autonomy instinct is the first motivation in evolution and has us focus on our needs as individuals. At the root of this instinct is the desire to maintain a self. This includes the strong drive of self-preservation that we all carry. Without a desire to maintain a constitutional pattern, or internal relationships and integrity of form, all holons would fall apart. Autonomy creates a sense of selfhood, of individuality, regardless of each holon's self-reflective capacity. This includes a felt, or subjective, sense of experience. Alfred North Whitehead, in his magnum opus *Process and Reality*, presents in a logical fashion that feeling is the primary way the universe transmits information. Feeling requires a subject, an experiencer, and as he describes it, feeling is how the whole communicates to each part. He

---

[23] Grof, *Modern Consciousness Research*, 29.

calls this process *prehension*, which is an instantaneous knowing prior to cognitive reflection.[24] This means—staying with the structure of a holarchy—the whole subconsciously influences the parts within its system. In *Science and the Modern World*, which consists of a series of eight lectures he delivered at Harvard in 1925, Whitehead writes that

> the plan of the *whole* influences the very characters of the various subordinates which enter into it. In the case of an animal, the mental states enter into the plan of the total organism and thus modify the plans of the successive subordinate organisms until the ultimate smallest organisms, such as electrons, are reached. Thus an electron within a living body is different from an electron outside it, by reason of the plan of the body. The electron blindly runs either within or without the body; but it runs within the body in accordance with its character within the body; that is to say, in accordance with the general plan of the body, and this plan includes the mental state.[25]

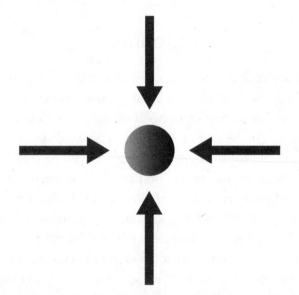

FIGURE 4. Autonomy. The picture shows energy going inward toward the self.

---

[24] Whitehead, *Science and the Modern World*, 73.

[25] Whitehead, 80.

This means one's autonomy is bound within the larger holon it is a part of, while at the same time, the sense of each "I" unconsciously feels all the wholes it encompasses.

Though granting any degree of subjectivity to something as rudimentary as an atom may seem ridiculous to a reductionist-materialist mindset, there have been many brilliant thinkers—from Bergson and Whitehead to Pierre Teilhard de Chardin and Sheldrake—who would agree.[26] Admitting that consciousness pervades the universe, which psychedelics seem to reveal to many explorers, could be seen as the most logical explanation as to why we humans have consciousness to begin with. Otherwise, one is left to conclude that subjectivity arises at some point out of a purely physical universe without reason.

Since autonomy exists as the foundational primordial need to maintain and stabilize an individual's existence, autonomy is the most urgent drive in life. This drive is clearly seen in Maslow's "general dynamic theory" and the first two levels of his famous hierarchy of needs (physiological and safety needs).[27] These drives, though expressed most vividly in humans, are evolutionary movements that run through the realm of biological life. Not only does each of the instincts become more ingrained but its expressions become richer as holons become more complex. The evolutionary self-preservation tendencies of fight, flight, freeze, and fawn that are found throughout the animal kingdom are expressions of the autonomy instinct and serve to preserve the self. The instinct is also deeper than simply psychological. In my definition, autonomy goes beyond self-governance and is the aspect of consciousness that focuses on oneself (this would neurologically correlate with the default-mode network), which includes self-preservation. Self-preservation includes psychological self-preservation (which is probably why the default-mode network is overdeveloped in people with chronic anxiety) and biological self-preservation. Autonomy

---

[26] Bergson, *Matter and Memory*; Whitehead, *Process and Reality*; Teilhard de Chardin, *Human Phenomenon*; R. Sheldrake, *Science Set Free*.

[27] Maslow, *Theory of Human Motivation*, 2.

is also the force that unconsciously preserves integrity of the body—such as breathing, circulating blood, and digesting.

Because of its necessity, autonomy is the primary instinct most often universally expressed by beings, but it can easily be worked on overdrive at the expense of the other natural instincts. Though this instinct has been and continues to be essential for existence, its overexpression at the expense of the other instincts brings out what we consider to be the worst of human qualities. Greed, pride, jealousy, hubris, cowardice, and self-ishness all come out of a wounded or grandiose sense of self and derive from feeling disconnected from others and a larger whole. Without a sense of self to protect or hoard for, none of what we experience as the negative and destructive expressions of human existence would exist, and yet without individuality, there would exist no human experience at all.

Autonomy is what shows up in the psychological landscape as the ego, and fear, anger, anxiety, and shame are the emotional expression of this instinct. At the human level of the holarchy, stress, fear, and pain can activate self-preservation, the autonomy instinct, in the form of defense mechanisms. In neuroscience terms, it is the default-mode network in the brain—the part that is activated when thinking about a sense of self.[28] Research shows that this is the part of the brain that psychedelics inhibit, which allows the experiences of the other instincts.[29]

Without autonomy as a primary function, holons would not have formed through the cosmic evolutionary journey, which requires collabo-ration and independence. When possible, in order to both individually and collectively heal and evolve, one needs to move away from overworking this instinctual drive for independence and enter into the vulnerability and maturity of conscious interdependence, which is already a potential of our larger holon's other quadrants. The autonomous drive must be balanced with our innate drive to seek connection. By easing our internal feelings of stress and deepening into feeling secure, we naturally move toward communion.

---

[28] Pollan, *How to Change Your Mind.*

[29] Anderson, "LSD May Chip Away."

FIGURE 5. Communion. In the image we see a holon moving to connect with other holons of the same depth.

Communion

Once individuals begin to form and then stabilize at the autonomous level, the next thing we see happen is that they instinctively seek to bond with other individuals. This is seen explicitly in Maslow's hierarchy of needs. Maslow writes:

> If both the physiological and the safety needs are fairly well gratified, then there will emerge the love and affection and belongingness needs, and the whole cycle already described will repeat itself with this new center. Now the person will feel keenly, as never before, the absence of friends, or a sweetheart, or a wife, or children. He will hunger for affectionate relations with people in general, namely, for a place in his group, and he will strive with great intensity to achieve this goal. He will want to attain this place more than anything else in the world and may even forget that once, when he was hungry, he sneered at love.[30]

Once the needs for physical security are established, humans seek to connect with other individuals both to secure a sense of safety and to experience love, which is an expression of the intersubjective/lower-left quadrant. This generally comes from an unconscious desire and a deep evolutionary motivation that runs through all creation. Protons, neutrons, and electrons bond in particular configurations to create atoms, building a community through a force of physics termed the strong nuclear force. Atoms, consisting of different amounts of protons, neutrons, and electrons, also begin to bond into larger wholes,

---

[30] Maslow, *Theory of Human Motivation*, 6–7.

creating communities within communities, families within families, through the weak nuclear force. The four fundamental physical forces of physics—gravity, electromagnetism, the weak nuclear force, and the strong nuclear force—are material manifestations of communion. They work to bring and bond physical bodies together. Mammals, with more complex forms of emotional attachment, feel longing, create sexual attraction, and even produce oxytocin to encourage bonding behavior. Communion is the cosmic glue that holds holons together through different forces of attraction.

Over the course of evolution—through learning, integration, and intelligent adaptation—the way communion occurs between individuals expresses itself in more complex ways. Attraction has intelligence embedded within the dynamic, as seen in the patterns or degrees of organization and connection. The holonic structure of the cosmos is evident at every level of existence. For example, molecules connect in geometric patterns; the attraction of gravity is mathematically correlated with mass and distance, while the internal pressure it causes within large cosmic bodies, stars, brings about a metamorphosis of new elements to continue a larger evolutionary process; the mating dance of many animals is infused with a somatic patterning, expressing rhythm through movement, and intelligence in its design and coordination; the sexual energy flowing through all bodies has a momentum flowing toward consummation. These are all processes orienting consciousness and attention toward a destination of unification that brings individuals, particles, and people into relationship through attractive forces.

A good example of the communion instinct is the relationship between children and their parents as described within the psychotherapeutic model of attachment theory.[31] The theory states that primary relational patterns are formed through the parent and child dynamic—specifically between the mother and the infant. Since an infant's survival, and therefore sense of autonomy, depend on the caregiver, trauma

---

[31] Levine and Heller, *Attached.*

forms if caregiving was not adequate. If the caregiver was adequate, the child develops a healthy and strong sense of self and feels generally more comfortable in connection. If the caregiving was not adequate, then it can cause arrested development when it comes to a healthy motivation toward communion. The child develops a pattern of anxiously looking for security through connection (anxious-ambivalent) or becomes overly autonomous (avoidant). If the child felt adequately loved and nurtured and had their needs met, they form a secure attachment style toward the world and other humans, decreasing the intensity of the autonomy instinct by letting their system know everything will be taken care of and that they are generally safe. If, early in life, our primary caregiver refused to give themselves to us or ignored our gestures of affection, we begin to feel anxiety, hate, and aggression that ultimately leads humans on a quest for power over others.[32] Unless healed, they project the patterning of their early environment and become unconsciously attracted to others that trigger their suppressed parts in the hopes that the psyche can reexperience the trauma and heal the initial wounds to free stuck energy.

At its highest expression, the emotional quality of the communal instinct is love. Love stands as the most fundamental attractive energy, of moving closer empathically, and bringing wholes together as parts of something more complex. At the rudimentary level it can be seen as the intersubjective empathic connective experience that systemically attracts all the parts of the cosmos together, which is an expression of their greater intersubjective connection that bonds the whole.[33] Communion creates interconnectivity, encouraging creativity to arise out of the complexity. When the conditions are right and one begins to feel safe and experiences a strong sense of self (autonomy) and feels a sufficient sense of love and belonging (communion) another instinct rises from our depths—transcendence.

---

[32] Rifkin, *Empathic Civilization*, 66.

[33] Swimme and Tucker, *Journey of the Universe*.

Transcendence

In Maslow's model of needs, the transcendence instinct is located in the other upper reaches of the hierarchy—the realms of self-esteem, self-actualization, and self-transcendence.[34] Though the transcendence instinct is present throughout life, it manifests most explicitly in mature forms, especially when one has already gained a strong, secure experience of self and feels a sense of meaning and purpose. These instinctual movements—first forming a self (autonomy), next forming relationships with other selves (communion), and then being of service to a greater whole (transcendence)—are all interdependent forces that arise out of each other and can be seen as the coming together of the different aspects of the quadrants.

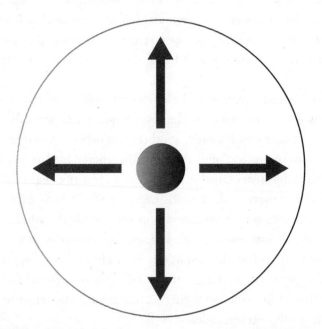

FIGURE 6. Transcendence. In the image we see a holon expanding toward that of the greater holon.

---

[34] Maslow, *Theory of Human Motivation*.

Maintaining the individual's autonomous forms, and then communing these forms into relationships, is not enough for a universe to evolve past the elementary particles. There is a creative motion that ultimately unites these bonded beings into newer levels of wholeness. Transcendence is the process of change, of movement and dynamism itself, ultimately organizing forms into creative and stable structures that continue the process of evolution into greater complexity and novelty. The universe drives toward greater degrees of unity, which means both deeper relationships and more expansive sense of selves. Not only did these instincts arise and form together, they cannot be completely separated. They are interdependent processes that coevolve with each other.

Transcendence is the evolutionary impulse ultimately striving to create higher levels of order and coherence. By doing so, it creates complexity in form and depth in consciousness. In humans, when accompanied with a sense of trust and satisfaction of the autonomous instinct and a feeling of love and social safety of the communal instinct, the transcendence instinct is normally experienced as intuition, creativity, curiosity, and the desire for exploration and learning. Being in touch with the transcendence instinct, while in alignment with autonomy and communion, gives one's life a sense of direction and organization. What psychologists have discovered time and time again is that once infants have bonded with their mothers and established safety, their curiosity leads them to explore their environment and eventually leave for another room outside the presence of the mother.[35] The child's first steps represent an emergent, developmental capacity arising from the transcendence instinct. In adults the instinct shows itself psychologically in the urge for progression, to mature, to evolve one's personality and understanding. Emotionally, it is experienced as curiosity, enchantment, awe, beauty, joy, bliss, potentiality, creativity, and religious feelings.

The transcendence instinct, which has developed into greater complexity and manifestations through a fourteen-billion-year developmental process it itself fueled, has many expressions. One important

---

[35] Rifkin, *Empathic Civilization*.

facet of transcendence is creativity—the quality of bringing something into existence that previously did not exist, further pushing the evolution of the universe. Normally, in the moments when one feels creative and full of inspiration, one also feels full of a real sense of self and a connection to something larger, indicating a fulfillment of both the autonomous and communal instincts. This shows the nested development of communion encompassing autonomy and transcendence encompassing communion. The transcendence instinct correlates with Whitehead's category of creativity, which he said is the category necessary to understand all other categories.[36] It is also the main evolutionary impulse in Terence McKenna's novelty theory, which states that the two main poles in the universe are those of habit and novelty, or newness.[37] McKenna says that the pace of novelty in the cosmos is accelerating as evolution moves toward greater complexity.[38] This evolutionary acceleration toward creative complexity is the focus of the last chapter of this book.

If the transcendence instinct is not active in our personal lives, we become stale, stagnant, and bored. Since all processes naturally move forth through time, without this drive we would not adapt to the movement, and we would stop changing and growing—and, evolutionarily speaking, would die. Here we can see the autonomy and transcendence instincts working in tandem—the autonomy drive calling forth action for self-preservation of form, which correlates with McKenna's notion of habit, and the transcendence instinct bringing us the power to find creative and novel ways to do so.

The transcendence instinct reveals itself most clearly in mystical states, which decades of scientific research has concluded are directly experienced by the majority of subjects who have taken psychedelics in clinical studies.[39] Michael Pollan, who did not consider himself spiritual

---

[36] Whitehead, *Process and Reality.*

[37] McKenna and McKenna, *Invisible Landscape.*

[38] T. McKenna, *Archaic Revival.*

[39] Pollan, *How to Change Your Mind.*

before experimenting with psychedelics, discovered after his psychedelic experiences that the "antonym for 'spiritual' might be 'egotistical.'"[40] Here one can see the contrast between transcendence and autonomy. The spiritual drive of transcendence can be seen in the diminished focus on one's self once a person reaches an adequate degree of functionality and can focus instead on a larger whole. This encourages them to expand their identity beyond the self. Wilber describes this well in his evolution of consciousness, as humans move from egocentric to ethnocentric to worldcentric to kosmocentric stages of identity.[41]

Dissolution

Dissolution correlates with the drive to die, break down, or kill. Generally, this is an instinct that becomes more active when the initial needs of autonomy, communion, and transcendence are not met. Destruction is necessary when a holon is not affirming the positive growth-oriented and life-affirming instincts of evolution. The wisdom of the higher holonic system knows to dissolve and recycle the energy of what does not serve it. Therefore, because this book is focused on evolution, it's the evolution affirming aspects we will be considering. Wilber writes: "If a holon fails to maintain its agency and its communions, then it can break down completely. When it does break down, it decomposes into its subholons: cells decompose into molecules, which break down into atoms . . . And this decomposition is 'self-dissolution,' or simply decomposing into subholons."[42] At a structural level of the cosmos, we can see that holons can break down: organisms die and can dissolve into molecules, which themselves can further dissolve into atoms. Even the process of eating food is of organisms dissolving other organisms into

---

[40] Pollan, *How to Change Your Mind*, 390.

[41] Wilber, *Integral Spirituality*; Wilber, *Integral Vision*.

[42] Wilber, *Brief History of Everything*, 19–20.

molecules necessary to maintain their own autonomy. Perhaps the focus of this instinct that I find most fascinating is how it expresses itself in the psychology of humans—for example, in part of the process of the spiritual journey known as "the dark night of the soul."

In his extraordinary book *Dark Night, Early Dawn*, Christopher Bache, who for three decades taught as a professor of religious studies in the Department of Philosophy and Religion at Youngstown State University and underwent a systematic and deep psychedelic exploration for two decades, writes about the dark night of the soul:

> In order to awaken to our true and essential condition, we must let fall from us everything that we thought we were or thought we needed in the most fundamental sense. In order to reach this naked condition, one must go through a transformational process that the Christian tradition calls the "dark night of the soul." The dark night is an arduous stage of spiritual purification in which the aspirant endures a variety of physical and psychological purifications, eventually undergoing a profound spiritual death and rebirth . . . There are no shortcuts through this night but there are more and less efficient ways of moving through it. Some methods intensify and accelerate the ordeal while others proceed at a gentler, more gradual pace. Psychedelic therapy is an example of the former; it intensifies the purification process and thus concentrates the dark night.[43]

He later continues:

> The dark night is the final stage of a long spiritual process in which our identity as a discrete self is challenged at its core and ultimately surrendered. It culminates in a spiritual death and rebirth that is more profound than mere physical death. According to most mystical traditions, physical death alone does not unravel our deepest instinct for living as a separate self (autonomy), and thus is usually followed by another birth. What dies in the dark night is precisely our deep attachment to separateness itself, and therefore the dark night

---

[43] Bache, *Dark Night, Early Dawn*, 15.

represents the culmination of many lifetimes of spiritual effort . . .
One's edges become softer and more porous, not in a pathological way
that erodes individual agency but in a way which opens one to a *felt*
connection with others and with the life-process itself. Self-interest is
not diminished but extended exponentially. One literally begins to live
a larger life.[44]

This part of the developmental process, known as the dark night of the
soul, is an expression of the dissolution instinct that disintegrates the
psychological structures and mental constructs within us that keep us
separate from living the deep experiential truth of our unity. This process may include surrendering the deep attachments associated with the
autonomy instinct, resulting in confronting the deep fear and depression
that come with letting go the parts of the self that we had identified with. Ultimately, the process is meant to purify our being, so that
we can release the aspects of our self that prevent us from living freer
lives and expressing the deeper essence of autonomy, communion, and
transcendence.

In *Beyond the Brain: Birth, Death and Transcendence in Psychotherapy*,
the psychedelic psychotherapist Stanislav Grof writes about the dark
night being a "death instinct":

The death instinct operates in the organism from the very beginning,
gradually converting it into an inorganic system. This destructive drive
can and must be partially diverted from its primary self-destructive
aim and be directed against another organism. It seems to be irrelevant
whether the death instinct is oriented towards objects in the external
world or against the organism itself, as long as it can fully achieve its
goal, which is to destroy.[45]

Grof, trained in Freudian psychology, writes of Freud: "In his later drastic theoretical revision, he considered various mental phenomena to

---

[44] Bache, 230–31.

[45] Grof, *Beyond the Brain*, 149.

be the products of conflict between Eros, the love instinct striving for union and the creation of higher units, and Thanatos, the death instinct, the purpose of which is destruction and return to the original inorganic condition."[46] Generally unconscious, an instinct exists in both the human mind and body to kill. We can divert that energy from ourselves to others, such as eating other beings, but eventually the dissolution instinct wins and breaks down our own body until we die and decompose back into nature.

In his book *The Ultimate Journey: Consciousness and the Mystery of Death*, Grof presents how the dissolution instinct, expressed in the form of dying, has been perceived and worked with by cultures throughout history. He points out that industrial societies have a disinterest about death in comparison to preindustrial societies, many of which intentionally integrated the dissolution instinct as part of their lives. "This disinterest is even more striking when we compare it to the attitude toward mortality found in preindustrial societies, where the approach to death and dying was diametrically different. Death dominated and captivated the imagination of people in ancient high cultures and provided inspiration for much of their art and architecture."[47] Grof continues to write about the varieties of rituals associated with dying found in cultures around the world and that shamans would practice dying in order to live consciously and prepare for its arrival. Toward the end of the book he presents several case histories of how psychedelics were used with cancer patients to help them come to terms with their death.

Dying itself serves the collective evolution of life. For example, the transformation of energy through the "death" of stars, when they explode energy and matter into space, allows the formation of new molecules that wouldn't otherwise exist and contribute to the formation of biological life. The death of the dinosaurs gave space for the further evolution of higher-order intelligence in the form of mammals to develop. Within

---

[46] Grof, 337.

[47] Grof, *Ultimate Journey*, 19.

our species, death allows the progress of perspective. As a generation dies, power is passed on to a new generation that may have developed different values. This enables the evolution of culture to occur more quickly. Our drive to eat also contains a desire both to destroy and to live. A crucial understanding here is that the plant kingdom has evolved in a synergistic relationship with animals to satisfy this instinct in a way that is symbiotic. For example, plants evolved fruit so that animals can spread its seeds, and the excrement from animals goes back into the earth as fertilizer, enriching the soil to grow plants and fungi. This synergy between plants, animal, and fungi is the focus of the next chapter.

The integral model, as summarized here, is helpful to more comprehensively understand the transformative power of psychedelics. Psychedelics diminish the focus on oneself (upper-left/subjective quadrant) and at the same time enable one to feel more connected to a greater whole by dissolving the default-mode network in the brain (upper-right/objective quadrant), allowing more of the brain to communicate as a whole. Psychologically, psychedelics free the evolutionary energy bound up with autonomy (the sense of self that correlates with the default-mode network) through a death-rebirth process.[48] Experiences of unity are the results of transcendence, of consciously merging with a greater holon (lower-left/intersubjective quadrant), which correlates with the more connected brain states. These unity states can be experiences of merging with one's environment, the planet, the solar system, or even the entire cosmos (lower-right/interobjective quadrant), and as Whitehead writes: "We must also allow the possibility that we can detect in ourselves direct aspects of the mentalities of higher organisms."[49]

---

[48] Grof, *Future of Psychology*.

[49] Whitehead, *Science and the Modern World*, 150.

3

AN ECOLOGY OF SYNERGY

I n *Darwin's Pharmacy: Sex, Plants, and the Evolution of the Noösphere,* Richard Doyle, professor of English at Pennsylvania State University, writes, "I have reviewed thousands of reports about psychedelic experience . . . and suggest that a signature of these varied and incessantly ineffable experiences has been what I call the 'ecodelic' insight: the sudden and absolute conviction that the psychonaut is involved in a densely interconnected ecosystem for which contemporary tactics of human identity are insufficient."[1] These findings support the assertion that the best way to understand both psychedelic experiences and the reason why psychedelics grow in our environment is with an integral understanding of living systems theory. This perspective—of an interconnected system that is pervaded by consciousness—is one that psychedelics themselves foster.

---

[1] Doyle, *Darwin's Pharmacy*, 20.

Gaia and Living Systems Theory

Using the understanding cultivated from the field of cybernetics, which would later be integrated into systems theory, the chemist James Lovelock first proposed the Gaia hypothesis in the 1970s to describe the self-regulating process between the gases in the atmosphere and the organisms on the planet in which they work together to maintain optimal temperature for life on Earth.[2] The hypothesis views the entirety of Earth through the metaphor of an organism. George Lakoff, professor of cognitive science and linguistics at UC Berkeley, and Mark Johnson, professor of liberal arts and sciences at the University of Oregon, argue in *Metaphors We Live By* that metaphors underlie all paradigms and that they form our primary way of thinking.[3] The philosopher of science Alfred North Whitehead writes in his beautiful and engaging work *Science and the Modern World* a reinterpretation of the scientific enterprise, of the "Philosophy of Organism."[4] He makes it clear that even at the most fundamental level of quantum particles, the universe comes closer to resembling an interconnected, holistic, and sentient organism rather than a mechanistic clockwork. The physicist Fritjof Capra also spends the entire first chapter of his refreshing book *The Hidden Connections: Integrating the Biological, Cognitive, and Social Dimensions of Life into a Science of Sustainability* illustrating how the image and dynamics of a biological cell, such as the interdependence of elements and cohesive organization, shed light on the structure of consciousness, the universe, and sustainable social organizations.[5] The Gaian perspective takes the metaphor of organism to a planetary level.

---

[2] Wiener, *Cybernetics*; Capra and Luisi, *Systems View of Life*; Lovelock, *Ages of Gaia*.

[3] Lakoff and Johnson, *Metaphors We Live By*.

[4] Whitehead, *Science and the Modern World*.

[5] Capra, *Hidden Connections*.

The evolutionary biologist Lynn Margulis helped Lovelock develop his hypothesis and writes:

> The term Gaia was suggested to Lovelock by the novelist William Golding, author of *Lord of the Flies*. In the early 1970s, they both lived in Bowerchalke, Wiltshire, England. Lovelock asked his neighbor whether he could replace the cumbersome phrase "a cybernetic system with homeostatic tendencies as detected by chemical anomalies in the Earth's atmosphere" with a term meaning "Earth." "I need a good four-letter word," he said. On walks around the countryside in that gorgeous part of southern England near the chalk downs, Golding suggested Gaia. The Ancient Greek word for "Mother Earth," *Gaia* provides an etymological root of many scientific terms, such as *geo*logy, *geo*metry, and Pan*gaea*.[6]

Tyler Volk, a New York University professor of biology and science director of environmental studies, writes in his 2003 book *Gaia's Body: Toward a Physiology of Earth*:

> I consider Gaia the interacting system of life, soil, atmosphere, and ocean. It is the largest level in the nesting of parts within wholes that encompasses—and thus transcends—living beings, a nesting that ranges from the molecules within cells all the way outward to the Gaian system itself. Like the interior of organisms, Gaia contains complex cycles and material transformations driven by biological energy. Indeed, Gaia's inclusion of life means that from some perspectives, it resembles life. But how Gaia differs from organisms turns out to be its glory. . . . Gaia exists on its own unique level of operating rules, a level surely as complex as that of organisms and therefore worthy of its own science—which Jim Lovelock calls geophysiology.[7]

From the perspective of Gaia theory, organisms participate in a planetary ecological regulating process, with every component of the larger

---

[6] Margulis, *Symbiotic Planet*, 118.

[7] Volk, *Gaia's Body*, xiii.

organism providing a necessary function within and for the whole. This chapter proposes that psychedelics are an integral part of these regulating processes.

A perspective that includes ecological regulatory processes will transform our understanding of the context in which life, including plant and fungi psychedelics, evolves—"the evolution," Volk writes, "from cell to complex body, but also as evolution within the larger entity. Gaia is and always was the context for life."[8] This is why the Gaian context is indispensable to understanding why psychedelics occur and their role within the larger holon. A particularly important concept in this understanding is that of symbiosis between animals—including humans—and psychedelic plants and fungi.

Symbiosis

Symbiosis can be described as the process of two autonomous beings coming into habitual communion.[9] The word *symbiosis* is of Greek origin and translates to "living together." It was first used in 1877 by mycologist Heinrich Anton de Bary to describe the mutual relationship in lichens (algae or bacteria with fungi) and then defined as the living together of unlike organisms in his 1879 monograph. The biological organisms in symbiotic relationship are known as symbionts and the close and long-term interactions formed can be mutual, commensalistic, or parasitic.

Many species that evolved in spatially close and long-term interactions with others began to not only form interdependent habits but also evolve in attunement to the processes of the organisms they interacted with. For example, many plants can only be pollinated by specific species of insects, and those insects evolved adaptive qualities to work with

---

[8] Volk, 247.

[9] Margulis, *Symbiotic Planet.*

those plants. This process, of comingled long-term relationships that gave birth to new species, is called symbiogenesis. It was first described by Russian botanist Konstantin Mereschkowski in 1905. Microbiological evidence for the process was discovered in 1967 by biologist Lynn Margulis, who became the strongest proponent for this understanding of evolution. In her work *Symbiotic Planet: A New View of Evolution*, she writes:

> Symbiogenesis, an evolutionary term, refers to the origin of new tissues, organs, organisms—even species—by establishment of long-term or permanent symbiosis. . . . Although Darwin entitled his magnum opus *On the Origin of Species*, the appearance of new species is scarcely even discussed in his book. . . . Symbiosis, and here I fully agree with Wallin, is crucial to an understanding of evolutionary novelty and the origin of species. Indeed, I believe the idea of species itself requires symbiosis . . . long-standing symbiosis led first to the evolution of complex cells and nuclei and from there to other organisms such as fungi, plants, and animals.[10]

The claim being made is that the primary drive of evolution comes from species interacting with other species. After all, much of the crucial interactions an organism has in an environment is with other organisms.

This process can be seen through the evolution of all holons at all levels: protons, neutrons, and electrons come together to birth varieties of atoms; different atomic elements configure in geometric ways to form molecules with unique properties; and some of those molecules form systemic processes within cellular membranes to form biological life. This development of symbiotic merging to create higher-order, more complex processes follows an action of evolution than has occurred since the Big Bang. Symbiosis has increasingly become accepted by the mainstream as a driving force of evolution.[11] Margulis writes that life did not thrive on the planet by combat—but by networking: "Symbiogenesis

---

[10] Margulis, 6.

[11] Margulis.

developed the Earth's terra into occupiable real estate."[12] The network, as Fritjof Capra and Pier Luigi Luisi describe in their book *The Systems View of Life: A Unifying Vision*, is the central pattern found in living systems.[13]

Revisioning Evolution

The integral perspective of evolution described so far includes consciousness and relationship as essential aspects of the evolutionary process. From such a perspective the subjective experience of holons is also evolving along with their physical structures. The outward metamorphosis correlates with inward transformation; all physiological changes, such as brain development, affect the experience of the subject, and vice versa. An integral perspective of evolution also means that development is a relational process. All holons are a part of interlinked ecological systems. Systems evolve together. Evolution, in terms of moving toward complexity, is a symbiotic process. The evolution of a species affects the evolution of all the other species in its ecology. An integral perspective of evolution encompasses the standard neo-Darwinian view but also includes consciousness as a critical component of the evolutionary process.

Integral theorist Ken Wilber, who went to graduate school for biochemistry, describes evolution from a perspective that includes consciousness. He shares that there is a difference in how integral theory views evolution compared with the standard neo-Darwinian perspective.[14] The standard Darwinian perspective states that for evolution to occur genetic material (DNA or RNA) needs a random or chance mutation in an extremely rare form that is not lethal (because virtually all

---

[12] Margulis, 107.

[13] Capra and Luisi, *Systems View of Life*.

[14] Wilber, *Religion of Tomorrow*, 217–18.

are), and it must contribute to the organism's capacity to successfully reproduce. Also needed with this incredibly rare mutation (or a series of them) is for it to simultaneously occur in a male organism *and* a female organism, and—even more unlikely—they must find each other and then mate. Then they must also tend the offspring until it mates and passes on the "evolved" material. All highly unlikely. Wilber states:

> For Integral Theory, every moment is a Neo-Whiteheadian "prehensive unification" (or what Integral Theory calls a "tetra-prehension," to indicate that this pretension, or "feeling," of the previous moment by the newly emerging moment occurs in all 4 quadrants). The point is that every moment, in every quadrant, passes on its basic form and qualities to the next moment, which embraces and enfolds those items (the "include" part of the "transcend and include"). As long as this new moment "fits" in all 4 quadrants ("tetra-prehension"), then it will be selected and carried forward in evolution, along with its new and more creative aspects. If it doesn't fit well in all quadrants (through "mutual resonance"), it will be extinguished, or become extinct, and simply cease to exist.[15]

What Wilber is saying is that chance mutation cannot describe the intelligence we see on this planet in all forms of life; a self-organizing process, like that described by an integral approach to living systems theory, does. The dominant modern evolutionary paradigm cannot make sense of why consciousness exists. Why would experience form out of atoms and molecules? Why does inorganic matter come to life in the form of a cell with an inherent drive for self-preservation? And then why do these cells learn to bond to form complex structures that house expanded experiences and developing identities, such as those found in humanity? Instead of claiming that consciousness accidentally arose at some point in the evolutionary process, it is perhaps far more logical, and simpler, to acknowledge that consciousness has been present in the evolutionary process all along.

---

[15] Wilber, 217–18.

The reductionist perspective of evolution leaves us with many anomalies. When one integrates into their understanding the idea that consciousness is found in all aspects of the cosmos, which is a natural conclusion when the universe is perceived through the lens of the metaphor of an organism (a multilayered, living network with self-organizing processes), it is possible to develop a far more coherent, explanatory picture of evolution. This is also a perspective that psychedelics themselves foster, as suggested by Doyle. The universe, and especially our experience of it, cannot adequately be explained by collapsing phenomena into the right-side, objective, quadrants of the integral model, describing the world through physical structures alone. By expanding our perspective of evolution to include consciousness, we make ontological space for the qualities of autonomy, communion, and transcendence that are seen throughout the evolutionary process. This includes a desire for self-preservation, the inherent need for symbiotic connection through food and mating, and the drive for species and individuals to expand.

Too much emphasis has been placed on the function of autonomy when it comes to describing evolution—such as in the concept of survival of the fittest. For example, Richard Dawkins's *The Selfish Gene* does a great job of proudly presenting the conventional Darwinian perspective and focuses on competition.[16] If we adopt an integral evolutionary perspective, which we can see in Maslow's hierarchy of needs, we can honor autonomy, which includes self-preservation, as part of the process. But we also understand communion as part of the process. The ability to coherently connect as a larger whole has made ants the most successful groups of insects, and the ability to coordinate into civilization has given humans more power than any other organisms we know.[17] It is humans' ability to communicate and work cohesively in groups that gave humans our evolutionary advantage.[18] "At the base of the creativity of all

---

[16] Dawkins, *Selfish Gene.*

[17] Rifkin, *Empathic Civilization.*

[18] Harari, *Sapiens*; Ryan and Jetha, *Sex at Dawn.*

large familiar forms of life, symbiosis generates novelty," Lynn Margulis writes.[19] Novelty is an expression the transcendence instinct, which shows just how transcendence arises out of the symbiotic communion instinct, which itself is the attractive pull that unites autonomous beings.

Fungi and Plants

Fungi, plants, and animals have developed deep, interdependent relationships that have influenced their biological evolution. Three billion years ago blue-green algae began to excrete oxygen, which transformed the atmosphere and eventually the biosphere, enabling the evolution of higher-order organisms. The entire animal kingdom depends on plants for food and oxygen, and the plant kingdom depends on fungi for nutrients.[20] Ninety percent of plants have formed symbiotic relationships with mycorrhizal fungi, and over 80 percent of plants would perish if deprived of these relationships.[21] Mycelium helped create the soil that enabled plants to evolve onto the land, and then the animals followed plants out of the oceans.

By its nature, mycelium—which is the largest part of the body of fungi and lives in the soil—is largely symbiotic and creates an interconnective structure between plants. In *Mycelium Running: How Mushrooms Can Help Save the World*, Paul Stamets, who has researched fungi for forty years, writes about the communication that mycelium fosters:

> I believe that mycelium is the neurological network of nature. Interlacing mosaics of mycelium infuse habitats with information-sharing membranes. These membranes are aware, react to change, and collectively have the long-term health of the host environment in mind. The mycelium stays in constant molecular communication with its

---

[19] Margulis, *Symbiotic Planet*, 9.

[20] Stamets, *Fantastic Fungi*.

[21] Margulis, *Symbiotic Planet*, 110.

environment, devising diverse enzymatic and chemical responses to complex challenges. These networks not only survive, but sometimes expand to thousands of acres in size, achieving the greatest mass of any individual organism on this planet.[22]

A single species of fungus can transport nutrients to several species of trees within many acres of forest in a continuous network of cells.[23] Through establishing mutually beneficial relationships with a wide variety of species of plants, fungi have secured a thriving, long-term existence and have become the largest organisms on the planet. For example, the *Armillaria ostoyae* fungus in the Malheur National Forest in Oregon covers almost four square miles, living mostly underground as mycelia.[24] It is estimated to be 2,400 years old but could be as old as 8,650 years, which would place it among the oldest living organisms on the planet. At a fundamental level, the vast majority of plants, including those that produce psychedelic compounds, are informed of their ecology through mycelium.

While plants evolved in direct symbiotic evolution with fungi, animals evolved to become dependent on plants. Reflecting on the symbiotic relationship between humans and plants, bestselling author Michael Pollan says:

> My premise is that some plants . . . have evolved to gratify our desires; that's their evolutionary strategy in order to get us to work for them, to move their genes around the world. The reason that plants have come to produce an astonishing array of molecules, that they've become nature's alchemists, is their immobility. What they've done is use chemicals, for the most part, instead of feet. They use molecules that either attract or repel other species for defense or as an aid in reproduction. And those plants that managed to put to work a particular

---

[22] Stamets, *Mycelium Running*, 2.

[23] Stamets, 24.

[24] Stamets.

animal with a very large brain, a tool-making capability and a propensity to do a lot of wandering around the world, have done very well. If these plants were naming the phenomenon they would call it "the domestication of humans."[25]

Terence McKenna also documents the relationship between plants and humans well in his book *Food of the Gods: The Search for the Original Tree of Knowledge: A Radical History of Plants, Drugs, and Human Evolution.* He shows how human interaction with different plant chemicals, such as caffeine, alcohol, and sugar, catalyzed entire epochs of human history, including the reemergence of slavery (to harvest sugar) and fueling the industrial revolution (coffee).[26]

In his best seller *The Botany of Desire: A Plant's-Eye View of the World,* Pollan shows the thriving evolutionary strategies of four plants—apples, marijuana, potatoes, and tulips—that by gratifying human desires have become some of the most successful species on the planet.[27] Because of our desire for beauty, the tulip has impelled humans to take it from Central Asia to all over the world; because of the human desire to alter consciousness, marijuana has impelled many people to risk their lives to grow it, and now many people convert their houses and warehouses into spa-like optimal conditions for the plant to thrive; by gratifying the desire for control over population, the potato has impelled itself out of South America and become a staple crop in many countries in just five hundred years; by gratifying a desire for sweetness, the apple, which evolved in the forests of Kazakhstan and used mammals to spread its seeds, has become the universal fruit. Such examples show fundamental symbiotic coevolutionary processes existing between plants and humanity.

In *Entangled Life: How Fungi Make Our Worlds, Change Our Minds and Shape Our Futures,* Merlin Sheldrake presents the relationship between

---

[25] Pollan and Davis, "Garden of the Wild," 90.

[26] T. McKenna, *Food of the Gods.*

[27] Pollan, *Botany of Desire.*

fungi and the rest of nature.[28] Merlin is the son of Rupert Sheldrake, the Cambridge theoretical biologist who constructed the morphic field theory. Rupert collaborated with psychedelic philosopher Terence McKenna and pioneer chaos mathematician Ralph Abraham as part of the Trialogues, legendary discussions that started at the Esalen Institute in California in 1989 and continued for a decade. Following in his father's footsteps, Sheldrake received a PhD from the University of Cambridge and deepened into his own life direction, focusing his doctoral work on underground fungal networks in tropical forests and participating in a clinical trial focused on the relationship between LSD and creativity. His unique biography brings a refreshing approach to the study of fungi. He writes:

> Fungi are everywhere but they are easy to miss. They are inside you and around you. They sustain you and all that you depend on. As you read these words, fungi are changing the way that life happens, as they have done for more than a billion years. They are eating rock, making soil, digesting pollutants, nourishing and killing plants, surviving in space, inducing visions, producing food, making medicines, manipulating animal behavior, and influencing the composition of the Earth's atmosphere. Fungi provide a key to understanding the planet on which we live, and the ways that we think, feel, and behave. Yet they live their lives largely hidden from view, and over ninety percent of their species remain undocumented. The more we learn about fungi, the less makes sense without them.[29]

Sheldrake notes that the symbiotic relationship between plants' roots and fungi is so evolutionarily entangled that fungi were likely the first form of root systems that enabled plant life to develop on land.[30]

---

[28] M. Sheldrake, *Entangled Life*.

[29] M. Sheldrake, 4.

[30] M. Sheldrake, 127.

Sheldrake also points out that science keeps discovering that fungi are more ancient than previously thought. In 2017 fossilized mycelial structures that formed 2.4 billion years ago were found; that is a billion years earlier than fungi were previously believed to have evolved.[31] Fungi have continued to increase in complexity over the course of evolution. The mycelial structures of fungi are now so vast and complex that some fungi contain tens of thousands of mating types, approximately equivalent to our sexes, and if they are genetically similar enough, the mycelium of some fungi fuse with other mycelial networks even if they aren't sexually compatible,[32] widening the reach of these intelligent and relational webs.

Of specific relevance in Sheldrake's work is his focus on psilocybin. "Psilocybin was produced by fungi for tens of millions of years before the genus *Homo* evolved," he writes. "The current best estimate puts the origin of the first 'magic' mushroom at around seventy-five million years ago,"[33] while human ancestors first appeared five to seven million years ago, and modern *Homo sapiens* only around 130,000 years ago. Sheldrake observes that given its astounding impact on human consciousness, psilocybin and its evolution have been understudied:

> Two studies published in 2018 suggest that psilocybin did provide a benefit to fungi that could make it. Analysis of the DNA of psilocybin-producing fungal species reveals that the ability to make psilocybin evolved more than once. More surprising was the finding that the cluster of genes needed to make psilocybin has jumped between fungal lineages by horizontal gene transfer several times over the course of its history. As we've seen, horizontal gene transfer is the process by which genes and the characteristic they underpin move between organisms without the need to have sex and produce offspring. It is an everyday occurrence in bacteria—and how antibiotic

---

[31] M. Sheldrake, 67.

[32] M. Sheldrake, 36.

[33] M. Sheldrake, 113.

resistance can spread rapidly through bacterial populations—but it is rare in mushroom-forming fungi. It is even more rare for complex clusters of metabolic genes to remain intact as they jump between species. The fact that psilocybin gene clusters remained in one piece as it moved around suggests that it provided a significant advantage to any fungi who expressed it. If it didn't, the trait would have quickly degenerated.[34]

The evolutionary benefit of psilocybin for the fungi that produce it is still up for debate, though Sheldrake suggests that the evolutionary value of psilocybin comes from its ability to influence animal behavior.[35]

Sheldrake investigates in depth how certain fungi affect animals, especially ants. He concludes that psilocybin likely didn't evolve as a deterrent for insects and other animals but instead as a lure, changing behavior in ways that benefits the fungus. "This sort of relationship-building enacts one of the oldest evolutionary maxims. If the word *cyborg*—short for 'cybernetic organism'—describes the fusion between a living organism and a piece of technology, then we, like all other lifeforms, are symborgs, or symbiotic organisms."[36]

Animals and Psychedelics

Psychedelic plants and fungi are abundant in nature and are psychoactive for many species of the animal kingdom.[37] In his 940-page, coffee-table-sized book *The Encyclopedia of Psychoactive Plants: Ethnopharmacology and Its Application*, Christian Rätsch, a doctor focusing on anthropology and ethnopharmacology, presents 750 genera and species (of the several thousand that are known) of psychoactive plants and fungi from around

---

[34] M. Sheldrake, 114.

[35] M. Sheldrake.

[36] M. Sheldrake, 92.

[37] Samorini, *Animals and Psychedelics*; Siegel, *Intoxication*.

the world.[38] *Psychoactive plants* refers to any plant that changes the mind, so that includes coffee, tea, cocoa, coca, tobacco, and poppy as well as psychedelics.

The field of ethnobotany, the study of plants and human culture, is still young. Collectively, humanity has not placed a lot of resources and attention on searching the world for psychoactive plants, though that is changing. In his 1996 book *Psilocybin Mushrooms of the World,* Paul Stamets identified approximately one hundred species of mushrooms containing psilocybin.[39] Now there are over two hundred identified species of psilocybin-containing mushrooms.

Anthropologist Jeremy Narby, who focused on ethnobotany during his Stanford doctoral work, writes, "Humans have long considered psychoactive plants as teachers that enhance healing, thinking, and perception,"[40] and archeological evidence shows that cultures around the world and throughout time have used psilocybin mushrooms.[41] Though humans and their ancestors have intentionally used psychoactive plants and fungi for perhaps millions of years (a focus of chapter 5), many other animals are also drawn toward psychoactive plants and fungi. In the book *Animals and Psychedelics: The Natural World and the Instinct to Alter Consciousness,* Italian ethnobotanist Giorgio Samorini documents countless cases from around the world in which species of animals eat certain plants and fungi that alter their consciousness: mules, donkeys, horses, cows, sheep, antelope, pigs, rabbits, and hens are drawn to the psychoactive locoweed from the legume family;[42] elephants are known to search out fermented fruit to get drunk and establish traditions of seasonal binges; cats crave catnip intoxication, eating the plants to get high and then rubbing their body all over the plant; Siberian reindeer

---

[38] Rätsch, *Encyclopedia of Psychoactive Plants.*

[39] Stamets, *Psilocybin Mushrooms of the World.*

[40] Narby and Huxley, *Shamans through Time,* ix.

[41] Metzner, *Sacred Mushroom of Visions*; Devereux, *Long Trip.*

[42] Samorini, *Animals and Psychedelics,* 18.

look for the *Amanita muscaria* mushroom and even drink each other's urine after they eat it to alter their consciousness; goats and dogs eat psilocybin mushrooms; robins fly seasonally to California to intoxicate themselves with holly berries; rats and pigs look for kava; cows, horses, deer, and monkeys sneak into cannabis farms looking for the plant; and insects of all kinds consistently search out psychoactive plants and fungi.[43] Samorini writes that "drug-induced alterations of consciousness preceded the origins of humans. Drugging oneself is a behavior that reaches across the entire process of animal evolution, from insects to animals to women to men."[44]

Ronald Siegel writes, "There is a natural force that motivates the pursuit of intoxication."[45] Siegel was a psychopharmacologist on the faculty of the Department of Psychiatry and Biobehavioral Sciences at the UCLA School of Medicine. In his book *Intoxication: The Universal Drive for Mind-Altering Substances*, he states:

> We have seen that intoxication with plant drugs and other psychoactive substances has occurred in almost every species throughout history. There is a pattern of drug-seeking and drug-taking behavior that is consistent across time and species. This behavior is similar for many animals because it has been shaped and guided by the same evolution and environment, the same plants and pressures. In considering an evolutionary explanation of the phenomenon, we might ask if intoxication is in some way beneficial to the species. After all, the pursuit of intoxication with drugs has no apparent survival value and in some situations has certainly contributed to many deaths . . . What then could be the evolutionary value of such a condition? One possibility is that the pursuit of intoxication is a side effect of a beneficial gene or genes. Intoxication with drugs is widespread in animals, especially mammals, and it seems plausible that in order to appear in so extensive a range of genetic contexts it was inextricably associated with something else that

---

[43] Samorini, 27, 32, 38, 41, 49, 59, 62.

[44] Samorini, 78.

[45] Siegel, *Intoxication*, 206.

An Ecology of Synergy

was of survival value. The universal pursuit of intoxication implies the existence of direct connections between the molecular chemistry of the drugs and the chemistry of the central nervous system, such as opiate receptors in the mammalian brain, a biological investment that is difficult to think of as arising by accident. We are organisms with chemical brains and drives that pit the chemistry of the individual against that of the environment. We have survived these interactions and learned to thrive on them.[46]

Similar to the reference Siegel makes to the opiate receptors, most psychedelic molecules lock into serotonin receptors, which are found in almost all animals.[47]

Similar to what Michael Pollan presents in *The Botany of Desire*, Siegel claims that drugs, like those derived from plants and fungi, have met a wide variety of our desires, such as "pleasure, relief from pain, mystical revelations, stimulation, relaxation, joy, ecstasy, self-understanding, escape, altered states of consciousness, or just a different feeling."[48] These are natural human desires, and psychoactive substances have served as a means to achieve these experiences. While it is still unknown if the molecules that cause intoxication directly influence genetic evolution, as Siegel suggests, they certainty meet psychological needs. The motivation for mind-alteration is so widespread throughout the animal kingdom that Siegel calls it "the fourth universal evolutionary drive," after hunger, thirst, and sex.

If we look at this fourth universal evolutionary drive of animals to alter their consciousness through the lens of integral theory, we can easily see it as an expression of the transcendence instinct, which includes the impulse for novelty. The normal state of consciousness is momentarily exchanged for a new experience of oneself and the world. Such experiences provide the possibility for creativity, enable new perspectives, and

---

[46] Siegel, 209.

[47] Buhner, *Plant Intelligence and the Imaginal Realm*.

[48] Siegel, *Intoxication*, 208.

therefore provide the capability for problem solving. Bob Montgomery, founder of the Botanical Preservation Corps, writes in the foreword titled "Evolution through Inebriation?" in *Animals and Psychedelics: The Natural World and the Instinct to Alter Consciousness*:

> Animals engage in intoxicating drug consumption. This fact forms one of the most provocative and original of Giorgio Samorini's insights: this moment of drug-induced inebriation produces *deschematizzazione*, or deconditioning, that allows for new behavioral ways to be established in a species.[49]

By momentarily clearing their habitual patterns of organization, animals are now partially free to self-organize in new ways, including the integration of new adaptive strategies.

Mycologists have found that, through a variety of chemical processes, fungi have directed the evolution of entire ecosystems.[50] Situating fungi within a Gaian context, Paul Stamets writes:

> Ecotheorist James Lovelock, together with Lynn Margulis, came up with the Gaia hypothesis, which postulated that the planet's biosphere intelligently piloted its course to sustain and breed new life. I see mycelium as the living network that manifests that natural intelligence imagined by Gaia theorists. The mycelium is an exposed sentient membrane, aware and responsive to changes in its environment . . . A complex and resourceful structure for sharing information, mycelium can adapt and evolve through the ever-changing forces of nature . . . These sensitive mycelial membranes act as a collective fungal consciousness. As mycelia's metabolisms surge, they emit attractants, imparting sweet fragrances to the forest and connecting ecosystems and their species with scent trails. Like a matrix, a biomolecular superhighway, the mycelium is in constant dialogue with the environment,

---

[49] Montgomery in Samorini, *Animals and Psychedelics*, ix.

[50] Stamets, *Mycelium Running*.

reacting to and governing the flow of essential nutrients, cycling through the food chain.[51]

If we consider integral theory's assertion that all matter has a subjective consciousness, an interpretation that can be drawn from the dynamics of fungi and other species is that fungi hold the long-term well-being of the ecosystem in their mind. The more harmonious diversity that exists in its ecosystem, the more resources are provided to the mycelium, allowing it to live a long life. Like the 2,400-acre mycelium net in Oregon existing in a symbiotic relationship with a rich, large tree forest, as long as the forest stays healthy, the fungal structure will continue to live and thrive.

The ethnopharmacologist Dennis McKenna, who did his postdoctoral work at the Department of Neurology at Stanford University School of Medicine, elaborates on the diverse and rich influential chemical processes occurring between the plant and animal kingdom:

> If we are going to think of plants as "messengers," we have to realize that the language they speak is a molecular language. Plants, unlike animals, are chemical virtuosos. They can photosynthesize: take sunlight, carbon dioxide, and simple elements from mineral sources and, from those basic elements, form complex organic compounds. Plants also go one step further and spin out a vast array of what used to be called "secondary" compounds with an enormous variety of structures, from alkaloids (like psychedelics) to terpenes and polypeptides. Animals adapt to their environment mainly through behavior. They can move around. They can flee in case of danger or move toward something they are attracted to—a potential mate or a food source, for instance. Plants can't move, so they substitute biosynthesis, chemical ability, for behavior. They have elaborated an enormous array of chemical compounds to help them achieve their goals . . . It's now understood that these chemicals are often messenger molecules that plants release into their environment to influence their interactions

---

[51] Stamets, 4.

with other organisms, be they other plants, or bacteria and fungi in the soil, or herbivorous animals or human beings that feed on them and use them in all sorts of ways.[52]

Research shows that chemicals are one of the most efficient ways nature has to reorient the behavior of a species. By seeing molecules as messengers, one may begin seeing chemicals as a language through which instructions and complex information can be transferred from plants and fungi into an animal's consciousness. Following this logic, the psychedelic molecules of fungi like psilocybin may serve as one of humanity's greatest options for cultivating an ecological consciousness to heal our planetary crisis.

The Ecological Self

In his five decades of guiding people through holotropic states of consciousness, Stanislav Grof has found patterns of phenomena such as the self becoming different people, animals, plants, the planet, and the universe, following the process of identity expansion presented by Ken Wilber as a movement from egocentric to ethnocentric to worldcentric to kosmocentric.[53] An egocentric self identifies primarily with one's body and biographical identity; an ethnocentric self expands to include other people that one may identify to be part of their same tribe or culture; a worldcentric self may move beyond culture to identify a humanness they see in themselves and all people in the world, or even deeper to see that all biological life on Earth shares similarities; and a kosmocentric self identifies with not only biological life and the physical realms of existence, but also spiritual realms, as one moves further into unity with all reality. As one's sense of self expands, the context through which they interpret information also enlarges.

---

[52] McKenna, McKenna, and Davis, "Plant Messengers," 63.

[53] Grof, *Way of the Psychonaut*, vols. 1 and 2; Wilber, *Integral Vision*.

For most people, their sense of identity is closely bound to their own body and remains within the realm of humanity. As such, there seems to be a strong belief that the boundaries of one's self end at one's skin. Our bodies, though, are open systems. At every moment we are in energetic exchange with our environment. Through our breath we constantly take in molecules that have been circulating through billions of beings for billions of years, and these molecules are made out of atoms that were once a part of stars. Through eating, the bodies of other organisms are integrated into ours. The water we depend on arrived through a long process of cycling through our world. Our body itself is composed of thirty-seven trillion cells and cycles through a continuous process of death and rebirth.

An identity that includes our body, but which does not include the environment that cocreates our body, leads toward a belief centered on autonomy, and in many ways this is a perspective that leaves us feeling isolated. Many of us do not realize we are also in communion with the environment, that our body is always making the environment a part of our self, and that by taking in the environment, both literally and through our senses, it influences our states of consciousness. The food we eat affects the neurotransmitters in our brain, which influence our mood and perception. The colors we see, including the beauty around us, affect our feelings and thoughts. By bringing in more of a nondual approach—in which the lines between inner/outer and self/other begin to dissolve, a perspective many meditative practices honor and that intentional psychedelic use cultivates—we begin to grasp that perhaps all the elements of the world are extensions of a larger self of which we are all a part.

One can call this expanded identity, in which one includes their individuality and their environment as an extended fundamental part of self, the *ecological self*. Kenny Ausubel, founder of the Bioneers Conference, shares how many cultures throughout history that held deep relationships with their environment developed this same orientation:

Many ancient indigenous traditions, as well as modern re-inventions of traditional knowledge, suggest that a special intelligence resides in certain sacred plants and organisms, including cacti and fungi. This "vegetable mind," they tell us, can open new and different ways of seeing the world that reveal the most basic of biological truths: As human beings, we are part of nature. We *are* the environment.[54]

Anecdotal evidence suggests that societies that have regularly taken psychedelic plants and fungi experience themselves much differently than those of us in our hyperautonomous modern Western culture. They tend to have a deeper relationship with nature and have a much more fluid sense of self, as their psychological consciousness has continually dissolved its boundaries and recognize the environment part of their consciousness.[55] Research shows that psychedelics allow people to experience themselves as being a part of a larger body and mind, which many, including myself, have reported to be the most profound and healing experiences of their lives. When a person realizes they are effortlessly part of a larger living whole they innately belong to, it can bring a feeling of safety, inclusion, and purpose. In these moments one's boundaries dissolve, and their individuality radiates as part of an interconnected pattern—a web of being—from which they grow.

The nitrogen cycle is an elegant model of how this ecological self works in the Gaian context. The nitrogen cycle is a biogeochemical cycle in which nitrogen, through biological and physiological processes, is transformed into several chemicals and cycles through land, water, and the atmosphere.[56] The nitrogen atoms cycle through the entire biosphere, and over billions of years, they have been recycled through plants, fungi, and animals. This interconnective atom, nitrogen, is present is every known naturally occurring psychedelic compound except those found in marijuana (which some people consider as a psychedelic)

---

[54] Ausubel as cited in Harpignies, *Visionary Plant Consciousness*, xi.

[55] Allen, *Maria Sabina*; Nour, Evans, and Carhart-Harris, "Psychedelics, Personality and Political Perspectives"; Walsh, *World of Shamanism*.

[56] Volk, *Gaia's Body*.

and *Salvia divinorum.*[57] This correlates to the most frequent psychedelic insight, as described by author and professor Richard Doyle, that the participant exists in an interconnected living system.

Another way to think of Richard Doyle's term *ecodelics*, compounds that catalyze or expand ecological awareness, is as Gaian molecules.[58] Many who have integrated these Gaian molecules into their life have experienced a profound level of connection with nature and have consequently oriented themselves toward becoming servants and protectors of nature. Many people who have experimented with psychedelics also became ecological activists. J. P. Harpignies, editor of the book *Visionary Plant Consciousness* and associate producer of the national Bioneers Conference, writes:

> While not often discussed, it is an undeniable fact that quite a few of the most dedicated environmental activists of our era were deeply affected by their experiences with psychoactive substances. In many cases, the encounters of these young people with hallucinogens in natural settings either triggered or enhanced powerful "biophilic" feelings—spiritual bonds with the natural world that set the tone for the rest of their lives.[59]

Paul Stamets shares how psychedelics give him a similar message:

> When I have ingested psychoactive plants and mushrooms, there is one message emanating from this world of plant spirit consciousness that comes to me loudly and clearly virtually every time. That message is that we are part of an "ecological consciousness," that the Earth is in peril, that time is short, and that we're part of a huge, universal biosystem. And I am far from alone. Many people who have taken these substances report receiving the same message . . . It is no accident that

---

[57] Schultes, Hofmann, and Rätsch, *Plants of the Gods*, 224.

[58] Doyle, *Darwin's Pharmacy.*

[59] Harpignies, ed., *Visionary Plant Consciousness*, 2.

they're producing compounds that stimulate consciousness: it's the way they speak to us and through us.[60]

After billions of years of refinement, these molecules may in fact be the most effective way for nature to pass critical information to its constituents.

"The consumption of psychedelic substances leads to an increased concern for nature and ecological issues," write Stanley Krippner and David Luke in a piece called "Psychedelics and Species Connectedness."[61] "Psychedelic substances may have provided a hidden resource to keep Homo sapiens from becoming so estranged from nature that the human species would contaminate, pollute, and ultimately destroy life on Earth."[62] This is echoed by Simon Powell in his book *Magic Mushroom Explorer: Psilocybin and the Awakening Earth*:

> What I can say for sure is that my experiences with psilocybin mushrooms certainly *felt* profoundly significant, particularly in terms of their ecopsychological impact, and that I therefore felt obliged to spread word of such a remarkable natural resource. These mushrooms really are a catalyst that can galvanize new ways of thinking and feeling and can help return the human race into harmony with the larger biospherical environment. If this sounds grandiose, then that is because the mushroom experience is so utterly compelling.[63]

If we are to adopt the integral model's assertion that all levels of existence contain degrees of consciousness, we can posit that Gaian molecules themselves are regulatory processes of the biosphere. Just as our bodies produce chemicals to bring us toward homeostasis, it is possible that psychedelics grow in the environment to influence behavior

---

[60] Harrison et al., "Plant Spirit," 138.

[61] Krippner and Luke, "Psychedelics and Species Connectedness," 238.

[62] Krippner and Luke, 243.

[63] Powell, *Magic Mushroom Explorer*, 4.

through increasing awareness that will compel species to favor ecological equilibrium. The development of psychedelics in nature may be a protective, and evolutionary, strategy of the Gaian system. This theory is further clarified when we look at it from a living systems perspective, which is a perspective that these Gaian molecules themselves facilitate.[64]

---

[64] Doyle, *Darwin's Pharmacy*.

PART II
The Past

4

EMERGENCE OF HUMANITY

N ow with the concepts of both integral theory and living systems theory in place, this chapter delves deep into the past and situates the story of evolution within an ecological framework. It begins with the Big Bang, goes slowly through primate evolution, and expands on the lifestyle of our hunter-gatherer ancestors. Chapter 5 is meant to overlay this one and will delve into the theory that our great ancestors' symbiotic evolutionary relationship to psilocybin mushrooms might have encouraged the lifestyle presented in this chapter, and it explores some of the major missing pieces that have remained a mystery in the general understanding of human evolution. These two chapters about the past will end with evidence of the premodern history of psychedelia, including the recognition that before the colonization by the Europeans, tens of millions of Indigenous Americans likely ingested psychedelics.

Big Bang to Primates

The universe began as an undifferentiated whole, the so-called Singularity. This initial singularity, a united energy, blossomed into beings. With the existence of individual nodes within the network came relational forces (gravity, the strong force, the weak force, and electromagnetism) that pulled the individual holons together. The initial wholeness still remains, only this large network that we call the universe has evolved through the forces of autonomy, communion, transcendence, and dissolution into individual nodes of experience and structure, pulling them into relationship, and then creating new nodes through these configurations.

The Big Bang, or Flaring Forth as cosmologist Brian Swimme calls it, sparked a decentralized network consisting of nodes that self-regulate and maintain their own form.[1] Atoms, for example, maintain their structure on their own. From a singularity of seemingly endless energy, a flaring forth fueled by quantum fluctuations caused a rapid expansion of space and time, allowing quantum particles to arise. Neil Shubin, professor of evolutionary biology at the University of Chicago, in his book *The Universe Within: Discovering the Common History of Rocks, Planets, and People* writes:

> A little over three minutes after the birth of the universe began the stirrings of one of the deepest patterns in the world, captured by the chart that is the source of either awe or angst for young science students—the periodic table. . . . There would only be three boxes in it: hydrogen, helium, and lithium.[2]

Within moments of the cataclysmic event that birthed existence, atomic nuclei formed as the sea of energy began to coalesce into protons and neutrons and then bonded these two entities into partnership. Half a

---

[1] Swimme and Berry, *Universe Story*.

[2] Shubin, *Universe Within*, 27.

million years later, electrons made their entrance to team up with the duo to create the first of the atoms. These atoms communed into clouds and then thirteen billion years ago began to collapse when these clouds reached a critical mass, creating stars, which began a process of transformative consequences.

After the first stars, which can be seen as a network of atoms, completed their life cycle, they pushed out newly formed atoms created by the process of nuclear fusion, and these emerging elements created even more complex solar systems. About four and a half billion years ago our sun, a second-generation star system, was born. Soon after, our solid Earth coalesced from the gas and dust left behind by prior stars. And, half a billion years after Earth's formation, biological entities emerged: cells— networks of processes inside of a membrane. Fed by the energy of the sun, the cells multiplied, and three billion years later, many formed symbiotic relationships with each other, eventually merging into multicellular systems. Sexual reproduction began over a billion years ago, which quickened the pace of evolution. The Cambrian explosion, blooming a diversity of life forms, took place 541 million years ago; then about 30 million years later the first eyes evolved and the first brains emerged in flatworms, which are the oldest living ancestors to all living bilateral animals.[3]

Between 1.3 and 2.4 billion years ago (new evidence suggests fungi developed almost a billion years earlier than previously suspected), fungi began to evolve onto land.[4] Then about 700 million years ago; after mycelium set the soil, the plants joined them.[5] About 10 million years later, the first jaws appear in fish. The book *Your Inner Fish: A Journey into the 3.5 Billion-Year History of the Human Body* chronicles evolutionary biologist Neil Shubin's journey of finding, in 2004, the fossils of the oldest vertebrate ancestor to come onto land, the *Tiktaalik roseae*, which

---

[3] American Association for the Advancement of Science, "Flatworms Are Oldest Living Ancestors."

[4] M. Sheldrake, *Entangled Life*.

[5] Stamets, *Mycelium Running*, 1.

stepped onto the Earth about 374 million years ago.[6] About 95 million years later, the first mammal-like creatures evolved.

The rise of the dinosaurs began 45 million years later. They roamed our planet for about 170 million years. The ability of humans to hear high-pitch noises comes from the ears of our rodent ancestors around 200 million years ago.[7] During the dinosaurs' reign, our rodent ancestors lived underground to avoid becoming prey. This is also when the first flowers evolved, attracting animals for the purpose of their own reproduction. Around 66 million years ago, a large asteroid impact, known as the K/T extinction event, wiped 75 percent of the plant and animal species, including the nonavian dinosaurs, off the planet. This set the stage for the flourishing of new forms of life. Fungi were one of the first forms of life to evolutionarily expand after the cataclysm.[8] The K/T impact darkened the skies with dust, killing most plant life, while mycelium, feeding off the decomposing organic material, thrived and spread across the planet, creating the foundation for future plant life to further develop.

Life in the Trees

For much of the time during the reign of the dinosaurs, our ancestors lived underground. One of the first animals that is considered a primate, the genus Purgatorius, took to the trees seventy million years ago, before the K/T impact.[9] Ten million years later, after the K/T impact, many more lemur-like animals took to the trees and eventually evolved into primates.[10] For approximately fifty million years,

---

[6] Shubin, *Your Inner Fish*.

[7] Shubin, *Universe Within*.

[8] Stamets, *Mycelium Running*, 2.

[9] Wright and Gynn, *Return to the Brain of Eden*, 90.

[10] Wayman, "Five Early Primates You Should Know."

these ancestors lived in the canopies of the trees and in that time underwent drastic evolutionary processes. Once their noses got off the ground, they began to lose much of their olfactory functions, and they started to climb up to the trees, where sight became more important. They needed to differentiate between colors, such as shades of brown and green in the wood and leaves of trees, and also expand the range of colors that their eyes registered so as to notice the different bright colors of fruits. "We humans are part of a lineage that has traded smell for sight. We now rely more on vision than smell, and this is reflected in our genome. In this trade-off, our sense of smell was deemphasized, and many of our olfactory genes became functionless," Shubin writes.[11]

This migration into the trees also meant a drastic change in diet. Whereas our rodent-like ancestors focused much more on insects and leafy greens, our primate ancestors began to focus on fruit. "All the early hominids and their great ape cousins were mainly fruit-eaters," Wright and Gynn write.[12] In their book they build a convincing case that it was a fruit diet that drastically enhanced our primate ancestors' brain development. They state:

> Species of primates that have a high percentage of fruit in their diet tend to have proportionally larger brains than do their cousins that eat a more leafy or omnivorous diet. These examples clearly show that changing from an insect-based diet to a fruit-based one is linked to an increase in brain size.[13]

Not only did this diet change the brains of our ancestors, it also changed their social behavior. Wright and Gynn dedicate a chapter to how this fruit diet might have impacted our hormonal system. "Pumping chemicals from the forest fruits into the hominid system," they

---

[11] Shubin, *Your Inner Fish*, 147.

[12] Wright and Gynn, *Return to the Brain of Eden*, 61.

[13] Wright and Gynn, 37.

note, "would have limited aggressive behavior. Steroids are linked to aggression, and as we have seen, many of the chemicals found in fruits suppress steroids."[14] It is possible that this suppression of steroids and corresponding less-aggressive behavior were a major factor in human development because, as noted in the previous chapter, it was the ability to cooperate, not competition, that gave humanity one of its main evolutionary advantages.

Looking at bonobos, who tie with chimpanzees as being humanity's genetically closest living relatives, we can perhaps glimpse a similar diet to that of our great ancestors:

> Primates, given a choice, will select fruit in preference to any other food. Fruit is rich, nutritious, and easily digestible food. If it is available, this is what all the great apes prefer to eat. However, other foods are eaten regularly. Our nearest relative, the bonobo, eats between 60 percent and 95 percent fruit, depending on the fruit productivity of its specific habitat. The rest of its diet comprises mostly shoots and herbs and a small amount of insects, eggs, and the occasional small mammal.[15]

This suggests that for about fifty million years our ancestors lived on a largely plant-based diet, which may have made them much less aggressive than most humans are now, since eating meat increases steroid intake.[16] During their time in the trees, which dwarfs the time of bipedal evolution, our ancestors lived largely carefree and playful lives. They had far fewer predators in the canopies, and food in the luscious rain forest was abundant. They likely spent most of their days socializing, resting, eating, and mating.[17]

---

[14] Wright and Gynn, 55.

[15] Wright and Gynn, 62.

[16] Wright and Gynn, 56.

[17] Ryan and Jetha, *Sex at Dawn*.

From the Trees to Planting Seeds

The human evolutionary trajectory parted with bonobos and chimpanzees around seven million years ago as changing weather patterns gradually forced our tree-dwelling ancestors to the forest floor. "In the forest the human brain was expanding and expanding at a phenomenal rate,"[18] write the authors of *Return to the Brain of Eden: Restoring the Connection between Neurochemistry and Consciousness*, but environmental changes eventually forced our ancestors to adapt. The luscious canopies they previously occupied turned into drier grasslands in only a few million years. During this transitional time, our ancestors again underwent dramatic evolutionary changes. Plant pharmacologist Dennis McKenna writes of this period:

> As a consequence dietary regimens shifted toward roots, tubers, grass seed, and a greater proportion of animal protein, triggering a reversal of the positive feedback loops that had sustained pineal potentiation and hemispheric integration in the paradisiacal, forest-dwelling golden age. Pineal dominance was disrupted by steroid-mediated, testosterone-driven function, primarily due to the reduced consumption of flavonoids and other steroid-inhibitory dietary factors. Changes in the dietary patterns that were forced on the population by this migration put an end to the rapid evolution of the human brain and triggered its devolution, ultimately resulting in the damaged human neural architecture that we suffer from today.[19]

The plant life in the forest began to transform according to weather patterns, and then so did the bodies, and minds, of our ancestors.

In her book *The Scars of Evolution: What Our Bodies Tell Us of Human Origins*, Elaine Morgan makes the case that bipedalism and loss of hair evolved in response to a flooded forest floor.[20] The Congo River basin,

---

[18] Wright and Gynn, *Return to the Brain of Eden*, 57.

[19] D. McKenna in Wright and Gynn, *Return to the Brain of Eden*, xii.

[20] Morgan, *Scars of Evolution*.

current home to our closest living relatives, seasonally floods, as do other forests such as the Amazon, which floods six months out of the year. Such a situation, which even occurs in dry regions, would have forced our ancestors to begin standing up, and the water would have assisted them in standing. The water would have aided this move upright, helping relieve the pressure from their spines to stand erect. The loss of hair may have occurred as a response to our body's need for vitamin D, which it gets from the sun. If our ancestors' bodies began to be immersed in water, with only the top of their heads receiving direct sunlight, then hair on most other parts of the body may have begun to fall off to allow more direct exposure between their skin and the sun.

When most of the large fruit-filled trees disappeared, our ancestors that depended on them likely began to roam the savanna to look for food, leading to a hunter and gatherer lifestyle.[21] Our ancestors eventually encountered herds of mammals that thrived on the grassland, which became quick sources of large amounts of calories. Other animals became available and highly efficient, long-lasting energy sources for our ancestors, and a chemical feedback loop began between our ancestors and animal protein. Animal protein increased their testosterone and steroid production, which in turn made our ancestors more aggressive than they once were, encouraging them to hunt even more. The chemical changes in their diet, in addition to the changes in their environment, caused dramatic changes over time in their behavior.

Our ancestors shared the planet about half the time, between the four million years since coming down from trees until the Agricultural Revolution, with other species of humans. Including us *Homo sapiens* (meaning "wise man"), there have been at least eight species of humans coexisting on the planet. "The truth is that from about two million years ago until about ten thousand years ago, the world was home, at one and the same time, to several human species," writes professor Yuval Noah Harari in his best-selling book *Sapiens: A Brief History*

---

[21] T. McKenna, *Food of the Gods.*

of Humankind.[22] Humans first evolved in East Africa from an earlier genus of primates. About two million years ago some of them migrated out of Africa and settled in Europe and Asia. The different environments caused a diversification into different species. *Homo neanderthalensis* (meaning "man from the Neander Valley") were more muscular than sapiens, lived in northern Eurasia, and were better suited for the Ice Age. *Homo erectus* ("upright man") lived for two million years in the border between Asia and Europe. *Homo soloensis* ("man from the Solo Valley") lived the Indonesian tropics. *Homo floresiensis* reached the small Indonesian island of Flores when the water was exceptionally low and, when the sea rose again, became trapped; the island's poor resources forced the humans into dwarfism, reaching a maximum height of three and a half feet and weighing fifty-five pounds. *Homo rudolfensis* ("man from Lake Rudolf") evolved in West Africa. *Homo ergaster* ("working man") lived in southern and western Africa. The fossils of *Homo denisova* were found in the Denisova Cave in Siberia in 2010, making them our newest known relative.

Most of our ancestors' time, and likely also that of our relatives within the genus of Homo, was spent in community. Sex played a major role in tribal bonding. As the authors Christopher Ryan and Cacilda Jetha point out in their book *Sex at Dawn: The Prehistoric Origins of Modern Sexuality*, our ancestors were largely orgiastic, openly having sex as a group and also each person having perhaps several mates, which allowed deep bonds to form in the group as a whole. Since they were naked, it was more comfortable to adapt to both the surfaces and weather of the environment by sleeping next to each other. They likely subscribed to a sexual orientation that more closely resembles modern-day polyamory than monogamy. Monogamy, the restriction of sexual activities to only one partner, is scarce in the animal kingdom. Only 3 percent of mammals are monogamous, and of all our primate relatives only the gibbons are monogamous.[23]

---

[22] Harari, *Sapiens*, 8.

[23] Ryan and Jetha, *Sex at Dawn*, 97, 64.

The dominant scientific paradigm generally considers chimpanzees to be our genetically closest living relatives and has studied them to understand human behavior, but this leaves out our equally closest genetic relatives, the bonobos, which can offer us additional insights into how some of our ancestors may have lived. Bonobos exhibit a polyamorous lifestyle, taking on several partners, of both sexes, within the community. Bonobo females have sex an average of twelve times a day.[24] Anthropologist Marvin Harris argues that the payoff of the bonobo lifestyle is "a more intense form of social cooperation between males and females, leading to a more intensely cooperative social group, a more secure milieu for rearing infants, and hence a higher degree of reproductive success for sexier males and females."[25] Biological anthropologist Helen Fisher writes that "bonobos engage in sex to ease tension, to stimulate sharing during meals, to reduce stress while traveling, and to reaffirm friendships during anxious reunions."[26] If we imagine the bonobos as nodes within a system, this lifestyle creates deep connection between many nodes in that system, which creates a more resilient network.

In a hunter and gatherer lifestyle, a different value system predominates than that in our present-day materialistic culture. Because they were often nomadic, one could only own as many material goods as one could carry, and sharing was likely mandatory, because the primary value in such a group is relationship, for through relationships one finds security.[27] In communal living the health of the individual is dependent on the well-being of the collective group. Sharing—of both resources and sexual partners—fosters social bonds and group health. Anthropologist Marshall Sahlins, in his book *Stone Age Economics*, writes: "If one

---

[24] Ryan and Jetha, *Sex at Dawn*, 12.

[25] Harris as cited in Ryan and Jetha, *Sex at Dawn*, 64.

[26] Fisher as cited in Ryan and Jetha, 73.

[27] Fisher as cited in Ryan and Jetha, 11; Harari, *Sapiens*.

is in danger, or needs food, the best source of security comes from other people in the tribe."[28] Ryan and Jetha state:

> In evolutionary terms, it would be hard to overstate the importance of such networks. After all, it was primarily such flexible, adaptive social groups (and the feedback loop of brain growth and language capacities that both allowed and resulted from them) that enabled our slow, weak, generally unimpressive species to survive and eventually dominate the entire planet. Without frequent S.E.Ex. [Socio-Erotic Exchanges], it's doubtful that foraging bands could have maintained social equilibrium and fecundity over the millennia. S.E.Ex. were crucial in binding adults into groups that cared communally for children of obscure or shared paternity, each child likely related to most or all of the men in the group (if not a father, certainly an uncle, cousin ...).[29]

As Ryan and Jetha illustrate in their book, many tribes and cultures around the world carry on similar lifestyles today and maintain rich and secure social dynamics.

This style of group bonding is also a perfect representation of the universal instincts described in integral theory. Each human is a relatively autonomous individual. They are pulled to communion with many members of the tribe in the form of sexual exchanges. When a woman birthed a child, no one knew precisely which man impregnated her, so the entire tribe treated the child as a child of the tribe. The child is then born from the tribe into a unitive embrace; though one mother birthed them, they were also the child of all the men. The child grows up identified with the tribe, establishing a secure feeling of belonging to a group far more substantial than the modern nuclear family unit.

Charles Darwin also believed that humans evolved in such conditions. In *The Descent of Man and Selection in Relation to Sex*, he writes:

---

[28] Sahlins, *Stone Age Economics*, 27.

[29] Ryan and Jetha, *Sex at Dawn*, 94.

It seems certain that the habit of marriage has been gradually developed and that almost promiscuous intercourse was once extremely
common throughout the world... present day tribes [exist where] all
the men and women in the tribe are husband and wives to each other...
Those who have most closely studied the subject, and whose judgment
is worth much more than mine, believe that communal marriage was
the original and universal form throughout the world. . . . The indirect
evidence in favor of this belief is extremely strong.[30]

One such contemporary group of people are the Mosuo, who live close
to Tibet and have hundreds of sexual relationships within their lives.[31]
From their perspective, monogamy seems inappropriate—to them one
does not have the right to restrict another's sexual freedom. Indeed,
the multiple sexual connections of our ancestral tribes would have supported the human need for belonging, as described in Maslow's hierarchy of needs, perhaps more so in comparison to monogamy, in which
individuals tend to isolate into pairs. This instinctual need for belonging,
according to Maslow, arises as soon as we secure our survival,[32] and,
as Peter Block points out in *Community: The Structure of Belonging*, is
the foundational quality necessary for sustainable group dynamics.[33]
The brain itself evolved to reward this bonding behavior—the more our
ancestors physically bonded with members in their tribe, the more their
bodies would have released the "love hormone" oxytocin, leading to a
feeling of well-being, and again encouraging a feedback loop between
their neurochemistry and physical connection.

Further strengthening the bonding instinct, humans are also wired to
be empathetic.[34] Mirror neurons found across the mammalian kingdom

---

[30] Darwin, *Descent of Man*, 360.

[31] Ryan and Jetha, *Sex at Dawn*, 129.

[32] Maslow, *Theory of Human Motivation*.

[33] Block, *Community*.

[34] Rifkin, *Empathic Civilization*.

can also be seen as empathy neurons, allowing us to instinctively feel in our body what someone else is feeling in theirs. In *The Empathic Civilization: The Race to Global Consciousness in a World in Crisis,* Jeremy Rifkin writes:

> Empathy is the psychological means by which we become part of other people's lives and share meaningful experiences. The very notion of transcendence means to reach beyond oneself, to participate with and belong to larger communities, to be embedded in more complex webs of meaning.[35]

Building on the work of researchers in the field of developmental psychology, Rifkin continues to state that the drive for destruction and unnecessary aggression arises from an infant's needs for connection being unmet by their parents.[36] In a tribal society, this destructive drive is less likely to arise, because there are greater opportunities for the child's needs getting met by the abundant population of adults that are taking care of the children. In a modern nuclear family, which is generally separated in its own house, the connection must come from just one father and one mother. In a tribe, this connection comes from likely all the men and likely all the women. Since pathologies tend to develop as a response to unmet innate need, the unavailability for parents to meet a child's emotional needs (even more so in today's demanding society) maybe the greatest source of neuroses in our species.[37] This is in alignment with attachment theory, as discussed in chapter 2.

The groundbreaking psychologist Wilhelm Reich might agree with the statement that our less sexually repressed ancestors held less neurosis than people today, and that there is a causal relationship between these phenomena. In an overview of Western psychology, Stanislav Grof writes of Reich that:

---

[35] Rifkin, 2.

[36] Rifkin.

[37] Wilber, *Integral Psychology.*

Maintaining Freud's main thesis concerning the paramount importance of sexual factors in the etiology of neurosis, he modified Freud's
concepts substantially by emphasizing "sex economy"—the balance
between energy charge and discharge, or sexual excitement and release.
According to Reich, the suppression of sexual feelings, together with
the characterological attitude that accompanies it, constitutes the true
neurosis; the clinical symptoms are only its overt manifestations.

The emotional traumas and sexual feelings are held in repression
by complex patterns of chronic muscular tensions—the "character
armor." The term "armoring" refers to the function of protecting the
individual against painful and threatening experiences from without
and within. For Reich, the critical factor that contributes to incom-
plete sexual orgasm and congestion of bioenergy is the repressive
influence of society. A neurotic individual maintains balance by bind-
ing his excess energy in muscular tensions, and thus limiting sexual
excitement ...

According to Reich, the goal of therapy was to ensure the patient
was capable of fully surrendering to the spontaneous and involuntary
movements of the body that are normally associated with the respiratory process. If this was accomplished, the respiratory waves produce
an undulating movement in the body that Reich called the "orgasm
reflex." He believes that those patients who achieve it in therapy are
then capable of surrendering fully in the sexual situation, reaching
a state of total satisfaction. The full orgasm discharges all the excess
energy of the organism, and the patient remains free of symptoms.[38]

Grof himself believes that there is validity to Reich's claims and situates
his understanding of this energy within a larger transpersonal context.
He believes these trapped energies could be accessed and freed through
the assistance of psychedelics, along with other forms of therapy. (Nearly
one in five women in the United States experience rape during their lifetime, and psychedelic-assisted psychotherapy might help heal one of the
most traumatic experiences occurring in our species.) Psychedelics might
have been more commonly used with our ancestors, making this form of

---

[38] Grof, *Way of the Psychonaut, Vol. 1*, 216–18.

healing more available. Our ancestors, though, may also have held less trauma than people today because they allowed their sexual energy to move more freely. They also likely held less shame about sexuality than people in modern society and experienced more opportunity to move the energy and heal through intimate encounters with each other.

Despite the deep ties that various forms of social and sexual bonding created, there likely came moments within the tribe, whether it be because of meeting maximum capacities of resources within the environment or because of political differences, when the tribe would split. In the best-selling book *The Tipping Point: How Little Things Can Make a Big Difference*, Malcom Gladwell makes a convincing case that a maximum population capacity for an intimate community is 150 people—this is known as Dunbar's number. Robert Dunbar is a British anthropologist who discovered a correlation between a primate's brain size and the average size of their social group. After 150 people it becomes hard for each person to personally know each other member.[39] When that occurs, a sense of safety and belonging, as well as cohesion, within the group begins to diminish. Yuval Noah Harari, in *Sapiens: A Brief History of Humankind*, agrees that the tipping point for a group was likely 150.[40] Below 150 people, Harari believes, gossip could hold the group social structure and that over that number communities need more structured levels of social organization. Before such levels were developed to create structure to the group, the group may have begun to organically split at 150 members. Harari writes:

> If a forager band split once every forty years and its splinter group migrated to a new territory sixty miles to the east, the distance from East Africa to China would have been covered in about 10,000 years. In some exceptional cases, when food sources were particularly rich, bands settled down in seasonal and even permanent camps.[41]

---

[39] Gladwell, *Tipping Point*.

[40] Harari, *Sapiens*, 27.

[41] Harari, 48.

This may have been the way groups navigated and then began spreading across the world, until the time of permanent settlements, which began with fishing cities and the invention of agriculture about twelve thousand years ago.

In *Sapiens* Harari describes how our hunter-gatherer ancestors lived during the roughly four million years between our primate ancestors coming down from the trees and learning to plant seeds, kicking off the Agricultural Revolution. In a chapter titled "A Day in the Life of Adam and Eve," Harari writes:

> The hunter-gatherer way of life differed significantly from region to region and from season to season, but on the whole foragers seem to have enjoyed a more comfortable and rewarding lifestyle than most of the peasants, shepherds, laborers and office clerks who followed in their footsteps.
>
> While people in today's affluent societies work an average of forty to forty-five hours a week, and people in the developing world work sixty and even eighty hours a week, hunter-gathers living today in the most inhospitable of habitats . . . work on average for just thirty-five to forty five hours a week. In normal times, this is enough to feed the band . . .
>
> The forager economy provided most people with more interesting lives than agriculture or industry do . . . They'd roam the nearby forests and meadows, gathering mushrooms, digging up edible roots, catching frogs and occasionally running away from tigers. By early afternoon, they were back at the camp to make lunch. That left them plenty of time to gossip, tell stories, play with the children and just hang out. Of course the tigers sometimes caught them, or a snake bit them, but on the other hand they didn't have to deal with automobile accidents and industrial pollution.
>
> In most places and at most times, foraging provided ideal nutrition. That is hardly surprising—this had been the human diet for hundreds of thousands of years, and the human body was well adapted to it. Evidence from fossilized skeletons indicates that ancient foragers were less likely to suffer from starvation or malnutrition, and were generally taller and healthier than their peasant descendants. Average life expectancy was apparently just thirty to forty years, but this was due largely to the high incidence of child mortality [the high

occurrence of deaths at birth has been included in the statistic of the average lifespan being around thirty, which paints an unrealistic picture that most adults died early]. Children who made it through the perilous first years had a good chance of reaching the age of sixty, and some even made it to their eighties ...

The wholesome and varied diet, the relatively short working week, and the rarity of infectious diseases have led many experts to define pre-agricultural societies as "the original affluent societies."[42]

Harari also makes sure that the readers are not left ignorantly idealistic about the forager lifestyle: "Though they lived better lives than most people in agricultural and industrial societies, their world could be harsh and unforgiving."[43] Child mortality rates were high, a small injury could mean death, and old or disabled people may have been killed or abandoned if they did not keep up with the tribe.

Starting seventy thousand years ago there occurred what Harari terms the "Cognitive Revolution," which he defines as

the point when history declared its independence from biology. Until the Cognitive Revolution, the doings of all human species belonged to the realm of biology. . . . From the Cognitive Revolution onwards, historical narratives replace biological theories as our primary means of explaining the development of Homo sapiens.[44]

This is when, according to mainstream anthropology, language evolved to the point of constructing myths, people began to create art, and culture directed human evolution. Shared myths create structured beliefs about the world and are able to tie together a large amount of people beyond blood kinship.[45] Religion, for example, enables tribes to unite under the

---

[42] Harari, 50–51.

[43] Harari, 52.

[44] Harari, 37.

[45] Beck and Cowan, *Spiral Dynamics*; Wilber, *Brief History of Everything*.

notion of gods or larger ideas. Before myths, tribes were largely held together by kinship. Now several tribes could come together, united under a perceived larger order. This organization paved the way for a rudimentary form of government to arise, and with more humans communing together, larger divisions of labor could form.

The next major revolution, the Agricultural Revolution, occurred sixty thousand years later, around 9000 BCE in the Middle East. It radically reshaped human life. Agriculture, the ability to grow and control food production, enabled humans to settle and accumulate material wealth over generations. In contrast, the hunter and gatherer lifestyle restricted material possessions to what one could carry. Once humans could accumulate and store goods, it also meant there was more worth stealing. For most of human history, it wasn't worth it for one tribe to attack another. The cost was too high for the goods the tribe was carrying, and most of the goods could also not be carried by the attacking tribe. After the Agricultural Revolution, a roving tribe might encounter a permanent settlement with housing as well as an entire season's worth of crops, resources that might be worth the risk involved in fighting for them. Before the Agricultural Revolution a tribe could flee if getting attacked, but a settlement is less likely to run away and more likely to engage in conflict to protect their home.

There is no doubt that the complex lives we have now would have not been possible without the Agricultural Revolution. But it can be argued that what humanity gave up in the process of this progress was substantial. Harari writes:

> The Agricultural Revolution certainly enlarged the sum total of food at the disposal of humankind, but the extra food did not translate into a better diet or more leisure. Rather, it translated into population explosions and pampered elites. The average farmer worked harder than the average forager, and got a worse diet in return. The Agricultural Revolution was history's biggest fraud.[46]

---

[46] Harari, *Sapiens*, 79.

The entire social structure of humanity began to change with the emergent capacities that came with the ability to grow food. As individuals received wealth from their parents and began to own property for the first time, it became important for men to know which children were their blood descendants, so that their legacy could be passed on. This eventually led to the idea of patriarchal marriage, where a man owned a wife so that he could be sure that she did not sleep with anyone else and he could be sure that the children were his. This is when our modern sense of monogamy might have arisen, which is the dominant relationship model in all industrialized nations that were enabled by the Agricultural Revolution.[47]

Though many historians may believe the Agricultural Revolution had the greatest impact on the evolution of humanity, it is possible there was something else working in tandem with these environmental and social factors, which may have had an even greater impact on humanity by shaping its consciousness—our ancestors' encounters and symbiotic relationship with psilocybin mushrooms.

---

[47] Harari, 79.

5

THE MYCELIAL MIND

Twenty-three species of primates, including that of our own, regularly eat fungi. The diet of the Goeldi's monkey of South America consists of up to 35 percent of the mushrooms.[1] The cap and stem formation makes mushrooms easy to spot and grab, and several species of primates are known to come down from the trees to grab mushrooms as soon as they fruit. Our human line of evolution has always been directly and indirectly in contact with mycelium, whether that underneath our feet or through the food on which we feast. In an anthology titled *Fantastic Fungi: How Mushrooms Can Heal, Shift Consciousness, and Save the Planet*, Paul Stamets writes, "That's mycelium, the network of fungal cells that permeates all landscapes. It is the foundation of the food web. It holds all life together."[2]

---

[1] MAPS, "Mycology of Consciousness," at 00:10:50.

[2] Stamets, *Fantastic Fungi*, 11.

In addition to providing energy in the form of food, mushrooms exhibit myriad other health benefits, including cognitive advantages. Stamets continues, "A 2017 study of eleven mushrooms, including maitake, cordyceps, and nine other edible and medicinal species, found that each one increased the production of specific nerve cells in the brain that could protect against both dementia and Alzheimer's."[3] Psilocybin mushrooms, as discussed in chapter 3, may have also provided our ancestors greater harmony with their environment. Stamets states, "I believe that habitats have immune systems just like people, and that mushroom mycelium is the molecular bridge between the two. Incorporating these fungi into our lives and our environment strengthens the defense of the entire ecosystem."[4] This relationship between our ancestors and fungi, including psychedelic fungi, likely began when our primate ancestors lived in the canopies, and use escalated when they were forced permanently out of the trees and then followed herds of game.

As mentioned, it was easy for our largely vegetarian primate ancestors to find the saucer-shaped mushrooms on the ground. Many mushrooms grow in clusters, making them obvious to foragers. The oldest cave paintings in the world depicting mushroom use are found in Africa, where humanity evolved, and are at least nine to twelve thousand years old.[5] Psilocybin mushrooms are the most common form of mushrooms found on the African savanna,[6] and until a couple million years ago, many of those areas were rain forest, with wetter climates that encouraged even more mushroom growth. Terence McKenna points out that it was almost inevitable for our ancestors to come across the mushrooms by the time they began to follow game.[7] Mushrooms are coprophilic and grow on dung such as that of the ungulates that roam the African

---

[3] Stamets, 76.

[4] Stamets, 115.

[5] Devereux, *Long Trip*.

[6] MAPS, "Mycology of Consciousness"; T. McKenna, *Food of the Gods*.

[7] T. McKenna, *Food of the Gods*.

savanna. These psychedelic fungi would have been regularly within our ancestors' tribal environment. As humans followed the tracks of wild game, they would come across the mushroom in the animals' footsteps.

Newly discovered genetic factors also support the high likelihood that our ancestors would have found and then sought out the mushroom. A gene named DRD4-7R (known as the wanderlust gene) has been found to affect levels of dopamine, our neurotransmitter linked to rewards and pleasure, and correlates to novelty-seeking personality traits.[8] Dopamine is quite a fascinating neurotransmitter. In the book *The Molecule of More: How a Single Chemical in Your Brain Drives Love, Sex, and Creativity—and Will Determine the Fate of the Human Race*, Lieberman and Long write: "Mammals, reptiles, birds, and fish all have this chemical inside their brains, but no creature has more of it than a human."[9] Dopamine is the molecule of motivation. The authors go on to say, "In a broad sense, saying something is 'important' is another way of saying it's linked to dopamine. Why? Because among the many things it does, dopamine is an early-warning system for the appearance of anything that can help us survive."[10] The DRD4-7R gene that affects dopamine is twice as likely to be found in the population diagnosed with attention deficit hyperactivity disorder (ADHD) and is believed to also have been present in humanity at least as far back as the hunter-gatherer period of our species.[11] The term *cognitive "disorder"* is highly misleading, however, as this mutation has brought about many evolutionary advantages, including character traits that well served hunter and gatherer societies but often prove difficult for individuals in modern society, as do most types of neurodivergence, or neurological patterning different from that of the average human.

---

[8] University of California, Irvine, "Disorder Related to Advantageous Gene."

[9] Lieberman and Long, *Molecule of More*, xvi.

[10] Lieberman and Long, 32

[11] Pearson, "Out-of-Africa Migration."

A 2019 study of people with ADHD found six core themes of positive traits (cognitive dynamism, courage, energy, humanity, resilience and transcendence),[12] and many scientists believe this gene was positively selected to move forward in our evolution.[13] These neurodivergent individuals might have been more courageous than others in their tribe and picked up a spear to defend their community when needed. The same individuals are also highly creative, as their minds are constantly seeking for novelty through both ideas and the environment. These individuals would have looked for new sources of food and eventually (and repeatedly) come across the mushroom. Even though the mushroom may have caused highly disorientating experiences, it would have given these individuals the experience of novelty that psilocybin offers, inspiring them to seek out the mushroom again. Because the gene mutation of ADHD affects dopamine production, these individuals actually seek stimulation in the form of novelty just to regulate their mood. People that carried this gene were likely catalysts for human migration and were likely the ones that came up with many of the inventions along the way.[14]

Given that the psilocybin mushrooms grew in our ancestors' environment for at least tens of millions of years, and that once they began to follow game for protein the chances of finding the psilocybin mushrooms largely increased, and also that there were probably members in the tribe who (once they found the mushroom) would regularly seek it out, it is likely that psilocybin mushrooms deeply influenced the consciousness, biology, and culture of our ancestors in profound and numerous ways.

In a section titled "The Real Missing Link" in *Food of the Gods*, Terence McKenna writes about the relationship between psilocybin and early humans:

---

[12] Sedgwick, Merwood, and Asherson, "Positive Aspects."

[13] Pearson, "Out-of-Africa Migration."

[14] Williams and Taylor, "Hyperactivity, Impulsivity and Cognitive Diversity."

My contention is that mutation-causing, psychoactive chemical compounds in the early human diet directly influenced the rapid reorganization of the brain's information-processing capacities. . . . The action of hallucinogens present in many common plants enhanced our information-processing activity, or environmental sensitivity, and thus contributed to the sudden expansion of the human brain size. At a later stage in the same process, hallucinogens acted as catalysts in the development of imagination, fueling the creation of internal stratagems and hopes that may well have synergized the emergence of language and religion.[15]

One way the brain's informational-processing capacities and environmental sensitivities, as McKenna puts it, might have been enhanced by psilocybin mushrooms was an improved ability to process visual information. Roland Fischer, a psychopharmacologist, conducted experiments with psilocybin in the 1970s and concluded that, at small doses, psilocybin increases visual acuity, most notably edge detection.[16] If our ancestors ate microdose amounts even without knowing they were psychoactive, even maybe a mushroom at a time, this increased vision could have been helpful as they swung from branch to branch. The psilocybin would have also made colors appear brighter and shapes better defined, which would have helped our ancestors both forage for food and detect predators, such as snakes camouflaged in the leaves.

Group Dynamics

As evolution moved forward, and especially when our ancestors took to the ground to track wild game and eventually domesticate cattle, dosage and also the effects of psilocybin on the population likely increased as people became more intentional about using the mushrooms for their

---

[15] T. McKenna, *Food of the Gods*, 24.

[16] Doyle, *Darwin's Pharmacy*, 34.

mind-altering benefits. An increased dose might also have led from just enhancing environmental awareness to affecting group dynamics, as Terence McKenna writes:

> At the first, low level of usage is the effect that Fischer noted: small amounts of psilocybin, consumed with no awareness of its psychoactivity while in the general act of browsing for food, and perhaps later consumed consciously, impart a noticeable increase in visual acuity, especially edge detection …
>
> Because psilocybin is a stimulant of the central nervous system, when taken in slightly larger doses, it tends to trigger restlessness and sexual arousal. Thus, at this second level of usage, by increasing instances of copulation, the mushroom directly favored human reproduction. The tendency to regulate and schedule sexual activity within the group, by linking it to the lunar cycle of the mushroom availability, may have been important as a first step toward ritual and religion. Certainly at the third and highest level of usage, religious concerns would be at the forefront of the tribe's consciousness, simply because of the power and strangeness of the experience itself.[17]

In these three stages of dosage one can clearly see the instincts of autonomy, communion, and transcendence. At the lowest dose, the heightening of one's strongest sense, vision, enables one to better scout for food and become aware of predators, therefore supporting an individual's survival. At the second stage of dosage, one begins to feel the need to physically connect with others and to copulate, encouraging greater degrees of communion. At the higher stages of dosage, both those needs begin to fall away, as one begins to feel connected to a much larger whole and move into a more visionary realm, connecting instead with a transcendental creativity.

Our ancestors, whether when living in trees or once they became bipedal, were considerably smaller in size and weight than humans are now. In working with participants, I have commonly seen that a small

---

[17] T. McKenna, *Food of the Gods*, 25.

amount of mushrooms stimulates sexual arousal. Eating just one or two mushrooms might have also stimulated arousal in our ancestors. Sexual arousal would have been more welcomed in preagricultural societies, as the boundaries of monogamy did not exist.[18] This behavior is in alignment with the sexual dynamics presented in the previous chapter. Psilocybin, which Metzner says at one point was called the love drug, acting as an aphrodisiac in the population would have supported considerable evolutionary effects.[19] Since individuals, and the tribe, that ate psilocybin mushrooms likely had a higher rate of copulation, they would have had a higher population growth than tribes that did not. Psilocybin acts a stimulant to the nervous system, and the extra energy would have led to tribal members exploring more areas and using more resources. The territory of the psilocybin-eating tribe might have expanded, while they also expanded their intelligence through the nootropic. These more hyperconnected and visually enhanced psilocybin-using groups would have had considerable creative advantages over many species in the environment.

A common question I hear in response to the psilocybin explanation of human evolution is, "If psilocybin encourages evolution, and it is freely available to all species of animals, then why is it that humans evolved to our developmental level of intelligence while other species have not?" Primates (specifically the groups humans evolved from) were likely more primed to receive fuller benefits from psilocybin compared to other species. As explained in chapter 4 and presented in Tony Wright and Graham Gynn's *Return to the Brain of Eden: Restoring the Connection Between Neurochemistry and Consciousness*, our ancestors had already undergone drastic evolutionary transformations due to the enormous environmental shifts of moving to the ground from living in the canopies over a fifty-million-year period of evolution. This radically changed both their bodies and diets,

---

[18] Ryan and Jetha, *Sex at Dawn*.

[19] Metzner, *Sacred Mushroom of Visions*, 34.

transmuting their neurochemistry and experience of the world. Some biological factors would have enabled greater benefits of psilocybin. For example, our ancestors became bipedal and developed opposable thumbs that evolved from grasping branches. These transformations allowed them to have tool-creating hands (as opposed to something like hoofs), which could be used alongside their emergent cognitive abilities that psilocybin might have catalyzed. The creativity inspired by psilocybin could have been used to make art or shape the environment, more so than animals whose bodies could not have allowed the ability to hold tools.

At higher doses, individuals would also have boundary-dissolving experiences, which Terence McKenna asserts are the most common properties of psychedelic experiences across all substances.[20] As Kotler and Wheal point out, the ability to dissolve individual boundaries is necessary for optimal group coordination.[21] The authors looked into the process of becoming a Navy SEAL and found that what is primarily tested for to become one of the most elite warriors in the country is the ability for members to dissolve their egos enough to work as a larger whole. Instead of being an alpha male, a Navy SEAL has the ability to enable the team to function almost like a single organism. In each moment-to-moment instance, the team may change leaders and then must trust that leader's direction. Each Navy SEAL must be able to feel and trust the shifts within the group. This is the communion and transcending ability of autonomous individuals becoming a part of a larger whole. The psilocybin mushroom may have enabled similar effects in our ancestors by loosening their ego grips and strengthening bonds within the group.

There is research that shows a correlation between psilocybin and an increase of empathy, which might have led to more harmonious group dynamics. One research study, based on responses from a total of

---

[20] T. McKenna, *Food of the Gods*.

[21] Kotler and Wheal, *Stealing Fire*.

1,266 participants, found that men who had tried LSD or mushrooms had decreased odds of using physical violence against their partner and reported better emotion regulation in comparison to men with no history of psychedelic use.[22] Another study, titled "Effects of Psilocybin on Empathy and Moral Decision-Making," that was published in the *International Journal of Neuropsychopharmacology* states:

> Empathy is important for the maintenance of social relationships and plays a crucial role in moral and prosocial behavior. This study investigated the acute effect of the serotonergic hallucinogen psilocybin in healthy human subjects on different facets of empathy and moral decision-making. Psilocybin significantly increased explicit and implicit emotional empathy, compared with placebo, whereas it did not affect cognitive empathy nor moral decision-making. These findings provide first evidence that psilocybin has distinct effects on social cognition by enhancing emotional empathy but not moral behavior. As the psychological effects of psilocybin are primarily mediated by serotonin (5-HT) 2A receptor activation and partially modulated by 5-HT1A receptor modulations, our findings suggest the implication of these receptor subtypes in everyday social experience. Therefore, targeting 5-HT2A/1A receptors may have potential beneficial effects in the treatment of mood disorders or psychopathy, which are characterized by deficits in social skills and in particular in the ability to feel with other people.[23]

The study is the first of its kind and shows that psilocybin increases the experience of empathy.

Societies that used psilocybin were likely more egalitarian,[24] and the lack of large-scale hierarchies in our tribal ancestors may have been what held them back from becoming what is considered more "culturally sophisticated." However, the lack of hierarchical rule also

---

[22] Burns, "Men Who Tried Psychedelics."

[23] Pokorny et al., "Effect of Psilocybin on Empathy," 748.

[24] T. McKenna, *Food of the Gods.*

meant that they likely experienced less repression and lived freer and happier lives. A paper titled "Psychedelics, Personality, and Political Perspectives," published in the *Journal of Psychoactive Drugs*, states, "Ego dissolution experienced during a participant's 'most intense' psychedelic experience positively predicted liberal political views, openness, and nature relatedness, and negatively predicted authoritarian political views."[25] Rather than climbing a never-ending social ladder and focusing on egotistical power, our tribal ancestors likely spent more time experiencing pleasure and growth through relationships and while enjoying tribal life.

Spirituality

Different degrees of dosage would have enhanced different instincts within consciousness. A small dose may have supported autonomous survival, while a slightly higher dose may have turned one's attention toward communion with others. At higher doses, one may not have been able to move around too much at all, taking away some capacities for self-preservation and connection, and instead immersing one in transcendental visionary experiences. Our ancestors might have begun constructing rituals, intentionally creating and planning a social container, for taking higher dosages. A handful of dried mushrooms is roughly five grams, which also approximately equals the amount used in the experiments studying psilocybin and mystical experiences. What fifty years of science has repeatedly found using this amount is that psilocybin can "safely and reliably 'occasion' a mystical experience."[26]

---

[25] Nour, Evans, and Carhart-Harris, "Psychedelics, Personality, and Political Perspectives," 1.

[26] Pollan, *How to Change Your Mind*, 10.

Gordon Wasson was the first to hypothesize that the very notion of God and the genesis of spirituality in humanity came from the bemushroomed experience. He writes:

As man emerged from his brutish past, thousands of years ago, there was a stage in the evolution of his awareness when the discovery of the mushroom with miraculous properties was a revelation to him, a veritable detonator to his soul, arousing in him sentiments of awe and reverence, and gentleness and love, to the highest pitch of which mankind is capable, all those sentiments and virtues that mankind has ever since regarded as the highest attributes of its kind. It made him see what this perishing mortal eye cannot see. How right the Greeks were to hedge about this Mystery, this imbibing of the potion with secrecy and surveillance! . . . Perhaps with all our modern knowledge we do not need the divine mushroom anymore. Or do we need them more than ever? Some are shocked that the key even to religion might be reduced to a mere drug.[27]

The potion that Wasson refers to in the quote is *kykeon*, a psychedelic drink used in the Greek Eleusinian Mysteries, which for millennia was perhaps taken by the citizens of Ancient Greece.[28] Gordon Wasson, Albert Hofmann, and Carl Ruck concluded after extensive research that the psychoactive element used in kykeon was ergot, a fungus that grows on rye that was used to derive LSD.[29]

If our ancestors consumed psilocybin mushrooms in Africa, and then elsewhere throughout the world, they would have been flooded with archetypal content that is characteristic of deep psychedelic experiences.[30] In trying to make sense of these experiences, they would have formed myths. These myths would have led to belief systems and

---

[27] Wasson, Hofmann, and Ruck, *Road to Eleusis*, 23.

[28] Kotler and Wheal, *Stealing Fire*, 1.

[29] Wasson, Hofmann, and Ruck, *Road to Eleusis*.

[30] Grof, *Modern Consciousness Research*; Grof, *Psychology of the Future*.

eventually religions. The Rigveda, humanity's oldest religious text, has hundreds of lines praising soma, in all likelihood an entheogenic plant or mushroom that allows one to commune with God. It was from the Rigveda that the entire Hindu religious tradition emerged—including its emphasis on practices like meditation. As Allan Badiner and Alex Grey present in *Zig Zag Zen*, meditation is something that even many people in the West felt inspired to take up as a lifelong practice after their experiences with psychedelics.[31]

The general consensus in academia is that practices we now categorize as shamanism were the first forms of human spirituality.[32] Shamanism— Earth- and plant-based practices (which sometimes use psychedelics and sometimes do not) grounded in an animist perspective—has been found on every continent on the planet, with the exclusion of Antarctica.[33] The animistic worldview, which holds that the world is alive and endowed with intelligence, would have been one supported and inspired by taking psilocybin mushrooms in nature.[34] As Simon Powell makes the case throughout his books *The Magic Mushroom Explorer* and *The Psilocybin Solution*, the natural world appears to come alive and communicate information directly to the subject about its essence when the subject looks at the world through the lens of a psilocybin catalyzed state of consciousness. John Rush, a professor of anthropology who has written eight texts in this field, states, "The use of plants and fungi as a conduit to the ancestors, eventually the gods, is an age-old tradition recognized by at least the Upper Paleolithic (c. 33KYA) and stretching perhaps millions of years into the distant past."[35] Such fungi and plants in our ancestors' environment would have been catalysts for the emergence of religious thought.

---

[31] Badiner and Grey, *Zig Zag Zen*.

[32] Devereux, *Long Trip*; Narby and Huxley, *Shamans through Time*; Walsh, *World of Shamanism*.

[33] Wilber, *Brief History of Everything*.

[34] T. McKenna, *Food of the Gods*.

[35] Rush, *Entheogens and the Development of Culture*, 3.

The idea that psychedelic plants and fungi might have been the very catalyst for the awakening of spirituality in humanity is integrating into academia. In the anthology *Entheogens and the Development of Culture*, Michael Winkelman, former president of the Anthropology of Consciousness section of the American Anthropological Association and the founding president of its Anthropology and Religion section, writes:

> Adaptations to the fungi in their environment . . . was a significant feature affecting hominin evolution. The psychoactive fungi that our foraging ancestors explored as possible food items in their environments exerted a selective influence on hominid evolution. Psychedelic mushrooms would have been invariably encountered in our ancestral past, especially in tropical regions, given their worldwide distribution. Species of mushrooms containing psilocybin have been found around the world. The worldwide distribution of neurotropic fungi used as sacraments in cultures around the world is good evidence that such substances altered consciousness in ways that induced spiritual experiences and contributed directly to the development of religious explanations and activities . . . These features of psilocybin-induced experiences are also central to shamanism. Since shamanism constitutes a primordial worldwide form of religious practice, this suggests that it was the effects of these substances that were responsible for the initial emergence of spirituality and the central alterations of consciousness institutionalized in shamanistic traditions around the world.[36]

David Kennedy, a professor of biological psychology in Europe, gives a similar statement:

> Contemporary scientific research shows that entheogens such as the hallucinogen psilocybin consistently engender altered states of consciousness that are described by consumers as mystical or spiritual and that often include experience of a "higher reality." They have this effect irrespective of the nature of the consumer's religious or spiritual

---

[36] Winkelman, "Altered Consciousness and Drugs," 37.

beliefs, or, indeed, lack of belief . . . it isn't difficult to conceive that entheogenic mystical experiences must have been interpreted by our distant ancestors as unveiling or confirming the existence of spirit worlds, gods, or an afterlife. In the light of this it seems reasonable to conclude that plant and fungal chemicals may well underlie the origin of many spiritual concepts. It also doesn't take a great leap of imagination to see the roots of our contemporary religions, including the dominant monotheistic religions, are firmly embedded in the soil of the polytheistic traditions that originated in plant-derived experiences.[37]

Perhaps part of why Western culture has taken so long to reach the possible conclusion that religion was originally inspired by psychoactive plants and fungi has to do with the bias of seeing itself as superior to other present and past cultures. In *Shamans through Time*, Jeremy Narby and Francis Huxley present how Western culture has looked at shamans throughout history.[38] Europe only began becoming aware of plant-based spiritual practices by medicine men and women about five hundred years ago. When Europeans reached the New World, they deemed Indigenous medicine men and women as devil worshippers. It is only recently that they have come to be regarded and revered as both healers and wisdom holders.

Terence McKenna discusses how mushrooms catalyzed the first forms of religions and how the knowledge of this was eventually lost.[39] He describes four stages through which this loss might have occurred. "With changes in climate, frequent, if not continual, low levels of mushroom ingestion gradually gave way to use that was merely seasonal."[40] The regions of Africa from where we evolved underwent dramatic environmental changes and had been much wetter throughout humanity's

---

[37] Kennedy, *Plants and the Human Brain*, 5.

[38] Narby and Huxley, *Shamans through Time*.

[39] T. McKenna, *Food of the Gods*.

[40] T. McKenna, 122.

prior evolution; in Roman times the upper desert region was referred to as the breadbasket of Rome. The second stage would have been a result of mushroom ecology becoming rarer, making mushrooms less plentiful, compelling shamans to want to create a reserve by drying the mushrooms and preserving them in honey. Honey ferments and turns into alcohol, so as mushrooms became more scarce, fewer were mixed in, and more honey would have been added to the mixture, and mushroom cults would have been replaced with cults of mead. In the third stage of this loss of shamanic knowledge, all that would be left were symbols. "Not only are psychoactive plants now out of the picture, but plants of any sort have disappeared, and in their place are esoteric teachings and dogma, rituals, stress on lineages, gestures, and cosmogonic diagrams."[41] The fourth stage is "the complete abandonment of even the pretense of remembering the felt experience of the mystery."[42] This last stage is "typified by secular scientism" and judging psychedelics as "evil and threatening to social values."[43] Hopefully, humans are now entering a fifth stage—integration—and will undergo what McKenna calls an Archaic Revival.[44]

The Expansion of the Mind: Art, Logic, and the Perception of Time

The oldest cave paintings in the world were inspired by shamanic states of consciousness, theorized David Lewis-Williams, an archeologist focused on the development of cognition who has won multiple international awards in his field. Author of over a dozen books on prehistoric people and art, Lewis-Williams presents scenarios of how prehistoric

---

[41] T. McKenna, 122.

[42] T. McKenna, 122.

[43] T. McKenna, 122.

[44] T. McKenna, *Archaic Revival.*

art in caves is remnant of rituals. Though his decades of research focused on South African and European cave art, his general theory on the formation of cave art can be applied to the prehistoric phenomenon around the world. The rituals would have been facilitated by the shaman and made use of altered states of consciousness that were likely catalyzed by several means—including breathing, drumming, and psychedelics. Participants of the rituals would experience visions, such as encounters with power animals, and they painted these visions directly on the walls.[45]

Building off the work of David Lewis-Williams that posits expanded states of consciousness ignited the creation of cave art, Graham Hancock, in his anthology titled *The Divine Spark: Psychedelics, Consciousness, and the Birth of Civilization*, writes:

> The appearance of the first great, fully representative symbolic art in caves and rock shelters between 40,000 and 30,000 years ago represents a spectacular enigma. That art, moreover, was already perfect and fully formed from the moment that it began to be created . . . And why was it accompanied by other significant changes in human behavior—including but not limited to better and more sophisticated stone and bone tools, better hunting strategies, and the first evidence of spiritual beliefs? . . . It is difficult to avoid the conclusion that whatever divine spark led our ancestors to start creating art caused all other changes as well.
>
> In other words, if we can explain the art, we can explain the origins of modern humanity. It is therefore of the greatest interest that such a theory has been proposed and does indeed completely explain the special characteristics of Stone Age art from as far afield as Europe, the Americas, Africa, and Australia, and moreover, why identical characteristics are found in the art produced by the shamans of surviving tribal cultures today. The theory was originally elaborated by Lewis-Williams and is now supported by a majority of archeologists and anthropologists. In brief, it proposes that the reason for the eerie similarities and universal themes linking all these different systems of art is that in every case—both ancient and modern and wherever in

---

[45] Lewis-Williams, *Conceiving God*, 225.

the world they are found—the shaman-artists responsible for them have previously experienced altered states of consciousness in which they had seen vivid hallucinations, and in every case their endeavor in making the art was to memorialize on the walls of rock shelters and caves the ephemeral images that they had seen in their visions. According to this neuropsychological theory, the different bodies of art have so many similarities because we all share the same neurology, and thus share many of the same experiences and visions in altered states of consciousness.[46]

This last sentence fits well with the notion covered later in this chapter (see "Psilocybin and Brain Development") that perhaps humans and their hominin ancestors had been taking psilocybin mushrooms, which stimulate neurogenesis, for the last several million years and therefore had similar neurological formations. Taking the neurotropic psilocybin at smaller supplemental doses would have integrally, both chemically and through the consciousness-expanding experiences, affected the evolution of human neurophysiology and mental capacities. Using the integral model described in chapter 2, changes in the upper-right/objective quadrant (like the brain) would also create changes in the upper-left/subjective quadrant (personal consciousness). As presented in chapter 3, evolution moves forward through the combination of all the quadrants together. In this case of cave art, humans are also transforming consciousness through art and culture, the lower-left/intersubjective quadrant, and reorganizing the environment and human systems for ritual, the lower-right/interobjective quadrant. The transformation of consciousness plays a large role in the evolution of consciousness, including brain development, and the use of consciousness-expanding plants and fungi might have drastically altered the formation of the human brain.

As the philosopher Ken Wilber frequently states, altered states become altered traits.[47] This evolution, which likely took place in Africa

---

[46] Hancock, *Divine Spark*, 6.

[47] Wilber, *Sex, Ecology, Spirituality*.

before the great migrations across the world, would have already been a part of every human being across the planet thirty to forty thousand years ago. What likely began prior to the emergence of cave art, which Yuval Noah Harari calls the "cognitive revolution,"[48] was the movement to the ritual use of psychedelics. Intentional ritual use of psychedelics likely included taking higher doses, as used in psychedelic ceremonies today. The caves and ritual containers would have given our ancestors a safer set and setting (a prepared state of mind and controlled environment) to work with these higher, visionary doses and possibly contributed to creative breakthroughs, both in art and tool making.

Tom Froese, who received his PhD in cognitive science and now serves as an editor of seven cognitive science journals, reaches a similar assessment as Hancock and Lewis-Williams. In an essay titled "Altered States and the Prehistoric Ritualization of the Modern Human Mind," Froese writes, "The similarities of the prehistoric patterns could thus be explained in terms of a common mechanism of altered states, for instance the workings of our species-specific brain."[49] Ffion Reynolds, who did her doctoral work on the Neolithic worldview, writes in an essay titled "Tracing Neolithic Worldviews: Shamanism, Irish Passage Tomb Art and Altered States of Consciousness" that "in the last 20 years or so, new interpretations regarding engraved art have emerged in which some imagery is associated with shamanism."[50] Irish tombs house more than a quarter of Europe's megalithic art, making them the highest concentration of megalithic art in the continent.[51] She writes, "It has been suggested that Neolithic Irish passage tombs, dating back to around five thousand years ago, were associated with a complex of consciousness-altering traditions, linked to the practice of shamanism. . . . Many authors working in archaeology and rock art studies, who suggest that

---

[48] Harari, *Sapiens*, 37.

[49] Froese, "Altered States and the Prehistoric Ritualization," 1.

[50] Reynolds, "Tracing Neolithic Worldviews," 13.

[51] Reynolds, 21.

shamanism may have existed during the Neolithic and before, also believe strongly that drugs may have been involved."[52]

Aside from artistic expression, other cognitive abilities of prehistoric humanity would have been influenced by psychedelic use. John Rush discusses the impact that psychedelics may have had on our ancestors' decision-making and problem-solving processes. In a chapter titled "Mind-Altering Substances, Decision Making, and Culture Building," he writes:

> The new model is more complicated but suggests there may be a deeper, neurochemical issue, an evolutionary leap away from all the other primates. That is to say, we purposely enhanced receptor sites in the brain, especially dopamine and serotonin, through the use of plants and fungi over a long period of time. The trade off for potential drug abuse was more creative thinking, or a leap in consciousness, and the development of primitive medicine wherein certain mind-altering plants and fungi silence fatigue, pain, or depression, while others promote hunger, expel parasites, and so on. Our ancestors selected for our neural hardware, and our propensity for seeking altered forms of consciousness, as a survival strategy, intimately bound to our decision-making processes, again going back perhaps a million years or more.[53]

The shaman played the role of the cosmologist, medicine man and woman, and the wisdom holder of the tribe. This distinct role in the group also was the point person that made group decisions, such as what direction the tribe should migrate to find a herd. In present-day entheogenic traditions, the medicine man or woman goes into altered states to harness power to overcome challenges for both themselves and the group.[54]

---

[52] Reynolds, 15, 22.

[53] Rush, *Entheogens and the Development of Culture*, 13.

[54] T. McKenna, *Food of the Gods*.

Steven Kotler and Jamie Wheal, the optimization experts who are responsible for the largest meta-analysis of creativity ever conducted, which included reviewing more than thirty thousand research papers, present how altered states of consciousness are being used today to bring out the best of people in a variety of fields.[55] "It's the story of an entirely new breed of Promethean upstart—Silicon Valley executives, members of the U.S. special forces, maverick scientists, to name only a few—who are using ecstatic techniques to alter consciousness and accelerate performance."[56] Enhanced abilities catalyzed by psychedelically inspired altered states, used by extreme athletes, business executives, scientists, and artists today, would have been just as true for our ancestors. A pivotal difference between those in the present and those in the past is that these psychedelic means of enhancements with plants and fungi would have been conventionally acceptable in the past.

Along with boosting energy and inspiring creativity, psychedelic experiences may have aided the evolution of the human capacity for logic, including mathematics, for two reasons. The first is that at deeper states of psilocybin experiences, and immediately on DMT (psilocybin builds on the chemical base structure of DMT, and is known as 4-PO-HO-DMT), a common trademark of the experience is to see geometric shapes. As presented in chapter 1, this experience is cross-cultural and is found throughout the psychedelic literature. One can think here of Platonic forms, a perspective that views mathematics as a universal and essential aspect of the cosmos that exists independent of the human mind.[57] There is no reason to believe that our ancestors would also not have been graced by the visualization of these shapes. Even Ralph Abraham, one of the founders of dynamic systems theory and chaos theory in mathematics, shared that psychedelics played a large role in his formulations.[58] Seeing

---

[55] Kotler and Wheal, *Stealing Fire*, 46.

[56] Kotler and Wheal, 4.

[57] Tarnas, *Passion of the Western Mind*.

[58] T. McKenna, Sheldrake, and Abraham, *Chaos, Creativity, and Cosmic Consciousness*.

perfectly shaped geometric objects, which rarely naturally occur in the physical world, may have inspired other mathematical capabilities within humans. It may not be coincidental that the Pythagoreans, who devoted themselves to mathematics and participated in the Eleusinian Mysteries, considered these shapes as expressions of the divine.

Another quality of consciousness that might have been expanded by psilocybin is the experience and understanding of time. It is common in psychedelic states, including those catalyzed by psilocybin, to experience an expanded sense of time.[59] There has only been one study on the topic, which was published as "Effects of Psilocybin on Time Perception and Temporal Control of Behavior in Humans" in the *International Journal of Psychopharmacology.* The experiment found that psilocybin significantly impacted the ability of participants to keep track of time.[60] The results indicate that the serotonin system is selectively involved in processing the passage of time when it comes to intervals that are longer than two to three seconds. It is common for one under the influence of psilocybin to experience large epochs of time, including becoming one with the Earth's entire evolutionary process. This pull of one's consciousness into deep history and the farthest imaginable possibilities of the future likely also occurred to our ancestors. The ability for humans to both imagine the future and a deep past is something that separates our consciousness from that of other animals, and that is integral to our ability to think logically. This stretching of the perception of time is necessary for logic. An essential aspect of logic is the mental process of imagining the unfolding of cause and effect that occurs throughout the passage of time. It appears that most other animals' mental life is one of living solely in the present moment, and they do not appear to possess imaginative capacities that come close to those of humans.

In *True Hallucinations: Being an Account of the Author's Extraordinary Adventures in the Devil's Paradise,* Terence McKenna offers some good

---

[59] Grof, *Way of the Psychonaut, Vol. 2.*

[60] Wittmann et al., "Effects of Psilocybin on Time Perception."

examples of the experience of time expansion on psychedelics by presenting psilocybin mushroom journeys of his brother, Dennis McKenna:

> Dennis's story was the classic description of a shamanic night jour-
> ney. He said that he had gone to the *chorro* and had meditated in the
> mission cemetery we had visited before. He had begun to return to
> camp when he confronted a particularly large *Inga* tree near where the
> path skirted the edge of the mission. On impulse, he had climbed it,
> aware as he did that the ascent of the world tree is the central motif
> of the Siberian shamanic journey. As he climbed the tree, he felt the
> flickering polarities of many archetypes, and as he reached the highest
> point in his ascent, something that he called "the vortex" opened ahead
> of him—a swirling, enormous doorway into time. He could see the
> Cyclopean megaliths of Stonehenge and beyond them, revolving at
> a different speed and at a higher plane, the outlines of the pyramids,
> gleaming and marble-faceted as they have not been since the days
> of pharaonic Egypt. And yet farther into the turbulent maw of the
> vortex, he saw mysteries that were ancient long before the advent of
> man—titanic archetypal forms on worlds unimagined by us, the arcane
> machineries of sentient agencies that swept through this part of the
> galaxy when our planet was young and its surface barely cooled. This
> machinery, this gibberish abysses, touched with the cold of interstellar
> space and aeon-consuming time, rushed down upon him. He fainted,
> and time—who can say how much time—passed by him.[61]

Terence McKenna continues:

> He seemed to be spread over so vast an amount of time and space that
> there was little to be identified out of the cosmic churning that he was
> undergoing. On that day, to even find our own galaxy in his mind had
> been impossible. On the second day, he awoke within the galaxy and
> his visions and fantasies remained within it. Had that been the only
> instance of his telescoping back into himself, it would not have been
> worth noting, but the fact was that each step of his return to a normal

---

[61] T. McKenna, *True Hallucinations*, 122.

state of mind was accomplished this way. The day after he reached the confines of the galaxy, he entered the solar system, condensing through its planets over several days until he identified only with Earth. Coalescing and condensing through the ecology of his home world, he came to think of himself as all humanity and was able to vividly relive all of its history. Later still, he became the embodiment of all the members of our vast and peculiar Irish family stretching back till before Judges had given us numbers or Leviticus committed Deuteronomy, as James Joyce put it. They were of all kinds and he played them all: hard-rock miners, a seventeenth-century cleric sweating beneath a burden of lust, bombastic patriarchs and thin-faced women one generation, and women with shoulders like field hands and tongues like hedge clippers the next. After a good bit of lolling around in those environs he was finally resolved down into our immediate family and progressed from there to confront and resolve the question of whether he was Dennis or Terence. Finally and thankfully, he came to rest with the realization that *he* was Dennis, returned from the edge of the universe of mind, restored and reborn, a shaman in the fullest sense of the word.[62]

These passages do illustrate a sense of linear consistency of events over a large period of time, and they show the vast ecological contexts with which a psychonaut can identify—as Dennis moves from first identifying with the whole cosmos, then evolving through this history of our planet, and surging through the logical unfolding of humanity until he reaches himself in the present moment.

A typical characteristic of psychedelic experiences, especially at medium to high doses, is that one experiences imaginal realms that are beyond what one normally sees, hears, tastes, touches, and smells in their environment. This imagination is crucial for symbolic thought, such as mathematics and sophisticated use of language. Our ancestors' imagination would have been expanded, and they would have seen things in their mind's eye that their physical eyes had never seen. Prolonged

---

[62] T. McKenna, 131.

use of psilocybin may have caused this ability, this inner "hallucination," to develop. The neural pathways that brought about this ability, and in many ways brought a greater capacity of creativity for humanity, may have been integrated into the evolution of our species. As discussed in the section on brain evolution, many pathways that are catalyzed by psilocybin stabilize, and this process of neuroplasticity might have given humans our current mental ability to hold parallel processes of seeing through our physical eyes and holding a visualization in our mind. This ability, which allows one to imaginatively see the future, is necessary for planning and is essential to the building of civilizations. Humans could see in their mind's eye houses, city layouts, and eventually complex systems. Even some of today's visionaries use psychedelics to enhance imaginative and complex processes. Peter Schwartz, a leading futurist and senior vice president for strategic planning at Salesforce, tells Michael Pollan that "several of the early computer engineers relied on LSD in designing circuit chips, especially in the years before they could be designed on computers."[63] Psilocybin has a similar molecular structure and neurological effect to that of LSD. The expansion of the perception of time may have increased the capacity of finding patterns for our ancestors, and, therefore, helped solve many of their problems. It could also have enhanced their creative capacities to create tools by helping them see in their mind's eye the potential of using objects to manipulate the world.

Paul Stamets had previously made it clear in his lectures that the idea of humanity evolving from a primate stage of consciousness to its current form because of the consumption of psilocybin mushroom is a hypothesis and not a theory.[64] A hypothesis is an assumption that one makes before any research has been completed. A theory is a principle set to explain phenomena already supported by data. In the summer of 2018 at the Lightning in a Bottle Festival, I asked Stamets: considering

---

[63] Pollan, *How to Change Your Mind*, 182.

[64] MAPS, "Mycology of Consciousness."

the MRI research, the cave paintings, and the widespread availability of psilocybin mushrooms, what else would it take for it to no longer be a hypothesis but to become a theory? He said a theory must be testable. He stated that if one could construct an experiment that shows that psilocybin could enhance our creative problem-solving abilities, then that would be enough. Until recently, due to legality it was difficult to conduct research into this area. But on February 26, 2019, an experiment titled "Sub-Acute Effects of Psilocybin on Empathy, Creative Thinking, and Subjective Well-Being" was published, saying:

> Results indicated that psilocybin enhanced divergent thinking and emotional empathy the morning after use. Enhancements in convergent thinking, valence-specific emotional empathy, and well-being persisted seven days after use. Sub-acute changes in empathy correlated with changes in well-being. The study demonstrates that a single administration of psilocybin in a social setting may be associated with sub-acute enhancement of creative thinking, empathy, and subjective well-being.[65]

The experiment used fifty-five participants, and the changes in creativity lasted at least a week for many. Another study, titled "Exploring the Effects of Microdosing Psychedelics on Creativity in an Open-Label Natural Setting" and published in the journal *Psychopharmacology,* also found that both convergent and divergent thinking performance improved with psilocybin.[66] During the Multidisciplinary Association for Psychedelic Studies (MAPS) Entheogeneration Speaker Series at Burning Man 2019, Paul Stamets gave a talk titled "The Mycology of Consciousness" and said he believes we now have enough scientific evidence to hold this explanation of human evolution as a theory.

---

[65] Mason et al., "Sub-Acute Effects of Psilocybin," 8.

[66] Prochazkova et al., "Exploring the Effect of Microdosing."

Before psychedelics became illegal, other experiments looking into the correlation between psychedelics and creativity reached similar conclusions in the 1960s. Michael Pollan writes:

> Working in groups of four, James Fadiman and Willis Hartman administered the same dose of LSD to artists, engineers, architects, and scientists, all of whom were somehow "stuck" in their work on a particular project . . . Subjects reported much greater fluidity in their thinking, as well as an enhanced ability to both visualize a problem and recontextualize it . . . Among their subjects were some of the visionaries who in the next few years would revolutionize computers.[67]

In the 1960s French scientists also administered psilocybin to artists to see how their painting styles would change.[68] Highly influenced by Freud and Jung, these scientists wanted to see if psilocybin allows one greater access to the unconscious and therefore into a wellspring of creativity. They found the artists all faced a similar challenge: deciding whether to control their experience and hold on to their own style or surrender and move toward more novel expression. Letcher writes, "Those that opted for the former seem to have gained little from the experience; those who opted for the latter, a great deal."[69] I imagine as psychedelics continue to gain acceptance in our modern culture, countless studies focusing on the intersection of creativity and psychedelics will emerge. More examples of how psychedelics have impacted individuals' creativity are presented in the next chapter.

---

[67] Pollan, *How to Change Your Mind*, 18.

[68] Letcher, *Shroom*, 188.

[69] Letcher, 190.

Language

Evolutionary biologist and anthropologist Robin Dunbar states in his book *Grooming, Gossip, and the Evolution of Language* that humans originally evolved language in order to gossip and maintain social cohesion.[70] Dunbar says that other primates spend 20 percent of their time grooming and live in groups of forty to fifty members. He speculates that when human group size began to grow, so that more than 30 percent of their time was required to be spent on social grooming in order to maintain secure cohesion, compromising the time for survival activities, our ancestors started to vocalize in order to connect more efficiently. In *Sapiens: A Brief History of Humankind*, Harari supports this perspective:

> Social cooperation is our key for survival and reproduction. It is not enough for individual men and women to know the whereabouts of lions and bison. It's much more important for them to know who in their band hates whom, who is sleeping with whom, who is honest, and who is a cheat.[71]

Rifkin states: "Studies for existing forager/hunter societies show that men and women spend, on average, about 25 percent of their day socializing."[72] Dunbar proposes that language enabled the expanded size of our ancestors' group from around 40 to 50 members to about 150 members. Dunbar notes that the size of the neocortex of the brains of mammals correlates with the size of their social group. In most mammals, the neocortex composes about 30 percent to 40 percent of brain volume. In comparison, it ranges from 50 percent in nonhuman primates to 80 percent in humans. This allows advanced social animals, such as ourselves, to keep track of each other's moods, feelings, and expectations in order to maintain proper social cohesion.

---

[70] Dunbar, *Grooming, Gossip, and the Evolution of Language.*

[71] Harari, *Sapiens*, 22.

[72] Rifkin, *Empathic Civilization*, 101.

The ability to vocalize meaning would have led to more extensive social relationships that had been previously limited by the physical energy and time it took to groom members of the tribe. It also would have transformed the coordination of a tribe into one more closely resembling that of a singular organism, since information could be transmitted through vocalization at once to everyone in the group. Here again one can see the dynamics of autonomy, communion, and transcendence: autonomous individuals communing with other individuals, transcending the boundaries of their consciousness by transmitting their experiences to one another through language, and feeling the larger wholeness of the group.

Dunbar's theory appears to be well accepted by the mainstream—academic sociologists, philosophers, and anthropologists are integrating his ideas in their efforts to make sense of human evolution. That being said, I would also like to present Terence McKenna's hypothesis on the emergence of language, which is a compelling argument:

> Our language-forming ability may have become active through the mutagenic influence of hallucinogens working directly on organelles that are concerned with the processing and generation of signals. These neural substructures are found in various portions of the brain, such as Broca's area, that govern speech formation. In other words, opening the valve that limits consciousness forces utterance, almost as if the word is a concretion of meaning previously felt but left unarticulated. This active impulse to speak, the "going forth of the word," is sensed and described in the cosmogonies of many people.
>
> Psilocybin specifically activates the areas of the brain concerned with processing signals. A common occurrence with psilocybin intoxication is spontaneous outbursts of poetry and other vocal activity such as speaking in tongues, though in a manner distinct from ordinary glossolalia. In cultures with a tradition of mushroom use, these phenomena have given rise to the notion of discourse with spirit doctors and supernatural allies. Researchers familiar with the territory agree that psilocybin has a profound catalytic effect on the linguistic impulse.[73]

---

[73] T. McKenna, *Food of the Gods*, 52–53.

McKenna's hypothesis is in harmony with Dunbar's work. Though glossolalia-like behavior (the phenomenon of people spontaneously speaking in what appears to be languages unknown to them) may have catalyzed the ability to vocalize meaning, day-to-day social interactions would have synergistically fostered further development of this ability. Socializing would likely have been the most common usage of language—just as it is today.

Glossolalia usually occurs in religious contexts and is found in virtually every tradition. In her book *Xenolinguistics: Psychedelics, Language, and the Evolution of Consciousness*, linguist Diana Reed Slattery writes about glossolalia and states:

> These utterances are often associated with altered states of consciousness. . . . It appears to be a broad, cross-cultural phenomenon of considerable antiquity. The appearance of glossolalic utterances in shamanic cultures relating to communication with spirits would indicate roots in the distant past.[74]

As an example, Fredrick Swain, a forty-year-old American who underwent a mushroom ceremony with Maria Sabina, says, "In that state of consciousness, tones came from my throat that are unimaginable to me, long sweet, beautiful exotic tones flowed out with strength and power, without effort."[75]

McKenna believed the emergence of language may have arisen through synesthesia, which is common in psychedelic experiences. The explanation that the emergence of language was the result of synesthesia is also believed by the neuroscientist V. S. Ramachandran and is supported by his research into synesthesia.[76] Some unitive experiences allow one to register sight, smell, taste, touch, feeling, and thought as a

---

[74] Slattery, *Xenolinguistics*, 229.

[75] Swain in Metzner, *Sacred Mushroom of Visions*, 206.

[76] Ramachandran and Hubbard, "Synaesthesia."

single phenomenon. In reference to Terence McKenna's hypothesis that synesthesia led to the formation of language, Pollan writes:

> This last hypothesis about the invention of language turns on the concept of synesthesia, the conflation of the senses that psychedelics are known to induce: under the influence of psilocybin, numbers can take on colors, colors attach to sounds, and so on. Language, he contends, represents as a special case of synesthesia, in which otherwise meaningless sounds become linked to concepts.[77]

Both synesthesia and glossolalia are emergent properties. Emergent properties are novel capacities that arise from the interaction of complex systems; biological life itself is an emergent property.[78] Synesthesia, the interaction of different systems within both consciousness and the brain, commonly occurs when using psilocybin mushrooms and may have led humans to intentionally associate sounds with specific meanings. These sounds were likely originally accompanied with physical gestures of expression, helping carry the meaning across from one individual to another, until the gestures were no longer necessary.

There may also have been a greater association between our visual sense and our ability to speak than is understood today. Diana Reed Slattery, who wrote her doctoral dissertation on visual languages that are experienced in psychedelic states, writes, "Psychedelic states of consciousness produce novel forms of language in some psychonauts, especially visual languages, and novel ideas about language."[79] Slattery also states:

> Beyond the ineffability barrier come reports of a wide variety of linguistic phenomena in altered states. Anthropologist Henry Munn studied the language used in ceremony by Maria Sabina and other

---

[77] Pollan, *How to Change Your Mind*, 115.

[78] Lobo, "Biological Complexity and Integrative Levels."

[79] Slattery, *Xenolinguistics*, xxix.

mushroom curanderos, describing natural language attaining heights of eloquence, what he calls "ecstatic significations." Stanley Kripper studied the distortion and rending of natural language that occurs at various stages in the psychedelic experience. Many researchers have noted the commonality of synesthesia in psychedelic experience where words or letters are linked to other sensory events.[80]

The small amount of research on psilocybin and linguistics seems to affirm the idea that psilocybin may have supported the development of linguistic capabilities in humans. It is worth noting that Terence McKenna, referred to as a "wordsmith" by nearly every book that references him, credits his own verbal capacities to his relationship with psilocybin mushrooms.

Slattery underwent four hundred psychedelic sessions within a ten-year period with the intention of studying a complex language that was being shown to her in those expanded states of consciousness. She writes:

> The speed of cognition increases greatly in altered states. Natural language is very slow software indeed viewed from an altered state of consciousness. Ideas are processed by associating them with words, the internal lexicon of natural language. In the high-dose psilocybin state, meanings converge or correlate. In altered states of consciousness, a single symbol can hold multiple meanings simultaneously instead of sequentially. Many paths of meaning can be held in the mind at once.[81]

The language she saw, which she named Glide, is a symbol system in which each character holds many meanings. She proposes that similar experiences may have encouraged our ancestors to create the first written languages.

She is not the only one to have experienced such an extensive relationship with novel languages in altered states. The visionary artist

---

[80] Slattery, 16.

[81] Slattery, 64.

Allyson Grey has been experiencing this phenomenon for over four decades. In the foreword to Slattery's book, Grey writes:

My most profound inner experiences told me to align with "the sacred." After years of art school training in sketch art, figure drawing, painting, and modeling, I chose to avoid any human depiction of the Divine. Secret Writing first appeared to me in 1971 during an LSD trip in my tiny Cambridge college room. . . . Deep into the trip, letter-forms and symbols from a language I did not recognize became visible skimming the surfaces of all objects in the room. Washing over the faces and figures, an array of secret symbols floated like infinite ribbons in mid-air, rimming the edges and surfaces of everything in the room. This secret writing communicated the ineffable in a spectral glowing array of light. Their meaning was holy and precious, unpronounceable and ineffable . . . I never renounced the sacrament and continued to sojourn. The letters continued to appear . . . When Alex found that the origin of the secret language came from LSD opening me to the Divine, he immediately recognized the significance of this mystic symbol outpouring as an essential expression of my psyche. Alex influences me to develop the secret writing personal symbol system that has become my signature work.[82]

In the same foreword, Alex Grey, her husband and fellow visionary artist, writes:

When we have tripped together, I've seen the letters on her [Allyson's] skin, moving in channels, flowing over the surface of her arm, her hand, her face. It hovered a bit above the surface, not like a tattoo that is embedded. It never stopped slowly moving. The letters were darkish grey like ink, but translucent. It felt like a flowing mystery language that points to something sacred. They came from the source of mystery like a calling card... Secret Language is a proto or meta text, an idea of text, a field of linguistic and creative expression, too sacred to have assigned meaning, a nameless presence. Fingers pointing to

---

[82] Grey, "Foreword: Visionary Language," xiv–xv.

the moon and not the moon. The language of God is a sacred secret language. . . . Seeing characters on the walls when you are tripping is like hieroglyphics. They are trying to speak to you through the ages, certainly representing intended linguistic communication, something important. On all temples where we see a foreign calligraphy, we intuit some resonance of the sacred without perceiving the translatable meaning.[83]

Translating this writing into art has become Allyson's life work.

The experience of connecting with the universal Logos, as McKenna and others refer to it, has been reported to happen audibly as well as visually.[84] Horace Beach, in his 1996 dissertation titled "Listening for the Logos: A Study of Reports of Audible Voices at High Doses of Psilocybin," sampled 128 participants. The data showed that almost 40 percent of the participants that had taken psilocybin in high doses reported experiencing voices.[85] Though his data showed that hearing voices happened to the participants with the use of many different psychedelics, a majority of participants indicated that they first heard the voice with mushrooms.[86] If our ancestors had taken psilocybin and heard voices, as well as seen symbols, it may have inspired them to speak and eventually write. One can also imagine that if a loud voice that felt all-knowing suddenly appeared in one's awareness and began talking, it would be interpreted as a higher power or mystical entity. This certainly goes along with Wasson's hypothesis that mushrooms were the original inspiration of our understanding of the Divine.[87]

Whether audible or visual, the experience is often one of information being transmitted from a larger awareness to the subject. This

---

[83] Grey, xvi–xvii.

[84] Tarnas, *Passion of the Western Mind*; T. McKenna, *Food of the Gods*.

[85] Beach as cited in Slattery, *Xenolinguistics*, 96.

[86] Beach, "Listening for the Logos."

[87] Wasson, *Soma: Divine Mushroom of Immortality*.

communication does not always occur in the same way as when humans speak to each other. As with many psychedelic experiences, people have described the experience of acquiring information in the psilocybin-expanded states as a kind of download—an entire gestalt of consciousness is instantaneously received like packets of information coming into a personal computer from a networked server. The information can often be intuitively understood at once, perhaps involving a glimpse into what mathematician and philosopher Alfred North Whitehead calls *prehension*.[88] Whitehead believed that all parts within the cosmos receive information from the whole through feeling and that this unitive information is felt by organisms before their process of cognition. This information, received and intuitively known in psychedelic states, then has to be cognitively unpacked and processed, integrated over hours or even years, in order to consciously grasp the details and meaning.

The term *download* is one that many psychonauts now use, and it may be the best metaphor currently available. Slattery describes this experience and defines the term in this context as

> the sudden arrival of a major organizing insight, the great aha! you never knew you were waiting for until it happened. Luminous, numinous, compelling, it can be invoked, but it cannot be programmed. And a download happens when you least expect it.

> What makes a download a download is the intensity of the experience. Intensity arises from the extreme compaction of densely interconnected knowledge. Intensity amplifies when a sense of potential access to any knowledge immerses one in infinite possibility. Infinite possibility, that is, if one can summon the wit to form a question under such extreme epistemological conditions. Epistemology, the study of knowledge and knowing, asks "What do I know, how do I know it, and how do I know that I know?" Applying a psychedelic to a mind in search of an answer is rather like setting Google loose on the Akashic

---

[88] Whitehead, *Science and the Modern World*; Whitehead, *Process and Reality*.

records. The impact of this single event triggered a sudden and irrevocable change in the course of my life. Downloads can do that.[89]

Downloads could be seen as a more holistic way to communicate information in comparison with a more linear style, like that of language. This kind of sudden understanding might be what some of the ancient Platonists called *anamnesis,* the remembering of things from a previous existence, such as one's consciousness previously consciously being part of a larger unity and remembering (re-membering) the information previously known from that larger state.[90] Like the art that appeared to come into reality almost fully formed at once,[91] language may have spontaneously developed in a short time during humanity's past and then rapidly developed.

Downloads entail that the received information already exists somewhere, such as a part of a larger consciousness already holding this information. Ancient Greek philosophers used the word *Logos* to describe a universal intellect. Heraclitus used it to mean a principle of order and knowledge. The Stoics used the term to mean the divine animating principle pervading the universe. "The universal Logos of Greek philosophy transcended all apparent oppositions and imperfections—the divine Reason ruling all humanity and the cosmos yet immanent in human reason and potentially available to every individual of whatever nation or people," the philosopher and historian Richard Tarnas writes.[92] McKenna also believed the Logos could be directly communed with and thought it was the best word that could describe what happens with regular use of high doses of psilocybin.[93] He states that through his psilocybin experiences the Logos would talk to and through him. Whether one calls it Logos or God, there is a common experience among users of psychedelics

---

[89] Slattery, *Xenolinguistics,* 23.

[90] Kotler and Wheal, *Stealing Fire,* 44.

[91] Hancock, *Divine Spark.*

[92] Tarnas, *Passion of the Western Mind,* 99–100.

[93] T. McKenna, *Archaic Revival.*

of communicating with a being from which one can directly receive the downpouring of symbols and hear a voice that feels connected to the whole cosmos and possesses all knowledge. Richard Doyle, who received his PhD from University California, Berkeley, for work on rhetoric and continued postdoctoral work at the Massachusetts Institute of Technology, also writes about the downpouring of linguistic capabilities as one connects with the Logos on psychedelics. In a chapter titled "Rhetorical Mycelium: Psychedelics as Eloquence Adjuncts?" he writes:

> Language itself seems to be activated by ecodelics, amplifying the abstract symbolization of alphabetic font to take on more explicit sensory context even as numerous writers attempt to compose any response adequate to the visions until they stop in recognition of the paradoxically "hopeless" task of transcribing the sensations into language.[94]

It is possible that our ancestors received downloads of knowledge and experienced a connection with the Logos that pushed them to expand their cognitive abilities until sounds, symbols, and meaning united, catalyzing a transcendence of our individual boundaries to share experiences with one another. Our ancestors may have transcended their personal limitations through the boundary-dissolving psychedelics to become a part of a larger awareness and then come back with the capacity of language, which brought greater communion with their tribe.

Psilocybin and Brain Development

"Evolutionary biologists have been long puzzled by what is perhaps the chief mystery of human origins: the explosive and rapid expansion of the human brain in size and complexity over a vanishingly small span of evolutionary time," neuropharmacologist Dennis McKenna writes.[95]

---

[94] Doyle, *Darwin's Pharmacy*, 120.

[95] D. McKenna, "Foreword," xii.

Over the last decade scientists have made significant strides in understanding psilocybin's effects on the brain, and though still in its infancy, this research may get us closer to solving this chief mystery of human evolution.

The experiential capacities of consciousness that psilocybin may have catalyzed in our ancestors would have had neurological correlations, and recent scientific research into psilocybin affirms this. Psilocybin, and other tryptamine psychedelics like LSD and ayahuasca, stimulates neurogenesis—the creation of new neurons—which scientists did not believe was possible before the 1990s.[96] A study supported by the University of California, Davis, Department of Biochemistry and Molecular Medicine, titled "Psychedelics Promote Structural and Functional Neural Plasticity," was published in *Cell Reports*, an open-access, peer-reviewed journal that focuses on cutting-edge research in biology. The study found that tryptamines—including psilocybin, LSD, and DMT—promote structural and functional plasticity in the brain. These serotonergic psychedelics showed robust increases in neuritogenesis, the process of forming new neurites (which develop into axons and dendrites). The changes in neuronal structure include increases in the numbers of synapses as well as expanding their functions. This research shows that psilocybin not only repairs broken neural networks but also works to grow new connections. It was found that, in rats, tryptamines increase spinogenesis, the development of dendritic spines in neurons. Dendritic atrophy, or decay or loss of dendrites, is a hallmark of depression, and the authors believe that the ability for psychedelics to catalyze spinogenesis might be a biological explanation for the effectiveness of psychedelics treating depression:

> The researchers did not do any human experiments, but experiments in both vertebrates and invertebrates showed psychedelics produced similar effects across species. This indicates the biological mechanisms

---

[96] Renter, "Grow and Repair Brain Cells"; Riba, "Ayahuasca Stimulates the Birth of New Brain Cells."

that respond to psychedelics have remained the same across eons of evolution and that psychedelics will likely have the same brain growth (neural plasticity) effects in humans.[97]

In the *Journal of Psychopharmacology*, the article "Serotonin and Brain Function: A Tale of Two Receptors" focuses on the receptors 5-HT1A and 5-HT2A, the serotonin sites that tryptamines lock into. The authors elaborate "on the remarkable psychological and functional plasticity associated with the acute 'psychedelic' state—as produced by psychedelic drugs such as LSD and psilocybin—and the enduring changes that appear to follow from exposure to these drugs' effects."[98] Psychedelics, the authors explain, stimulate positive effects on the hormones that regulate mood and aggression, while also encouraging neuroplasticity. Findings in a more recent study on psilocybin, published in October 2017 in *Scientific Reports*, used fMRI brain scans. The scans showed that psilocybin reduces activity in the amygdala, the part of the brain associated with processing fear and anxiety. The reduction of activity in the amygdala allows for more overall interconnectivity within the brain. The study was conducted on nineteen volunteers suffering with depression; half showed improvement in brain activity that was correlated with relief of their depressive symptoms for five weeks after just one psilocybin session.[99]

Almost all life on the planet uses serotonin, not just the human brain. Stephan Buhner, author of twenty-one books on nature, writes:

> Serotonin, or 5-HT, is a very ancient molecule, first appearing eons ago in aerobic unicellular organisms. As with all Gaian innovations, future complexities of form and function built upon this early discovery . . . Bacteria use the molecule; so do all fungi, plants, insects,

---

[97] Ly et al., "Structural and Functional Neural Plasticity," 11.

[98] Carhart-Harris and Nutt, "Serotonin and Brain Function," 1092.

[99] Carhart-Harris et al., "Psilocybin for Treatment-Resistant Depression."

and animals. It is very deeply interwoven into the Gaian system and all its neural functioning.[100]

The chemical plays an essential role in regulating consciousness, and it is a compound that the tryptamine psychedelics closely resemble. In an essay titled "Altered Consciousness and Drugs in Human Evolution," Michael Winkelman, a professor and author of many publications exploring the intersection of shamanism and evolution, writes that a "wide range of evidence indicates that the role of serotonin in support of higher cognitive functions was modified in the course of human evolution."[101] This means that something changed the human serotonergic system.

Winkelman goes on to state that tryptamine psychedelics bind to human serotonin receptor sites 2.5 to 4 times more than those of chimpanzees.[102] Humanity's evolution diverged from that of chimpanzees six million years ago. The psilocybin explanation of human evolution includes the claim that the difference between the serotonergic system of humans and chimps may also explain the development of humanity's higher-order cognitive processes. Winkelman's findings are congruent with Pollan's research. Pollan concludes:

> The group of tryptamines we call the "classical psychedelics" have a strong affinity with one particular type of serotonin receptor, called 5-HT2A. These receptors are found in large numbers in the human cortex, the outermost, and evolutionarily most recent, layer of the brain. Basically, the psychedelics resemble serotonin closely enough that they can attach themselves to this receptor site in such a way as to activate it to do various things. . . . Curiously LSD has an even stronger affinity with the 5-HT2A receptor—is "stickier"—than serotonin

---

[100] Buhner, *Plant Intelligence*, 180.

[101] Winkelman, "Altered Consciousness and Drugs in Human Evolution," 35.

[102] Winkelman, 36.

itself, making this an instance simulacrum is more convincing, chemically, than the original.[103]

This suggests that the cortex evolved to work with something that chemically resembles LSD. Psilocybin is molecularly close to LSD and plentiful in the landscape where our ancestors evolved. It is also found on every continent but Antarctica, with over two hundred species of fungus producing it worldwide.

The following statement is an essential reasoning at the core of this book: changes in consciousness and the brain catalyzed by psilocybin stabilized over time, and as new neurons formed in individuals, and as these individuals later birthed new humans, some these traits of consciousness expansion and brain development were passed on epigenetically. Bruce Lipton, an award-winning biologist whose pioneering research on cloned human stem cells and genetics was a presage to the field of epigenetics, writes:

> Gene-as-destiny theorists have obviously ignored hundred-year-old science about enucleated cells, but they cannot ignore new research that undermines their beliefs in genetic determinism. While the Human Genome Project was making headlines, a group of scientists were inaugurating a new, revolutionary field in biology called *epigenetics*. The science of epigenetics, which literally means "control above genetics," profoundly changes our understanding of how life is controlled. In the last decade, epigenetic research has established that DNA blueprints passed down through genes are not set in concrete at birth. Genes are not destiny! Environmental influences, including nutrition, stress and emotions, can modify these genes, without changing their basic blueprint. And those modifications, epigeneticists have discovered, can be passed on to future generations as surely as DNA blueprints are passed on via the Double Helix.[104]

---

[103] Pollan, *How to Change Your Mind*, 292.

[104] Lipton, *Biology of Belief*, 67.

For example, trauma can be passed down over generations. The same goes for the expansion of consciousness. Psilocybin can be seen as a type of nutrient that promotes brain growth, and the expansive emotional states it catalyzes are all elements that fit into the description of what influences epigenetic inheritance. The neurogenesis and brain hyperconnectivity catalyzed by psilocybin might have also led to the formation of more serotonin receptors so that humans could make more use of the medicine. This explains why our species, whose ancestors might have eaten psilocybin mushrooms throughout a long evolutionary process, have more 5-HT2A serotonin receptors than our primate relatives. Over the course of hundreds of thousands or millions of years, many of these receptor sites integrated into the biology of our species. The development of these receptor sites over the last several million years also explains why humans have a much greater sensitivity to tryptamines in comparison to other animals, including the ability to experience the wide range of consciousness-expanding effects that they catalyze. Over generations, both the brain and consciousness of our species began to expand.

Thanks to cutting-edge brain scans carried out by the Beckley Foundation and Imperial College London, scientists have begun mapping the physiology of a number of psychedelic states. Recent studies employing brain imaging have provided ample evidence that psilocybin and LSD deregulate the brain's default-mode network, which scientists have associated with the ego state of consciousness.[105] Dissolving the default-mode network's thought patterns allows flashes of insight to manifest in conscious awareness. Scientists found that some of the neuronal connections correlated with psychedelic states of consciousness are stabilized and permanently integrated into an individual's physiology after they returned to their normal state of consciousness.[106] If our ancestors underwent an experience like this countless times, by picking up the mushrooms in their environment and eating them during the

---

[105] Cormier, "How LSD Affects Consciousness"; Keim, "How Magic Mushrooms Rearrange Your Brain"; Anderson, "LSD May Chip Away."

[106] Carhart-Harris and Nutt, "Serotonin and Brain Function."

four million years they were bipedal in Africa, this may help explain the evolution of the human brain.

Michael Pollan devotes a chapter to some of the recent neuroscience research into psychedelics. Pollan interviewed the scientists who are responsible for taking the first fMRI brain scans of participants taking psilocybin and LSD and who discovered that psychedelics dissolve the default-mode network. Pollan writes:

> This is why some neuroscientists call it "the me network." If a researcher gives you a list of adjectives and asks you to consider how they apply to you, it is your default mode network that leaps into action . . . Nodes in the default mode network are thought to be responsible for autobiographical memory, the material from which we compose the story of who we are, by linking our past experiences with what happens to us and with projections of our future goals …
>
> Perhaps the most striking discovery of Carhart-Harris's first experiment was that the steepest drops in default mode network activity correlated with his volunteers' subjective experience of "ego dissolution." ("I existed only as an idea or concept," one volunteer reported. Recalled another, "I didn't know where I ended and my surroundings began.") The more precipitous the drop-off in blood flow and oxygen consumption in the default network, the more likely a volunteer was to report the loss of a sense of self.
>
> Shortly after Carhart-Harris published his results in a 2012 paper in *PNAS* ("Neural Correlates of the Psychedelic State as Determined by fMRI Studies with Psilocybin"), Judson Brewer, a researcher at Yale who was using fMRI to study the brains of experienced meditators, noticed that his scans and Robin's looked remarkably alike. The transcendence of self reported by expert meditators showed up on fMRIs as a quieting of the default mode network. It appears that when activity in the default mode falls off precipitously, the ego temporarily vanishes, and the usual boundaries we experience between self and world, subject and object, all melt away.[107]

---

[107] Pollan, *How to Change Your Mind*, 304–05.

This resonates with Terence McKenna's hypothesis that psilocybin worked to minimize the growth of the ego in our ancestors and enabled them to stay in relative harmony with each other and nature for millennia.

By calming down the default-mode network, the rest of the brain moves into a more hyperconnected state, as shown in the fMRI images. David Nutt, a neuropsychopharmacologist at Imperial College London, claims that in the default-mode network "we've found the neural correlate for repression."[108] Psilocybin reduces blood flow to certain parts of the brain, such as the thalamus, enabling "a state of unconstrained cognition" by other parts of the brain.[109] In *Plants and the Human Brain*, David Kennedy, the director of the Brain, Performance, and Nutrition Research Centre at Northumbria University, writes, "Intriguingly, these findings map quite nicely onto Aldous Huxley's metaphor that hallucinogens function by removing the constraints imposed on reality by the 'reducing valve' of the brain, ultimately flinging open William Blake's 'doors of perception.'"[110] The hyperconnected physiological configurations that take place within the brain may be linked to the subjective experiences of unity reported by participants during psychedelic sessions. Robin Carhart-Harris believes that when the influence of the default-mode network declines, so does one's sense of separateness from nature. His team at the Imperial College London tested volunteers on a standard psychological scale to measure their sense of connection to nature and found that psychedelic experience raised participant's scores.[111] This correlates the proposition in chapter 3 that natural psychedelics partly evolved as ecological regulators.

Evidence for our ancestors' relationship with psilocybin mushrooms, as explained by archeological evidence, neurology, and the psychological

---

[108] Nutt in Pollan, *How to Change Your Mind*, 307.

[109] Kennedy, *Plants and the Human Brain*, 106.

[110] Kennedy, 106.

[111] Pollan, *How to Change Your Mind*, 315–16.

enhancements that would have benefited their tribal society, have been elucidated in this chapter. Upcoming studies may offer additional evidence for the evolutionary advantages psilocybin would have given for our ancestors. As their website states, Beckley Foundation has a study planned at Maastricht University that uses MRI spectroscopy and fMRI to examine if psilocybin increases creativity. The relationship between psilocybin and creativity would give a biological explanation for many of the advancements in humanity, such as innovations in tools and art. These sudden jumps in human innovation could be correlated with other behavior, such as beginning of the ritual use of psychedelics, which likely involved taking higher doses for the intent of exploration. Some of the neuronal structures that represent the emergent creative capacities catalyzed in our ancestors by psilocybin would still be present in the physiology of their descendants, by both the process of natural selection (such as choosing creative individuals as mates) and through epigenetics. A positive finding would be congruent with all the neuroscience research to date on psychedelics. There is ample evidence, as presented in the next chapter ("Creativity, Healing, and Economics"), supporting the notion that the neurophysiological correlations between psilocybin and creativity will continue to be found. Studies on psilocybin and creativity, grounded in neuroscience, will add further support to the theory that human evolution was catalyzed through a relationship with psilocybin mushrooms over millions of years in Africa.

Contrasts with Other Theories of Human Evolution

This section on the past has introduced three major claims about human evolution that differ from mainstream theories, namely that our ancestors were largely plant-based, that they were largely nonmonogamous, and that psilocybin mushrooms catalyzed brain evolution and consciousness. The first two claims have been discussed by researchers for at least a century and do have some, if not widespread, support. Aside from milk during infancy, a plant-based diet is the predominant diet of all the largest land-based animals that have ever existed.[112] Even during Darwin's time, leading anthropologists believed that our ancient ancestors were nonmonogamous and that a more polyamorous lifestyle would have had many tribal benefits.[113] In *Sapiens: A Brief History of Humankind*, Yuval Noah Harari explains how the movement toward monogamy has been incongruent with evolutionary biology:

> The proponents of this "ancient commune" theory argue that the frequent infidelities that characterize modern marriages, and the high rates of divorce, not to mention the cornucopia of psychological complexes from which both children and adults suffer, all result from forcing humans to live in nuclear families and monogamous relationships that are incompatible with our biological software.[114]

Agriculture shifted humanity toward monogamy, so as to secure the heir of material possessions and property, and also gave humanity the crops to raise animals and supply meat on a scale previously unimaginable.

These two claims, vegetarianism and nonmonogamous bonding, would also lend support to the psilocybin mushroom theory. Our ancestors, having largely plant-based diets, would have looked for readily and easily available sources of food in the form of plants and fungi that they could simply pick up and eat. Given that psilocybin mushrooms are the most plentiful mushrooms in the African savanna, it is likely that they would have eaten the mushroom over the course of millions of years. A polyamorous style of relating may have also been encouraged by the boundary-dissolving, creative novelty-seeking behavior supported by the psilocybin. As discussed in chapter 1, the greatest change in personality found with the use of psilocybin is the trait defined as *openness*, which correlates with creativity and the acceptance of new ideas,

---

[112] Berson, *Meat Question*; Wright and Gynn, *Return to the Brain of Eden*.

[113] Ryan and Jetha, *Sex at Dawn*.

[114] Harari, *Sapiens*, 42.

and this orientation of openness might have been present in their relationships. Our modern culture (the most meat-heavy in history, with a belief that humans are naturally monogamous, even in the face of rising divorce rates and promiscuity) perhaps feels threatened because these ideas challenge the status quo and the security of the identity of what it is to be human. That these compelling interpretations of our history have yet to be included as part of the conventional human story is likely due to cultural bias and our own fear.

In *Fantastic Fungi: How Mushrooms Can Heal, Shift Consciousness, and Save the Planet*, Dennis McKenna presents the psilocybin mushroom explanation of human emergence. Andrew Weil offers the following counterpoint in another essay:

> I don't buy the "stoned ape" hypothesis and never have. The perceptual distortions and sensory scrambling that psychedelics cause would be a fatal risk in developing species, making you more vulnerable to being eaten by a predator or dying accidentally. I think human beings had to wait until there was some minimal level of civilization and protection in which you had the luxury of space and time to safely explore such experiences.
>
> Human beings are capable of experiencing and appreciating the mystery of the wonder of the divine without substances. You look up at the night sky or observe birth and death, and you're starkly confronted with the mystery in which we live. I think there are all sorts of reasons throughout history as to why the brain has increased in size. Even before there were primates, the brain was developing and growing without any dependence on psychedelic substances.[115]

The inclusion of Weil's viewpoint in the volume provides a balancing perspective, though ample evidence is presented to counter his standard understanding of our ancestors. Psilocybin, at lower doses, would have increased our chances of survival by enhancing our senses, increasing cognition, and leading to greater copulation. All this while it interconnected

---

[115] Weil, "Stoned Ape Theory—Not," 155.

our brain and increased the number of neurons over millions of years; just as our digestive system has evolved to absorb specific nutrients in our diet, our brain and serotonin receptors in our gut probably evolved to do the same. Our primate ancestors also lived within large groups, which would have provided safety and, as mentioned, primates spend a great deal of their time leisurely socializing. It is unlikely that our ancestors were living on the edge at every moment. Though there are certainly scenarios in which a primate ancestor might have ingested a debilitating amount of mushrooms, they would have quickly learned the proper dosage. Most journeys would have lasted about four hours, but our ancestors slept longer than that every day, leaving them far more vulnerable than any impairment caused by occasional psilocybin. It is important to note again that decades of research shows that many other animals use plants, fungi, and even other animals to alter their consciousness.[116] Chemically altering consciousness is common throughout the animal kingdom, and there is no evidence that it causes any kind of evolutionary disadvantages that would bring a species to extinction. Intentional larger-dose ceremonies most likely occurred once our ancestors developed ritual containers, giving rise to the first expressions of religion.

Diet, including the chemicals that enter our body, has always played perhaps the most dramatic role in evolution—whether that be root systems of a plant, the digestive systems within all of life, or the speed of animals to catch their prey. These are not just substances, as Weil states, but compounds that evolved in symbiotic relationship in our environment. It is true that other mammalian brains were evolving larger in size to previous reptilian ancestors, but what likely caused this growth in size was their ability to connect, to move deeper into communion, with other members of their group. A great portion of our newly evolved human brain is devoted to language and creativity, and it is perhaps these abilities, which helps us to more deeply connect with other people that psilocybin may have catalyzed. As studies have shown, psilocybin increases our experience of empathy, and this could have led to deeper group bonding and therefore survival.

---

[116] Siegel, *Intoxication*; Samorini, *Animals and Psychedelics*.

There exists an enormous cultural bias against most substances that alter consciousness, reinforced by religion and law for thousands of years.[117] This bias has also prevented people from entertaining the idea that what accelerated the expansion of consciousness in human brain development was a psychoactive fungus in our ancestors' diet. Academia (with its own conventional culture that seeks security and prestige) has largely been unaware of the theory or has discarded it without much thought. This is not unlike when psychedelics were deemed illegal without looking at the thousands of scientific papers written on the topic. Once psychedelics became illegal, academia dropped almost all interest in the subject. Ralph Metzner, who did his doctoral work at Harvard and postdoctoral research at Yale, writes about the mushroom theory and the difficulty academia has had entertaining the theory:

> While this thesis has been generally treated with disdain, or else ignored, by the academic establishment, it is interesting that there isn't really a good alternative theory of the development of language or higher intelligence; furthermore, establishment academics are not likely to be familiar with the nature of psychedelic experience . . . In favor of the idea that mind-expanding plants may have had some role (if not the only one) [in our evolution] are (1) laboratory evidence that psilocybin and other psychedelics lower sensory thresholds, i.e., heighten acuity of sense perception, which would confer a direct adaptive advantage; (2) evidence from subjective experience accounts, as in this book and elsewhere, that psychedelic mushrooms heighten cognitive awareness and linguistic fluidity . . . (3) heightened problem-solving ability, with adaptive advantages, is also suggested by the effective use of psychedelic drugs in psychotherapy and shamanic divination; (4) studies of brain areas activated during psilocybin states that show major activity in the frontal cortex, the area most involved in processing complex perception and thoughts.[118]

---

[117] Kotler and Wheal, *Stealing Fire*, 51–69.

[118] Metzner, *Sacred Mushroom of Visions*, 40.

The lack of prehistoric psychedelic use being integrated into our understanding of human evolution in academics is echoed by professor of anthropology John Rush:

> These substances were paramount in importance and their neglect in mainstream academia robs the research of important insights around the human condition and how we reached this point in history . . . The importance of mind-altering substances, as noted in the art forms around the world since the Upper-Paleolithic, cannot be overstated. These substances are paramount in ritual context, both rites of intensification and rites of passage, as well as in prophecy, which resulted in decision making affecting millions and millions of people. There is a great deal of art available showing mushrooms and other plants.[119]

The well-titled *National Geographic* article "12 Theories of How We Became Human, and Why They're All Wrong" lists the major contending theories of human evolution.[120] I will briefly explore two plausible and popular theories presenting the conditions that may have catalyzed the emergence of humans found in the article. The first of these claims holds that the interplay of tools, the environment, and our awareness created a learning feedback loop that expanded consciousness; the second theory states that the use of fire to cook food acted as external stomach, and the physiological energy freed from digestion went to fuel brain development. However, neither humans' increased intake of cooked food nor the accelerated use of increasingly complex technology has affected the ratio between the higher-functioning neocortex and evolutionarily older parts of the brain. Actually, the human brain size has shrunk since the Agricultural Revolution.[121] As Wright and Gynn

---

[119] Rush, *Entheogens and the Development of Culture*, 20–21.

[120] Strauss, "12 Theories."

[121] Hawks, "How Has the Human Brain Evolved?"; McAuliffe, "Why Are Our Brains Shrinking?"

point out, "There is some evidence that our brains are still shrinking and that they may have done so over the last ten thousand years by as much as 5 percent."[122] Humans are consuming more calories than ever before and have more technology than our ancestors could have ever imagined, and yet our brain size has decreased.

One plausible reason for the decrease in brain size is that humans stopped taking mushrooms after the Agricultural Revolution, which is around the same time as brain size began to shrink. As Harari points out, "fungi were too elusive" to become domesticated and incorporated into the Agricultural Revolution.[123] I propose that it was during the Agricultural Revolution, when generations mostly ate what they grew, that the greater part of humanity lost its relationship with psychoactive plants and fungi. Only in the last half century have humans learned how to cultivate psilocybin mushrooms through the techniques that Terence and Dennis McKenna discovered and then published under pseudonyms.[124] During the Agricultural Revolution, people began to move from nature-based spirituality to organized religion, which generally includes a social hierarchy. The focus moved away from the environment, including plants and fungi, and toward culture. Psilocybin, as a serotonergic agent, was needed to further brain development, and without psilocybin as a neurotropic spurring the growth of neurons and extending the length and connection of dendrites, neurons begin to atrophy. What in the brain has likely been strengthened is the default-mode network, associated with an overdeveloped self-conscious attention on oneself, which has increased the sense of depression and anxiety in our society and repressed our creativity and sexual energy.[125]

Meanwhile, psilocybin can be interpreted as brain food, as it stimulates brain growth, complexity, and plasticity. The mushroom theory

---

[122] Wright and Gynn, *Return to the Brain of Eden*, 57.

[123] Harari, *Sapiens*, 78.

[124] Oss and Oeric, *Psilocybin Magic Mushroom Grower's Guide*.

[125] Ryan, *Civilized to Death*.

does not rule out that multiple factors played a role in the acceleration of human evolution. Rather, it adds to humanity's understanding of its own evolution by specifying that consciousness-expanding experiences, catalyzed by the nootropic psilocybin, stimulated growth and novel neuronal connections in the brain, and that this process might have played a pivotal role in human development. Our ancestors eating psychedelic mushrooms does not take away the impact that tool making or learning to start fires might have had on our biology; instead the theory says that the creative sparks of the psychedelic state might have played a part in the origins and developments of these behaviors.

Humanity's Long Psychedelic History

Aside from the focus on evolution, psychedelics had tremendous cultural impact on prehistoric societies. In *The Long Trip: A Prehistory of Psychedelia*, Paul Devereux writes, "The ritual use of hallucinogens . . . harks back to Paleolithic and Mesolithic shamanism."[126] Since the cognitive revolution, sixty to seventy thousand years ago, artifacts implying and confirming prehistoric psychedelics use have been found worldwide. In a chapter titled "Drawing Conclusions on the Wall," Devereux lays out the work of Lewis-Williams and a dozen other archaeologists and analyzes how many of the oldest artworks depicted on rocks around the world correspond with the visual and psychological effects psychedelics would have had on the artists. Much of humanity's earliest art depicts geometric symbols, wavy lines, spirals, and human-animal hybrids, and these are consistent with that of cross-cultural psychedelic experiences worldwide. Medicinal psychedelic use may even have extended beyond our own species within our genus. A sixty-thousand-year-old burial of a Neanderthal man has been found in northern Iraq. With him was placed pollen from eight different plants that have been used for healing. The Neanderthal man

---

[126] Devereux, *Long Trip*, 108.

was likely a medicine man, and the pollen may have been part of his medicinal kit. Devereux writes, "If herbalism was practiced, then the knowledge of psychoactivity in the plant world was also almost certainly known."[127]

Since eating mushrooms requires no tools, the next best historical evidence inferring mushroom use is the art that conveys reverence for them. Much of this creative expression has been in the form of art on caves and rocks that depicts mushrooms. David Kennedy writes:

> Cave murals in the Spanish Sierra de las Cuerdas mountains dating 4000–6000 BC similarly appear to depict "Psilocybe hispanica," a hallucinogenic mushroom unique to the Pyrenees. Representations of mushrooms crop up as far afield as the easternmost tip of Siberia, where the Chukchi Eskimos' word for intoxication literally translates to "bemushroomed." A plethora of indirect evidence drawn from sculptures, reliefs, hieroglyphs, jewelry, clothing, and burial practices also suggest the widespread use of mushrooms such as "Psilocybe cubensis" in the religious practices of the early Egyptians.[128]

The most well-known mushroom cave art is found in Tassili, Africa, in modern-day Algeria; it is between nine and eleven thousand years old and depicts a shaman with mushrooms growing on his body.[129] Rock art has been found in Siberia depicting humanoid mushrooms, which the Russian archeologist N. N. Dikov dates back to the Bronze Age, between 3000 BCE and 1200 BCE.[130] Evidence of mushroom motifs engraved into bronze razors and rocks of mushroom cults exist in Norway, Denmark, and Sweden.[131]

---

[127] Devereux, 62.

[128] Kennedy, *Plants and the Human Brain*, 116.

[129] Metzner, *Sacred Mushroom of Visions*.

[130] Devereux, *Long Trip*, 68.

[131] Devereux, 69.

Statues are another way that societies have left indications of psychedelic mushroom use. About three hundred stone mushroom sculptures have been found in the Americas; some of them date back three thousand years. Similar stones have been found in Guatemala, Mexico, Honduras, and El Salvador.[132] Currently, the mycologist Paul Stamets is taking care of eighteen of these precious relics.[133] Mushrooms made of ceramics have also been found in a two-thousand-year-old tomb in Mexico.[134] And large mushroom statues have been found on the island of Nias, off the coast of Sumatra, in three uninhabited villages.[135] On the undersides of these three-foot-tall stones, where the spores would come out of mushrooms, are delicate carvings depicting geometric lines.

Mushroom cultures have existed on almost every continent, and there are still Indigenous mushroom societies living today, with the Mexican Mazatecs being the most well known. Two tribes in New Guinea, the Kiambi and the Kuma, use mushrooms to alter their states of consciousness. The Igorot, the aboriginal Malayan inhabitants of the Philippine island Luzon, continue to use mushrooms for rites of passage. In northwestern Canada, the Dogrib people in the Mackenzie Mountains use mushrooms as sacraments. Another North American tribe, the Ojibwa of Michigan, use the *Amanita muscaria* psychedelic mushroom in an ancient annual ritual.[136]

As writing developed, around 3200 BCE, people also expressed their reverence for psychedelics in text. The Rigveda, the earliest written work that shaped the Hindu tradition, is the world's oldest religious text. In it are over 1,000 hymns, 120 of which are devoted to a psychedelic called soma.[137] There is reason to believe that soma, the psychedelic referred to

---

[132] Devereux, 109.

[133] Stamets, *Mycelium Running*.

[134] Devereux, *Long Trip*, 115.

[135] Devereux, 96.

[136] Devereux, 95, 96, 115, 116.

[137] Devereux, 73.

as bringing one closer to God, is a mushroom. In seven lines of the text soma is described as "the Not-Born Single-Foot." Mushrooms appear to form mysteriously overnight, without the need for seeds or another plant. To our ancestors, they would seem to appear out of nowhere and rapidly grow full-sized within a couple days. Nowhere in the Rigveda does it mention leaves, branches, blossoms, seeds, or roots, again reinforcing the notion that it was a psychoactive mushroom. What kind of mushroom this might have been has been debated for decades. Gordon Wasson proposed that it was the *Amanita muscaria*.[138] Terence McKenna revived an idea that was first proposed in 1981 by two mycologists, R. Schroeder and G. Guzman, that soma was a psilocybin mushroom.[139] In Persian pre-Islamic Zoroastrian texts are references to *Haoma*, a word likely bearing a similar root to soma, as the roots of the Farsi language are similar to those of Sanskrit, the language of the Rigveda. *Haoma* is said to be a plant, which is what mushrooms were called at the time, that brings "healing, victory, salvation, and protection."[140]

In the West the civilization most known to have made use of psychedelics is the Ancient Greeks, who produced a large annual festival called the Eleusinian Mysteries. The city of Eleusis arose as a settlement between 1580 BCE and 1500 BCE.[141] "If Athens of the fifth and fourth centuries BC was the true source of Western life in the twenty-first century, then Eleusis was our first, undisputed spiritual capital," Brian Muraresku writes in his 2020 best seller *The Immortality Key: The Secret History of the Religion with No Name*, based on twelve years of scholarly research into the Eleusinian Mysteries and its ceremonial use of a psychedelic sacrament.[142] The Mysteries were a ten-day ritual that ran for at least a thousand years and were open to almost

---

[138] Wasson, *Soma*.

[139] Devereux, *Long Trip*, 78.

[140] Devereux, 76.

[141] Devereux, 81.

[142] Muraresku, *Immortality Key*, 25.

everyone.[143] Most citizens in Greece attended at least once in their life. During the ritual, participants drank a psychoactive brew called kykeon. It is likely that Pythagoras, Plato, Socrates, Aristotle, and other philosophers that inspired Western civilization drank the psychoactive substance. Kotler and Wheal write, "Foundational notions like Plato's world of forms and Pythagoras's music of the spheres were informed by these rites."[144] The ingredients remained a mystery, and disclosing the recipe or taking kykeon out of the ritual was punishable by death. Hofmann, Wasson, and Ruck spent years researching what kykeon could have been composed of and shared their research in the book *The Road to Eleusis*. The researchers, later backed up by Muraresku, deduced that the psychoactive ingredients were ergot and alcohol.[145] Ergot, the fungus from which LSD is derived, grows on rye, and rye is used to make beer.

After *The Road to Eleusis* was published, Terence McKenna again revived another theory, one proposed by the poet-scholar Robert Graves in 1964, that the ingredient in kykeon was perhaps *Stropharia cubensis*, a common psilocybin mushroom. The Greeks sculpted artwork that support both theories; there are depictions of mushrooms as well as wheat. Whatever the exact substance might have been, psychedelic states appear to have had a deep impact on the direct formation of Western culture until the decimation of these sacred rites of passage. Muraresku, a scholar of history and ancient languages, writes at length on how these ceremonies involving kykeon might have created early Christianity. Books—such as *The Sacred Mushroom and the Cross* by John Allegro and *The Psychedelic Gospels: The Secret History of Hallucinogens in Christianity* by Jerry and Julie Brown—have been dedicated to exploring the hypothesis that it was mushrooms that played an essential role in early Christianity. Whether it was ergot or psilocybin mushrooms that

---

[143] Muraresku, 25.

[144] Kotler and Wheal, *Stealing Fire*, 2.

[145] Wasson, Hofmann, and Ruck, *Road to Eleusis*.

were used in the kykeon brew, these rights of passage had considerable impact on Western culture. Muraresku notes how this important and influential time in Western history has been intentionally almost erased:

> When the once hallowed walls of Eleusis were trampled in AD 395, the Visigoths may have placed the dynamite, but the Church lit the fuse. Following Constantine's blessing earlier in the century, Emperor Theodosius had already made Christianity the official state religion of the Roman Empire in AD 380. Twelve years later he proclaimed the Mysteries illegal, drawing a line in the sand. Civilization would eventually reap the secular benefits of all things Greek, but from then on, Christianity would serve as the default faith of the Western world. When it came to spiritual matters, best to pretend those Greek infidels and their satanic rituals never existed. For a secret religion like Eleusis that refused to keep written records, the extinction was swift and thorough. Before the end of the fourth century AD, total victory was declared by the early Church Father Saint John Chrysostom: "The tradition of the forefathers has been destroyed, the deep rooted custom has been torn out, the tyranny of joy [and] the accursed festivals . . . have been obliterated just like smoke."[146]

Just a few generations after the declaration making the Mysteries illegal, Europe fell into the period that came to be known as the Dark Ages, a time marked by frequent warfare and intellectual darkness that lasted from about 476 CE to 800 CE. Though the exact ingredients of kykeon may never be known, as is the case with soma, what is known through several written cultural references at the time is that these two cultures, which influenced many of the major traditions in the world, were heavily inspired by the naturally growing psychedelic substances in their environments.

The psychedelic theory of human evolution may have come to the forefront of science a century ago, perhaps maybe only decades after Darwin's ideas, if awareness of the mushrooms had previously existed in

---

[146] Muraresku, *Immortality Key*, 32–33.

our culture. Unfortunately, as will be presented, knowledge of the mushroom was deliberately suppressed. In the Americas, entire civilizations honored and praised psychedelics until the Spanish conquistadors were ordered to eradicate them.[147] Metzner writes, "The suppression of the visionary mushroom cult by the Spanish clergy was effective and complete. For four centuries it disappeared from the memory of the general and scholarly public."[148]

For Western culture, the earliest reported descriptions of psilocybin mushroom use in the New World were from the Spaniards, years before the full Spanish invasion.[149] The Aztecs and Toltecs had elaborate rituals focused on the use of psilocybin mushrooms, and some of the instructions of these rituals have survived. Tom Lane, in *Sacred Mushroom Rituals: The Search for the Blood of Quetzalcoatl*, tries to bring some of these rituals to light. At the time of the Aztecs, a Spaniard commented in writing about the celebrations at the coronation of Montezuma II and wrote of everyone eating mushrooms. This is also confirmed by the writing of Spanish clergy. Tezozomoc, a Mesoamerican leader, told them: "They take these hallucinations as divine notices, revelations of the future, and augury of things to come."[150] In *Plants of the Gods: Their Sacred, Healing, and Hallucinogenic Powers*, Schultes, Hofmann, and Rätsch write:

> When the Spaniards conquered Mexico, they were aghast to find the natives worshipping their deities with the help of inebriating plants: Peyotl, Ololiuqui, Teonanácatl. The mushrooms were especially offensive to the European ecclesiastical authorities, and they set out to eradicate their use in religious practices.[151]

---

[147] Goldsmith, *Psychedelic Healing*, 87.

[148] Metzner, *Sacred Mushroom of Visions*, 16.

[149] DeKorne, *Psychedelic Shamanism*, 173.

[150] Stafford, *Psychedelics Encyclopedia*, 275.

[151] Schultes, Hofmann, and Rätsch, *Plants of the Gods*, 156.

In an essay titled "The Genesis of a Mushroom/Venus Religion in Mesoamerica," the scholars Carl de Borhegyi and Suzanne de Borhegyi-Forrest present several writings from the Spanish Church written at the time of Spain's conquest of the Americas.[152] One clergy member who recorded the use of mushrooms in the Americas was Franciscan friar Bernardino de Sahagun. In a multivolume work that he wrote between 1547 and 1582, titled *Historia general de las cosas de la Nueva España* (which translates to "general history of things in New Spain"), he writes:

> Toltecs were above all thinkers for they originated the year count, the day count; they established the way in which the night, the day, would work; which sign was good, favorable; and which was evil, the day sign of wild beasts. All their discoveries formed the book for interpreting dreams . . . Through sacred mushroom rituals priests summoned the deities of creations to manifest themselves in the underworld where life regenerates from death.[153]

He also wrote about the Aztecs:

> For four days there was feasting and celebration and then on the fourth day came the coronation of Montezuma II . . . At the very first, mushrooms had been served. They ate them at the time when the shell trumpets were blown. They ate no more food; they only drank chocolate during the night, and they ate the mushrooms with honey.[154]

This wasn't the only documented event where the Spaniards saw the Aztecs taking mushrooms on political occasions. The Dominican friar Diego Duran wrote of a particular instance in 1481 where mushrooms were given to Aztec guests:

---

[152] de Borhegyi and de Borhegyi-Forrest, "Genesis of a Mushroom."

[153] de Sahagun as cited in de Borhegyi and de Borhegyi-Forrest, "Genesis of a Mushroom," 455.

[154] de Sahagun as cited in de Borhegyi and de Borhegyi-Forrest, 455.

And all the lords and grandees of the provinces rose and, to solemnise further festivities, they all ate of some woodland mushrooms, which they say make you lose your senses, and thus they sallied forth all primed for the dance.[155]

The Aztecs had an annual ritual called the Feast of Revelations, in which captured prisoners of rival tribes were pardoned and "magnanimously regaled with mushrooms."[156] Toribio de Benavente, another Spanish Franciscan missionary, wrote:

They had another way of drunkenness . . . and it was with some fungi or small mushrooms, which exist in this land as in Castillo; but those of this land are of such a kind that eaten raw and being bitter they . . . eat with them with a little bees honey; and a while later they would see a thousand visions, especially serpents, and as they would be out of their senses, it would seem to them that their legs and bodies were full of worms eating them alive . . . These mushrooms, they called in their language teonanácatl, which means "flesh of God" or the devil, whom they worshiped.[157]

These chronicles were written by clergy that came to the Americas with the conquistadors, observers biased by their agenda of colonization and beliefs in Christian supremacy. There were people, such as Bartolome de las Casas, a Spanish missionary and bishop, who tried to oppose the Spanish oppression and enslavement of the Indigenous peoples in the Americas, but overall most of the history of the invasion was written by the same people who are responsible for the greatest ethnocide in human history. The Christian clergy certainly did not have the context to understand what they were seeing. For example, bodies shaking on mushrooms, which they interpret as a kind of possession by the devil,

---

[155] Duran as cited in Letcher, *Shroom*, 74.

[156] Letcher, 75.

[157] De Benavente as cited in de Borhegyi and de Borhegyi-Forrest, 455–56.

is a common occurrence of cathartic somatic release, which is a natural part of the healing process.

In a chapter titled "Towards an Exploration of the Mind of a Conquered Continent: Shamanism, Sacred Plants and Amerindian Epistemology," Luis Eduardo Luna, who received a doctorate in comparative religion and authored three texts on shamanism, writes: "The conquest of the Americas by the empires of Europe nearly resulted in the total loss of the cultural, technical, and intellectual achievements of one third of the population of the world of that time."[158] The natives' books, art, and temples were destroyed, and "their knowledge treated as the work of Satan."[159] Luna writes that "the indigenous population was condemned to humiliation, subjugation, and poverty, barely surviving history's greatest ethnocide."[160]

One Latin American population that survived the almost complete eradication of mushroom rituals by the conquistadors is the Mazatec, in what is now southern Mexico. There are three important reasons the Mazatec mushroom culture may have survived through the brutal ethnocide from the invading Europeans. First, the Mazatec lived in high and remote mountains in Mexico. Second, they are a matriarchal culture, and most Mazatec medicine people are women. Christian clergy, coming from a patriarchal culture, believed all people in positions of spiritual power should be men, so they perhaps overlooked these powerful women in their attempts to silence a community's most influential people. In matriarchal cultures worldwide power is often balanced between males and females.[161] In my discussion with the Mazatec and their representatives, I learned that the conquistadors went after the men who held public positions of the medicine man, though they ignored the female facilitators, who

---

[158] Luna, "Mind of a Conquered Continent," 31.

[159] Luna, 32.

[160] Luna, 33.

[161] Ryan and Jetha, *Sex at Dawn*.

carried out most of the ceremonies for families within private houses. The third reason was the integration of Guadalupe, representing the Virgin Mary, as their primary spiritual icon. The Aztecs had an earth goddess named Coatlicue who they believed was the mother of creation. The clergy mistook the name for that of Guadeloupe, a city in France named after the Virgin Mary, the mother of Christ, and conquistadors eventually perhaps believed the natives were praying to the same figure, and counted their religious conversion as complete. Juan Diego, an Aztec peasant, reportedly showed a vision of Guadalupe that appeared on a robe to the archbishop in 1531, which the Church accepted as a sign that the Indigenous were also the children of God. The Church then halted the genocide of Indigenous people and their medicine people, allowing the more remote communities to continue many of their traditional practices.

While I was exploring the Museum of Anthropology in Mexico City, the stark contrast between psychedelic societies before and after the European invasion and American civilizations that followed became even more evident to me. The Maya, Aztec, and Toltec peoples—all of whom held rich psychedelic cultures—had aesthetics that were multilayered in symbolism and meaning that mirror the visionary art inspired by psychedelics today. Their statues are intricate, with deities such as snakes with wings, the mother goddess with a belt of serpents, and humans with ecstatic expressions of the divine. Evidence shows they had a complex and perhaps deeper relationship with death than cultures in the West, which tend to fear and repress all thought of death. While human sacrifice was a part of many ancient Indigenous Mexican and Central American cultures, it's important to understand that they did not perceive death in a similar way to those of us in the West. Public sport games were played where the winners of the game were sacrificed as a reward, which they saw as an honor. The Mayan cosmology held nature and the divine, animal and human, life and death as dimensions inextricably interwoven in ongoing existence. With Christianity, the cosmos became more anthropocentric. People began to pray only to the divine in human form, whether that be Jesus,

Mary, or God the Father. This is in contrast to the original Americans, and Indigenous societies throughout the world, who prayed to animals and plants; the moon, sun, and earth; and various natural phenomena. This spiritual shift is perhaps partly responsible for the great division between humanity and the planet that is at the roots of our ecological crisis. But there is an effort in Western culture to revive and reclaim the Mother Earth archetype by embracing of the concept of Gaia, the Greek name of the earth goddess. And there are still Mazatec and others throughout the globe who are committed to maintaining their traditions and connection to the earth.

The Mazatec mushroom culture today is alive and well. In my journey to visit the Mazatec people, I was surprised to see just how much mushrooms are celebrated in their society. Dozens of mushroom murals exist in the city center of Huautla de Jimenez alone. The entrance of the city of Huautla de Jimenez—which adopted the official name Pueblo Magico (Magical Village)—says "welcome" with mushrooms on both sides of the name. Next to the welcome sign is a sculpture of a mushroom approximately twelve feet tall with a statue of Maria Sabina, who has become the most celebrated person in town and gained almost the status of a saint, with her arms open in welcome. The people of the town still use mushroom rituals for healing ceremonies, and the mushrooms themselves are held as sacred. Tens of thousands of Mazatecs throughout southern Mexico still practice the ancient traditions, living peaceful, spiritual rich lives in balance with their environment.

As someone who is half Mexican myself, sharing roots with the native people of Latin America, I have found incredible meaning and empowerment in claiming my psychedelic heritage. Humans came to the Americas around twenty thousand years ago, developing rich cultures centered in deep Earth-based spirituality that worked in partnership with plant allies communicating through expanded states of consciousness. Around five hundred years ago Europeans came and deliberately pulled Americans from these cultural roots. Because it was so long ago, with so much oral tradition lost and so many artifacts destroyed, Latin

Americans are largely unaware of their spiritual history, only looking as far back as Catholicism for their foundation. But our roots go much deeper than those planted by our colonizers, and perhaps owning these psychedelic roots can be a way for two entire continents of American natives to reclaim their power.

PART III
The Future

6

CREATIVITY, HEALING, AND ECONOMICS

P sychedelics have influenced art, science, philosophy, religion, and social rights movements, and the impact of psychedelics is likely only to expand in the coming years. Within a decade, there could be hundreds and maybe thousands of psychedelic psychotherapy and retreat centers around the world. As shown in the last chapter, if psychedelics had an enormous impact in past societies where psychedelics were integrated into culture, then we may see a renaissance in our own cultures, a rebirth to heal the parts of society—from politics and economics to mental health and religion—that have been moving toward decay. In his book *Psychedelic Healing: The Promise of Entheogens for Psychotherapy and Spiritual Development*, the psychologist Neal Goldsmith also writes about the societal changes this could bring:

> Psychedelics are a catalyzing issue . . . over time their reintegration
> into psychiatry will have an enormous, transformative effect on society

as a whole. Psychedelics have the potential to bring science and spirituality into realignment and return us to our healthiest psychospiritual roots.[1]

Depending on one's culture and how far back one draws for context, psychospiritual roots can mean different things to different people. As already has been covered, psychedelics may have inspired humanity's first form of spirituality, can be found at the origin of Western culture with the Greeks, and may lay at the roots of Christianity. Outside the Christian context, psychedelics influenced the formation of the Hindu tradition by the writings of the Rigvedas, played a role in Islam with *Haoma*, and have formed the spiritual basis for many Indigenous lineages across the Americas. As psychedelics reintegrate into Western culture, there might be an expansion of consciousness that has the potential to influence many fields in the near future—including psychotherapy, art, science, philosophy, and even economics.

Psychotherapy and Guides

The occupations of psychedelic psychotherapist and medicine guide can be seen as modern expressions of the shaman, so it can be helpful to place these increasingly growing professions within the historical context of shamanism. The anthropologist Michael Brown writes, somewhat drolly: "Anthropologists are fond of reminding their students that shamanism, not prostitution, is the world's oldest profession."[2] The anthropologists Jeremy Narby and Francis Huxley do an excellent job of presenting a chronology of the developing Western perspective on shamanism in *Shamans through Time: 500 Years on the Path to Knowledge*. The book consists of sixty-four texts written over the last five centuries that show how shamans have been perceived by Western culture. Europeans

---

[1] Goldsmith, *Psychedelic Healing*, 171.

[2] M. Brown, "Dark Side of the Shaman," 251.

first categorized shamans as devil worshippers, then as imposters and charlatans, followed by an anthropological perspective that perceived them as protopsychiatrists for their society. Eventually, many anthropologists began participating in medicine ceremonies with medicine men and women, and now finally the shaman has generally been elevated to the status of a wisdom holder.[3]

The first mention of shamanism from a European perspective came from Christian clergy. In 1557 Andre Thevet, a French Franciscan priest who was the first to introduce tobacco to France, wrote about the dangers of investigating nature—God's personal knowledge realm—too deeply:

> The Americans are not the first to practice abusive magic; before them, it was familiar to several nations, back to the time of Our Lord, who erased and abolished the power that Satan exercised over human kind. It is therefore not without reason that it is forbidden by the scripture. Of this magic we find two main kinds, one by which one communicates with evil spirits, the other which gives intelligence about the most secret things of nature. It is true that one is more vicious than the other, but both are full of curiosity. When we have all the things we need and when we understand as much as God enables us to, what need is there to research with too much curiosity into the secrets of nature and other things, knowledge of which Our Lord has reserved for Himself? Such curiosities indicate an imperfect judgement, ignorance, and a lack of faith and good religion. Even more abused are the simple people who believe such impostures. I cannot cease to wonder how it is that in a land of law and police, one allows to proliferate like filth a bunch of old witches who put herbs on their arms, hang written words around their necks, and many mysteries, in ceremonies to cure fevers and other things, which are only true idolatry, and worthy of great punishment.[4]

---

[3] Narby and Huxley, *Shamans through Time*.

[4] Thevet, "Ministers of the Devil," 14–15.

The religious authorities believed they already held the absolute perspective and that any other point of view, indeed curiosity itself, must be punished. To them, shamans were worth killing.

The first time the word *shaman* was used in a published text was in 1672; Avvakum Petrovich, leader of a conservative clergy in Russia, referred to a Siberian "villain of a magician who calls demons."[5] The shift into the Enlightenment, which held reason as supreme, in the eighteenth century categorized shamans as impostors, which was only a slight improvement:

> This was a relatively progressive view in those days. Previous observers had mainly perceived such people as "agents of the Devil"—a serious charge in the times of witch-hunting. By judging shamans as imposters, Enlightenment observers implied that shamans did not really communicate with the Devil. This took away the witch-hunters' justification for executing people.[6]

Denis Diderot, philosopher and editor of the *Encyclopédie*, one of the key texts of the Enlightenment, saw the shaman as a juggler who "sometimes is quite close to the mark."[7]

In 1908 Roland Dixon, an American anthropologist, extended the definition of shamanism beyond that of a charlatan, though not in a flattering way. He included anyone relating to the supernatural:

> In any study of the religious beliefs and ceremonials of savage or semi-civilized peoples, either special or comparative, the shaman stands easily as one of the foremost figures. On almost every side of their religious life his influence makes itself felt, and his importance reaches out beyond the limits of religion into the domain of social life and organization and government control. By some the term shaman is confined, and perhaps rightly, within somewhat narrow limits; if I may

---

[5] Petrovich, "Shaman," 18.

[6] Narby and Huxley, *Shamans through Time*, 21.

[7] Diderot as cited in Narby and Huxley, 34.

be pardoned the liberty, I shall here extend rather the strict meaning of the term, and shall use it as applying to that motley class of persons, found in every savage community, who are supposed to have closer relations with the supernatural than other men, and who, according as they use the advantages of their position in one way or another, are the progenitors alike of the physician and the sorcerer, the prophet, the teacher, and the priest.[8]

As the field of psychology developed in the West over the following century, shamans became compared more to psychiatrists than to sorcerers of the spirit world. In 1949 the French anthropologist Claude Levi-Strauss pointed out common ground between psychoanalysis and shamanism. He writes that the shaman was someone in Indigenous cultures who seeks to bring consciousness to the unconscious:

The shaman provides the sick woman with a language, by means of which unexpressed, and otherwise inexpressible, psychic states can be immediately expressed. And it is the transition to this verbal expression—at the same time making it possible to undergo in an ordered and intelligible form a real experience that would otherwise be chaotic and inexpressible—which induces the release of the physiological process, that is, the reorganization, in a favorable direction, of the process to which the sick woman is subjected. In this respect, the shamanic cure lies on the borderline between our contemporary physical medicine and such psychological therapies as psychoanalysis. Its originality stems from the application to an organic condition of a method related to psychotherapy. How is this possible? A closer comparison between shamanism and psychoanalysis—which in our view implies no slight to psychoanalysis—will enable us to clarify this point.

In both cases the purpose is to bring to a conscious level conflicts and resistances which have remained unconscious, owing . . . to their repression by other psychological forces . . . this knowledge makes possible a specific experience, in the course of which conflicts materialize

---

[8] Dixon as cited in Narby and Huxley, 64.

in an order and on a level permitting their free development and leading to their resolution.[9]

In this passage we see the similarity between the shaman and the psychoanalyst—an aspect of their role is to help the client make sense of their experience. Once a client is able to articulate and express their experience, they can take a leap forward in becoming free of their unconscious processes. One notable difference is that a shaman actively guides their subject while a psychoanalyst generally just listens and reflects back.[10]

The American anthropologist Marlene Dobkin de Rios, who has studied the use of psychedelic plants in the Amazon for three decades, points out that as shamanism became popular with the counterculture, many shamanic retreat centers opened up as tourist traps.[11] While historically the shaman underwent rigorous training, rites of passage, and a lifelong commitment of responsibility to their social role, now anyone can position themselves as a shaman or medicine guide without being vetted by a community.[12] Now more than ever, the shaman, along with the medicine guide and psychedelic psychotherapist, needs a code of ethics perhaps similar to that of other therapeutic professionals. In "Shamans and Ethics in a Global World," the American anthropologist Eleanor Ott writes about the challenges of today's shamans, who are often distant from the deep culture and in fact could serve society in other professions:

> Until recently the shaman was the heartbeat of a tightly knit indigenous or traditional community that integrated the social and spiritual, material and mythic realms . . . Today many who dub themselves shamans no longer belong to a culture or community embedded in such a shamanic perspective, but rather come from the present generation of

---

[9] Levi-Strauss as cited in Narby and Huxley, 109.

[10] Narby and Huxley, 76.

[11] De Rios in Narby and Huxley, 227.

[12] Narby and Huxley, 107.

those primarily searching to find themselves. Thus, many of the new shamans are ill-equipped to engage in their practice of working with clients who come to them with a variety of physical, psychic, and spiritual ailments. The traditional indigenous shaman has the accumulated cultural experience and wisdom of generations of healers connected to a cosmology that gives meaning to both the illness and the shaman's processes of curing them. By contrast, many of the new shamans have but limited knowledge of any cosmology that could inform them and surround them with a sense of rootedness and ultimate meaning. Many of them received but limited training, some only from second- or third-hand sources.

The challenge for the new shaman today, if there indeed should be new shamans, is to maintain a strong personal ethical balance, free of self-delusion. This requires wisdom and knowledge and a lifetime commitment to this awesome responsibility. For some few this may be possible. For most, it is better to use their abilities in more contained but equally effective ways, as doctors, psychotherapists, teachers, artists, writers, priests.[13]

As the passage suggests, for most psychedelic practitioners today perhaps the title of *psychedelic psychotherapist* or *medicine guide* is more fitting. This also helps resolve the issue of cultural appropriation, since many practitioners may not be part of a lineage or have grounding in any real heritage.

Having a guide trained in Western psychotherapy and other modalities of healing, along with trainings influenced by Indigenous practices, can be truly helpful. Michael Pollan writes about his benefit from, and concern about, doing a guided journey:

Taking psilocybin on a guided journey, however, is a fundamentally different experience from the scare stories usually depicted. Many of these guides are highly skilled and use time-tested protocols for safety and comfort. My concern is that if demand for these experiences

---

[13] Ott, "Shamans and Ethics in a Global World," 280–85.

exceeds the supply of these underground professionals, the potential for things to go wrong goes up.[14]

Francoise Bourzat spent decades working with expanded states of consciousness and training within the lineage of the Mazatecs, learning everything she could from elders and wisdom holders within the tradition. In an effort to train and inform people interested in the emerging position of being a guide, she, with the help of Kristina Hunter, wrote *Consciousness Medicine: Indigenous Wisdom, Entheogens, and Expanded States of Consciousness for Healing and Growth*. Bourzat writes: "Consciousness Medicine is the art and science of exploring the infinite dimensions and manifestations of consciousness—the foundation of life. Consciousness Medicine uses varied theories, tools, and techniques to access specific states of expanded consciousness."[15] When she says "expanded states of consciousness," she is referring to all holotropic states of consciousness that can be entered through breathwork, drumming, dance, meditation, and other means, as well as through psychedelics. She writes that

> expanded states of consciousness tend to open people up to a level of deeply visceral and direct experience that is difficult, if not impossible, to reach through regular therapy. It is my experience that the healing accessed in expanded states goes swiftly to the core of the issue needing attention, making it an extremely effective modality. It is especially useful for addressing preverbal trauma, which talk therapy can barely access. However, it also means that this therapeutic approach calls for an extra level of caution and attention with aftercare and integration.[16]

---

[14] Pollan in Stamets, *Fantastic Fungi*, 122.

[15] Bourzat and Hunter, *Consciousness Medicine*, 16.

[16] Bourzat and Hunter, 33.

She goes on to point out the integral importance of a guide when working with expanded states of consciousness:

> A guide is someone who walks ahead and knows the territory, aware of the potential perils of the terrain. Like the jungle, our inner self is an environment full of beautiful complexity. In many cultures, rituals that invoke expanded states of consciousness for transformation and healing are guided. An appropriate guide is trained in specific techniques that aid the experience of inner exploration.[17]

As psychedelics move toward both decriminalization and legalization, the professions of the psychedelic psychotherapist and medicine guide may undergo an unprecedented acceleration of growth. *Consciousness Medicine* is helpful for everyone stepping into these positions, as it stresses the importance of both preparation and integration and bridges the world between Indigenous and psychotherapeutic practices, as well as for people interested in exploring psychedelics and clients of these psychotherapists/guides.

One of the most popular texts in the arena of psychedelic medicine work is James Fadiman's *The Psychedelic Explorer's Guide: Safe, Therapeutic, and Sacred Journeys.* It is an essential read for guides and serious psychonauts. Fadiman's credentials are impressive: undergraduate work at Harvard, graduate work at Stanford, former president of the Institute of Noetic Sciences, and cofounder of the Institute of Transpersonal Psychology (which is now called Sofia University). More importantly, he was a part of the team at the International Foundation for Advanced Study during the 1960s in Menlo Park, California. Their research using psychedelics included subjects who were some of the most brilliant minds that played key roles in the development of Silicon Valley. Having over five decades of experience in the cross-section of psychology and psychedelics, Fadiman is an authority in the field and presents a thorough approach to psychedelic psychotherapy—including detailed

---

[17] Bourzat and Hunter, 40.

checklists, a presentation of all the scientific data his team harvested, and an expansive history of the field from someone who was socially well-connected through its development. The first two chapters of the book, along with his checklist, have been integrated into the Guild of Guides training manual, an underground manual for practitioners that offer psychedelic psychotherapy.[18]

Neal Goldsmith's *Psychedelic Healing: The Promise of Entheogens for Psychotherapy and Spiritual Development* also emphasizes safety when using psychedelics. Goldsmith completed his federally funded dissertation at Princeton and was a deputy principal investigator for a four-year, nationwide study on mental health policies. The following are Neal Goldsmith's "Ten Lessons of Psychedelic Psychotherapy," as found in his book:

Lesson 1: Each Drug Has a Specific Effect

Lesson 2: Setting Can Strongly Influence State of Mind and Thus Outcome

Lesson 3: Mindset Can Scuttle a Beautiful Context or Transcend a Hellish One

Lesson 4: In General, Dose Determines a Mild or Extreme Experience, Although It Can Be Less Important Than Set and Setting

Lesson 5: Preparation and Knowledge Can Enable Lasting Value

Lesson 6: Ritual Can Transmit Prior Wisdom and Guide Successful Practice

Lesson 7: Support from Experienced Guides Reduces Fear and Increases Benefit

Lesson 8: Reentry to a Supportive Community Context Aids Retention

---

[18] Fadiman, *Psychedelic Explorer's Guide*, 251.

Lesson 9: Accompanying Depth Psychotherapy (If Needed) and Ongoing Spiritual Practice Offer the Main Opportunity for Lasting Growth

Lesson 10: A Revised Worldview Is Both a Requirement for and a Result of Integrated Psychedelic Practice[19]

Goldsmith shares on the process of set and setting:

> Open-Mindedness and a willingness to surrender to the process, confidence in the people and surroundings, and a motivation to learn and heal . . . are all associated with a successful outcome . . . Mindset is perhaps the single most important factor in determining the outcome of a psychedelic experience.[20]

As psychedelics move toward legalization, the process of working with set and setting—mindset, education, environment, and trained guides and therapists—will likely be refined. In the centers that emerge, it will be essential that they have careful protocols and trained facilitators.

A container where a trained facilitator is taking responsibility for the participant while the participant voyages is imperative. A strong dose of psilocybin can be uncomfortable, though with the right guidance, that discomfort can be enriching and beneficial. It is common for one to feel anxiety as the medicine is coming on, and while the journey may be difficult, the struggle can be transformative, leading to an increased sense of strength and humility. Dark emotions and challenging archetypal content can emerge in psychedelic states.[21] Hidden trauma, anxiety, fear, and primal power can surge to the surface. A grounded lifeline to a sober reality, in the form of a trusted guide or therapist, is invaluable.

A chapter outlining the role of the guide is included in the classic book *The Varieties of Psychedelic Experience* by Robert Masters and Jean

---

[19] Goldsmith, *Psychedelic Healing*.

[20] Goldsmith, 113.

[21] Bache, *Dark Night, Early Dawn*.

Houston. The authors legally worked with psychedelics before these medicines became Schedule 1 substances. They were both also pioneers in the field of transpersonal psychology and founders of the Human Potential Movement. Following is an excerpt, explaining some of the training that is important for a guide to have, from the chapter titled "The Guide":

> The master guide will never be much more common than is the master poet. But the guide, even now, should have certain minimal qualifications; and, as our knowledge increases, psychedelic guide training should become far more thorough and effective and the personal qualities and talents desirable in the guide much better understood than is possible at this time.
>
> Apart from his specialty as a therapist or whatever, the guide should have a broad educational background including a good practical knowledge of human psychology. He should be mentally and emotionally stable and possess the capacity to stimulate feelings of security and trust in the subjects. And his experience as a guide should be sufficient to enable him to cope with emergencies . . . the guide [must] have received some training in this specialty. It implies as well that the guide has himself been a subject, preferable on several occasions—that is, that the guide has experienced the drugs and so is able to understand the experience of the subject.
>
> Ideally, the psychedelic guide will have two (if not more) specialties. First, he will be a psychotherapist, educator, anthropologist, whatever. Second, he will be a psychedelic guide . . . Mature, intelligent individuals with widely divergent interests and talents as well as different specific professional training will be needed if the psychedelic experience is ever to yield up all the treasures it promises.
>
> Moreover, in addition to his specialties, it is highly desirable that each guide possess a broad background especially including knowledge of history, literature, philosophy, mythology, art, and religion. Materials from all of these fields, and from others, emerge in many of the sessions and the guide must recognize the materials if he is to be of maximum effectiveness.[22]

---

[22] Masters and Houston, *Varieties of Psychedelic Experience*, 131–32.

The relationship between the explorer and the guide acts as a tether for the explorer. The strength of this tether is based on trust. Before undergoing a psychedelic session, the practitioner and participant need good agreements between themselves to help build trust. These can be taken from Leo Zeff, the psychologist that first introduced MDMA into psychotherapy. Zeff's story is documented in the biographical book *The Secret Chief Revealed*, written by pioneer psychedelic researcher Myron Stolaroff; "The Secret Chief" is a name given to Zeff by Terence McKenna. Sasha Shulgin, the famed chemist known as "the Godfather of MDMA," introduced Zeff to MDMA in the 1970s. Zeff was already an elderly man who was ready to retire until he found the deeply therapeutic potential of psychedelics. During the '70s and '80s he worked with about four thousand individuals, including training about one hundred therapists, and played an important role in the underground psychedelic psychotherapy movement, where people risked their freedom to heal others.

Zeff developed a protocol during this time and asked all participants to make the following five agreements before each journey: 1) the participant agrees to not leave the space during the journey; 2) the participant agrees to not cause physical harm to themselves, the practitioner, or the environment; 3) the participant agrees that they will not reveal who they worked with or the location of the space without clearance; 4) the participant agrees that there won't be sexual touching between the practitioner and participant during the journey; and 5) the participant agrees that if the practitioner should tell them to stop a behavior during the session, they will obey.[23] These agreements can help deepen the trust between practitioner and participant and help make a safe container—leading to a more fruitful session. The more trust and comfort are established, the further the explorer can go. Without trust, the explorer will feel held back and will focus on safety instead of surrendering and exploring. As shared previously in regard to the instincts, once the autonomy and communion safety needs are met, transcendence becomes more possible and available.

---

[23] Stolaroff, *Secret Chief Revealed*, 68.

Trust—softening the autonomy needs while remaining in communion—takes time to develop, and there is a way to expedite the emotional process with the help of MDMA. In a therapeutic container, MDMA reliably produces feelings of love and well-being. MAPS projects that MDMA will be medically legal soon, and it will serve as an excellent aid in introducing subjects into expanded states of consciousness. With the right dose and setting, MDMA is consistently safe and produces positive experiences.[24] MDMA enables people with no prior altered-state experience to ease into expanded states of consciousness and develop a positive association with shifting states. Proven to produce numerous psychological benefits, including the reduction of fear, MDMA offers a graceful entrance to deeper exploration.[25] The molecule and its effect on our biology have been heavily studied, and clinical trials have been carried out with positive results that show MDMA is helpful in the treatment of depression, posttraumatic stress disorder, and schizophrenia.[26] MAPS has led the way in the MDMA research, bringing it into Phase III testing for severe posttraumatic stress disorder, which will be conducted at sixteen different sites.[27] The military veteran population has a lot to gain from MDMA, as posttraumatic stress disorder contributes to about eighteen US veteran suicides per day.[28] This crisis has led to people from across the political spectrum to support MDMA research.

Julie Holland, a medical doctor on the faculty of the New York University School of Medicine, in *Ecstasy: The Complete Guide: A Comprehensive Look at the Risks and Benefits of MDMA*, states that the simple availability of self-acceptance and self-love can be a breakthrough:

---

[24] Holland, *Ecstasy: The Complete Guide.*

[25] Holland.

[26] Holland.

[27] Multidisciplinary Association for Psychedelic Studies, "MAPS' Phase 3 Trial."

[28] US Department of Veterans Affairs, *Veteran Suicide Prevention Annual Report.*

At higher doses of MDMA, that feeling of satiety becomes a fortified self-image, a sense of enhanced capacity and strength. Taking that effect a step further, it becomes euphoria, intense self-love and self-acceptance. This is why experiences with MDMA can be so curative. Having feelings of confidence and self-worth can be invaluable during psychotherapy, allowing for the exploration of painful material. Lessening anxiety to explore core issues or repressed memories, and feeling calm in the face of what would typically be considered threatening, can help accomplish a great deal in therapy. Experiencing these feelings of self-love and acceptance, sometimes for the first time in years, can be therapeutic all on its own.[29]

In addition, MDMA tends to dissolve one's feelings of fear and fills one with feelings of love. This freedom from fear has the potential of bringing greater balance and clarity to a person's consciousness, allowing them to view events in their life more objectively and empathically. For these reasons it has been extremely helpful in couples therapy, treating posttraumatic stress disorder, and possibly social anxiety. One study, published in the September 2018 issue of *Psychopharmacology*, focused on treating social anxiety in autistic adults. It found that most of the participants experienced increased feelings of empathy and connectedness and reported an easier time communicating.[30] Another study, published the same month in *Current Biology*, found similar effects when administering MDMA to octopuses. When given MDMA, the normally solitary creature displayed less symptoms of fear and showed an increase in prosocial behavior.[31]

MDMA treatments, along with preparation and integration sessions, might prove to be beneficial before beginning psilocybin-assisted psychotherapy. The experience MDMA offers can establish deep trust between the therapist and client, providing a stronger sense of safety

---

[29] Holland, *Ecstasy*, 90.

[30] Danforth et al., "MDMA-Assisted Psychotherapy with Autistic Adults."

[31] Klein, "Octopuses Reached Out for a Hug."

in the psilocybin session. MDMA would also support one in releasing trauma, which we all carry to some degree, before entering deeper into the transpersonal states that psilocybin catalyzes.

People with heart conditions and on SSRIs need to consult with a health professional before using MDMA. Since MDMA may become legal before psilocybin, this protocol can be integrated as soon as psilocybin-assisted psychotherapy is legalized. Professional assistance and ethical responsibility are important in administering MDMA. Unlike psilocybin, MDMA can be toxic and has the potential for addiction.

Intentional care to create a safe container for a psilocybin journey is especially necessary because these experiences are known for bringing shadow material to the surface. The shadow, a term coined by Carl Jung, refers to the repressed parts of one's psyche.[32] In *Decomposing the Shadow: Lessons from the Psilocybin Mushroom*, James Jesso writes about the connection between the shadow and the self:

> Psilocybin mushrooms guide us into a state of increased emotional awareness, and in doing so, are able to bring us into direct encounter with the *shadow*. During these encounters with the *shadow*, the mushrooms can guide us into the emotional roots of *self* where the hard truth of psycho-emotional wounds can be faced directly, released, and healed.[33]

Jesso draws a metaphorical link between the role fungi play in nature and the effects of psilocybin on the psyche. In nature, fungi are decomposers. They break down the nutrients of bodies that have died to create energy for plants. Without fungi, plants and animals would not exist. Fungi exist at the thresholds of death and birth in the natural world. Jesso states:

---

[32] Campbell, *Portable Jung*.

[33] Jesso, *Decomposing the Shadow*, 69.

By guiding us into the *emotive-psychosynthesis* of emotional repression, it *decomposes the shadow* and unlocks the nutrients contained within it to feed the soil of psychospiritual growth. They take us on a journey through and beyond the death and decay of repression, into the fertile grounds of budding maturity, courage, and confidence. Through breaking down the emotional blockages that hinder us, the psilocybin experience guides us through the *shadow* and beyond, into the empowerment of personal responsibility and psychospiritual maturity. It helps us learn the ability to *surrender* ourselves into the honesty of dark emotional experiences without projection, assures us we are capable of going further, and enables us to see the true strength residing within the release of personal blockages. It exposes us to the crucial understanding that the *shadow* can be one of our greatest spiritual tools once we learn to navigate it. If founded on respect and the intention of healing, a practice with the psilocybin mushroom can bring about a full and successful integration of a fragmented emotional existence into an expression of a *whole self*.[34]

The integration of shadow material is essential to one's sense of wholeness, and as Stanislav Grof points out, psychedelics can catalyze holotropic states of consciousness that organically move through the shadow toward this wholeness.[35]

After decades of working with altered states of consciousness, Stanislav Grof shares that holotropic states follow an experiential logic rather than a linear logic. This means that content that arises in the psyche is linked by emotional charge rather than events that occurred sequentially through time.

Holotropic states tend to engage something like an "inner radar," that automatically brings into consciousness the contents from the unconscious that have the strongest emotional charge, are most psychodynamically relevant at the time, and most readily available for conscious

---

[34] Jesso, 72.

[35] Grof, *Psychology of the Future*.

processing . . . Once a client enters a holotropic state, the material for processing is chosen quite automatically. As long as the client keeps the experience internalized, the best we can do as therapists is to accept and support what is happening, whether or not it is constant with our theoretical concepts and expectations.[36]

This process is seen clearly in Grof's model of the basic perinatal matrices (BPMs). BPM is a model that Grof constructed based on archetypal patterns he detected in his years of working with clients in holotropic states.[37] The BPMs are four experiential stages, which usually involve transpersonal material, that are grounded in the birth process. Following is my summarization of each stage:

BPM I corresponds to the period of gestation prior to the onset of labor. The participant in this stage may experience nourishment, ease, and a sense of unity. There might be archetypal content that represents an oceanic oneness. This can be a heavenly state, unless there was trauma when the child was actually in the womb. In that case, the shadow can be experienced as a poisonous womb (especially if the mother was intoxicated during pregnancy), drowning, and engulfment.

BPM II corresponds to the period of labor when the cervix is still closed. The womb that once nourished the child is now the environment that crushes it. The womb is all the child has known up to this point, and so it seems that the painful experience will go on forever. The archetypal theme of eternal damnation is a quality of this state. One is in hell, frustrated, and in despair. Depression is a characteristic of this state. One feels trapped without the possibility of escape.

BPM III begins when the cervix opens and so a way out has appeared. Archetypal themes of power and sex arise, as now the fetus has to

---

[36] Grof, 28.

[37] Grof, 169.

make its way through the birth canal to survive. Experiences of passion and anger, as well as animalistic themes may emerge. Through tooth and claw, one must survive. Screaming, growling, and bursts of somatic movement may come through. If one moves fully through this stage, the depression and fear of BPM II turns into empowerment at BPM III.

BPM IV corresponds to actual delivery. The participant has gone through an ego-death, moved through tribulations, and is still alive. The experience is one of liberation. Symbolically, the infant has been birthed into a new world and sense of self. Experiences of enlightenment and wakefulness are typical of this stage. Archetypal contents of resurrection and feelings of wholeness may occur. Generally, one may leave feeling like a solid and strong individual.

The process may not always occur in sequence and at times may toggle back and forth, such as between BPM II and BPM III before breaking through to BPM IV in a later session.[38] Though this process may seem difficult, it also cultivates courage, strength, vulnerability, and trust in one's self.

The death-rebirth process is ever-expanding, as one evolves from shedding biographical conditioning toward transpersonal transparency of a deeper essence. Christopher Bache, in *Dark Night, Early Dawn: Steps to a Deep Ecology of Mind*, shares his twenty-year journey of presenting his psychedelic experiences through the lens of Grof's model. Bache noticed that he would process heavy materials for about four journeys before finally breaking through and reaping rewards in a fifth journey. One way to interpret this process is the dissolution instinct working to dissolve psychological structures that hold one back from greater autonomy, communion, and transcendence. Some of these structures are barriers that contain the shadow, repressed parts of oneself. These unconscious barriers form a separation between one's conscious self and material that has not integrated into one's personality. The

---

[38] Bache, *Dark Night, Early Dawn*.

dissolution of these boundaries may force repressed material to rise to the surface for integration. Over the years, Bache's death-rebirth experiences transformed from the personal into collective death-rebirth experiences, where he became groups of people, then all humanity, and even the planet as a whole.

About deeply transformative and evolutionary experiences such as this, the integral philosopher Ken Wilber notes the importance of interpretation:

> All depth must be interpreted. And how we interpret depth is crucially important for the birth of that depth itself. New depth allows us new interpretation; the new interpretations cocreate and give birth to that depth, help unpack that depth. Unpacking the depth is the emergence of that depth.[39]

Experiencing novelty and accurately translating it into language is a process of evolution. Therefore, we need clear models and maps to navigate and interpret this space, and the works of Grof and Bache are attempts at describing these far-reaching dynamics of consciousness.

A well-thought-out, thorough text for someone contemplating undergoing a psychedelic experience—whether in a therapeutic or ceremonial setting—is Kile Ortigo's *Beyond the Narrow Life: A Guide for Psychedelic Integration and Existential Exploration*. Ortigo received his doctorate in clinical psychology and is a graduate of the psychedelic-assisted psychotherapy certificate training at the California Institute of Integral Studies. The book itself is structured like a journey—preparing the subject before the journey, working with trials, tribulations, and death-rebirth experiences that can take place in expanded states of consciousness, and then integrating the journey. Ortigo covers a lot of material relevant for psychedelic experiences in this book, including going over major models in psychology, designing worksheets for the participant that encourage growth and exploration, and leading the curious explorer into deep waters

---

[39] Wilber, *Sex, Ecology, Spirituality*, 522.

by offering existential questions. The book itself might serve as a guide for those who desire to self-explore (in places that legally permit psychedelic use) but cannot afford or may not have access to skilled professionals.

Though our Western culture is formulating containers for psychedelic experiences, along with trying to strategize appropriate ways to use these medicines, some groups have engaged with these expanded states of consciousness as a central aspect of their culture over millennia. In the Mazatec tradition, families eat mushrooms together, and members begin taking mushrooms at a young age.[40] The anthropologist Henry Munn writes: "Usually several members of a family eat the mushrooms together: it is not uncommon for a father, mother, children, uncles, and aunts to all participate in these transformations of the mind that elevate consciousness onto a higher plane."[41] Western society, which until recently has largely seen psilocybin mushrooms as purely recreational drugs, may be appalled by families coming together to take a psychedelic substance, unable to see the potential of these expansive states to heal fractured relationships and conjure experiences of internal and relational unity. Our Western society, including the field of psychology, can learn much from some of these psychedelic Indigenous traditions, just as they perhaps have things to learn from us.

Psychedelics are versatile, and one's relationship to them can take many forms. In addition to the in-depth journeys explored earlier, psychedelics may also be experienced in microdose regimens. A microdose is a subperceptual amount of a psychedelic. This is about ten micrograms of LSD or five to ten milligrams for psilocybin mushrooms.[42] This lower amount can create an *enhanced* state of consciousness rather than an *expanded* state of consciousness. James Fadiman popularized microdosing in *The Psychedelic Explorer's Guide: Safe, Therapeutic, and Sacred Journeys*, where he notes that microdosing isn't something new:

---

[40] Jesso, *Decomposing the Shadow*, 15.

[41] Munn, *Mushrooms of Language*.

[42] Fadiman, *Psychedelic Explorer's Guide*, 198.

Indigenous cultures have known about and used sub-perceptual doses of different psychedelics for centuries. Until recently, this knowledge has been overlooked. After being involved in research on sub-perceptual doses for over a year, I found myself embarrassed at my own cultural bias as I came to realize I had ignored the obvious, and that indigenous healers or shamans, working with their own psychedelic plants, have systemically and fully explored every dose level.[43]

Fadiman currently continues his research on microdosing, with over 1,500 participants having reported their experiences following the protocol that he lists on his website.[44] This involves taking a microdose supplement on day one, followed by two days not taking it, before taking it again on the fourth day. After a month of this practice, subjects share their experiences, which are then analyzed and integrated into the larger data. This is the protocol that author and former University of California, Berkeley, law professor Ayelet Waldman used and wrote about in her book *A Really Good Day: How Microdosing Made a Mega Difference in My Mood, My Marriage, and My Life.*[45] Albert Hofmann, the pharmacologist who first synthesized both LSD and psilocybin and lived to the age of 102, is said to have microdosed for the last twenty years of his life, and he proposed that microdosing psychedelics could be a better alternative to Ritalin.[46] As mentioned earlier in this book, those with attention deficit disorder tend to have well-developed imaginations and also seek more stimulation than those with a regular neurological profile.[47] A subperceptual dose of LSD could act as a stimulant, like Adderall, and also enhance these

[43] Fadiman, 198–99.

[44] www.JamesFadiman.com

[45] Waldman, *Really Good Day.*

[46] Fadiman, *Psychedelic Explorer's Guide,* 204.

[47] Maté, *Scattered*; Maté, *In the Realm of Hungry Ghosts.*

people's innate abilities to be able to better contribute their visionary gifts to society.

The mycologist Paul Stamets created a microdose recommendation and made it public during a presentation at the 2017 MAPS Psychedelic Science Conference, which was the largest conference on psychedelic science to date. Stamets recommends creating a supplement that contains both psilocybin and lion's mane mushrooms, since both catalyze the growth of new neurons. Niacin (also known as vitamin B3) could be added, which opens the blood vessels in the body and causes a warm flush. The dilation of the blood vessels could help the psilocybin and lion's mane circulate through the body, while the flush causes uncomfortable irritation that turns skin red in more than small amounts. Because of the niacin, this formula, if it ever were to be prescribed, would act as a safe deterrent for anyone taking more than the recommended dosage of a microdose with the intention of having a psychedelic experience.

There are several forms of educational organizations offering lectures, practices, and other resources on psychedelics. North Star started an ethics pledge, where organizations and individuals working within the field of psychedelics pledge to seven principles (Start Within, Study the Traditions, Build Trust, Consider the Gravity, Focus on Process, Create Equality and Justice, and Pay It Forward), in order to create a standard of ethics in the field of psychedelic business.[48] Lucid News: Psychedelics, Consciousness, Technologies, and the Future of Wellness was launched in 2020 to bring ethical and transparent journalism to the expanding field of psychedelics.[49] Other notable sources of psychedelic news are *Psychedelic Times* and *Psychedelics Today*, which have created integration journals that can be purchased on Amazon.[50] George Lake, a lawyer and author of the book

---

[48] www.NorthStar.guide/EthicsPledge

[49] www.Lucid.news

[50] www.PsychedelicTimes.com; www.PsychedelicsToday.com; Buller and Moore, *Integration Workbook*; Buller and Moore, *Navigating Psychedelics*.

Psychedelics in Mental Health Series: Psilocybin, also wrote *The Law of Entheogenic Churches in the United States* in order to empower people in the Unites States to open legal churches in order protect their psychedelic practices.[51] For people who live in areas that have decriminalized the use of natural psychedelics, MycoRising offers quality online and in-person workshops to educate the public on private mushroom cultivation.[52] Integration Communications was launched in 2020 to provide integrity focused public relations to projects stepping into the field of psychedelics.[53] The Center for Consciousness Medicine emerged in 2019 to offer guide trainings without the use of psychedelics and will soon have an international and legal psychedelic psychotherapy and medicine guide training.[54] Inaura, an online platform to help people find guides of all kinds—from bodyworks and therapists to alternative healers and psychedelic integration counselors—was created in 2021.[55] The California Institute of Integral Studies has for years now offered a Certificate in Psychedelic-Assisted Therapies and Research.[56] PsiloHealth is in the process of creating psychedelic sitter courses.[57] Atman Retreat has enabled people to fly into Jamaica for legal, safe, and quality psilocybin ceremonies.[58] The San Francisco Psychedelic Society, Psychedelic Seminars, Entheogenic Research Integration Education (ERIE), and Mt. Tam Integration have been serving the Bay Area for several years with psychedelic education and

---

[51] Lake, *Mental Health Series: Psilocybin*; Lake, *Law of Entheogenic Churches*.

[52] www.MycoRisingFungi.com

[53] www.IntegrationCommunication.com

[54] www.CenterforCM.com

[55] www.Inaura.com

[56] www.CIIS.edu/Research-Centers/Center-for-Psychedelic-Therapies-and-Research

[57] www.PsiloHealth.co

[58] www.AtmanRetreat.com

integration and have now all brought offerings online.[59] Mt. Tam Integration launched an annual online Psilocybin Summit with over 4,000 people signing up for the 2020 summit.[60] Members of some of these organizations launched the Decriminalize Nature movement, which has now gone nationwide.[61] Aaron Paul Orsini, author of *Autism on Acid: How LSD Helped Me Understand, Navigate, Alter and Appreciate My Autistic Perceptions*, cofounded the Autistic Psychedelic Community, an online community where neurodivergent people can learn from and support each other through their psychedelic explorations.[62] The Multidisciplinary Association for Psychedelic Studies has offered the Zendo Project, psychedelic harm reduction and education, at several festivals including Burning Man and Lightning in a Bottle, which together total about 100,000 participants each year.[63]

I lead a free and public monthly online group with the San Francisco Psychedelic Society (SFPS) called Developing a Relationship with Sacred Mushrooms to create a safe space for integration, asking questions, and community building. SFPS is the largest psychedelic society in the United States and has grown into having an incredible global outreach by fully making its services and offerings available online. Access to psychedelic psychotherapists and medicine guides may not be available to everyone, especially those in low-income communities who cannot afford such services and often suffer the most, and some of these previous sources offer them the fundamental knowledge required for these populations to begin healing themselves. To help people navigate psychedelic experiences, the Fireside Project has launched an app

[59] www.PsychedelicSocietySF.org; www.PsychSems.com; www.ERIEvision.org; www.TamIntegration.com

[60] www.PsilocybinSummit.com

[61] www.DecriminalizeNature.org

[62] Orsini, *Autism on Acid*; www.AutisticPsychedelic.com

[63] www.MAPS.org; www.ZendoProject.com

and free around-the-clock service that makes a psychedelic peer support line available.[64]

Public offerings about psychedelic education and support are increasing, and the pace with which such organizations are forming will only quicken once psychedelics are legalized for therapeutic use. Therapeutic psychedelic experiences have the potential to heal treatment-resistant conditions, accelerate growth, transform lives, and inspire deep creativity within individuals—even giving them the experiences of being reborn. Collectively, we might undergo a second *renaissance*, which in French literally translates to "rebirth."

Visionary Art and Culture

This section presents examples of contemporary artists who have been impacted by psychedelics and in turn have publicly come out in support of psychedelics through their art. These artists' works serve as cultural points of reference for people describing their psychedelic experiences, which often include a flurry of aesthetic inspiration and expression. In visionary doses (about 5 dried grams of psilocybin mushrooms or 300 micrograms of LSD), psychedelics can conjure visionary states of consciousness with detailed images, sounds, and sensations connected through multilayered meaning that are often incredibly emotionally and spiritually moving. As archeological evidence suggests, psychedelics may have served as muses that inspired the imagination of humanity at least since the emergence of cave art.[65] "Songs, music, and decorative art of many traditional societies are said to originate with hallucinogenic experience,"[66] writes author and researcher Paul Devereux, and it is no

---

[64] www.FireSideProject.org

[65] Lewis-Williams, *Conceiving God*, 225; Hancock, *Divine Spark*.

[66] Devereux, *Long Trip*, 246.

secret that psychedelics inspired many of the great works of music, film, literature, and visual art of the 1960s and 1970s.

The term *visionary art* was coined in 1990 to describe art inspired by psychedelics. When Alex Grey was choosing a title for his first book, *Sacred Mirrors: The Visionary Art of Alex Grey*, his publisher (Simon & Schuster) offered the term *visionary* instead of *psychedelic*, stating that it might speak to a wider audience.[67] Laurence Caruana, another visionary artist, defines the artistic movement in his 2010 book *The First Manifesto of Visionary Art*:

> Visionary art is as ancient as the shaman's first etchings on cavern walls or the mysterious spirals carved on megalithic stones. Our art manifests itself among the Egyptians, Mesopotamians, Minoans, and ancient Greeks. In Middle America, it uprose among the Olmecs, Mayans, and Aztecs.[68]

Caruana briefly describes the intent of visionary art to bring to the visual realm the experience of the unseen:

> Art of the Visionary attempts to show what lies *beyond* the boundary of our sight. Through dream, trance, or other altered states, the artist attempts to *see the unseen*—attaining a visionary state that transcends our regular modes of perception. The task awaiting him, thereafter, is to communicate his vision in a form recognizable to "everyday sight."
>
> All visionary artists are united by this spirit of on-going experimentation. And their works bear testimony to those mind-altering, soul-shattering but potentially enlightening experiences which may transpire over the course of each experiment . . . The aim of these experiments is to bring alternative states of consciousness to reality. Or rather, to bear witness to other realities which are made evident in alternative states of consciousness.[69]

---

[67] Grey, *Sacred Mirrors*; Oroc, *New Psychedelic Revolution*.

[68] Caruana, *First Manifesto of Visionary Art*, 7.

[69] Caruana, 1–2.

When describing the books that have inspired many young visionary artists, Caruana writes:

> A quick glimpse at the books lying around the studio of many third generation Visionaries will no doubt reveal at least one or two titles by Ken Wilber or Stanislav Grof—the former a philosopher of the transpersonal, the latter its foremost psychologist.[70]

Both the foreword to Alex Grey's book *The Mission of Art* and a chapter in *Sacred Mirrors: The Visionary Art of Alex Grey* were written by Ken Wilber. As an expression of his esteem, Alex Grey produced artistic portraits of both Ken Wilber and Stanislav Grof.

As an ode to the feminine, David Jay Brown and Rebecca Ann Hill produced *Women of Visionary Art*, showcasing women artists in the field. Brown, who had produced several books on psychedelics, writes:

> One of the biggest criticisms I've received about my five previously published interview books is that, in those collected dialogues and trialogues, the men disproportionately outnumber the women so I have long wanted to do a collection that was composed exclusively of interviews with brilliant and remarkable women.[71]

The interviews are thorough and focus on how psychedelic experiences, dreams, and spiritual beliefs influence the work of these artists, many of whom are masters of their techniques, as each woman shares how her personal transcendental experiences give shape to her visionary art.

Stanislav Grof has written his own book, *Modern Consciousness Research and the Understanding of Art*, on the intersection of art and psychedelics. He dedicates a large portion of the book to the artist H. R. Giger, who passed away in May 2014. Giger was an Academy Award–winning artist (of *Alien* fame) and a friend of Grof's. For decades, Giger

---

[70] Caruana, 44.

[71] Brown and Hill, *Women of Visionary Art*, 6.

translated the deep and dark layers—of both his psyche and the collective unconscious—into exquisite visual work. In the book, Grof uses the lens of psychoanalysis to see Giger's life and work, pointing out the archetypal imagery and expressions of the basic perinatal matrices in Giger's art.[72] Giger himself was influenced by both psychedelics and his dreams, with his paintings holding deeply, psychically charged content. Of Giger, the psychologist Timothy Leary said: "In Giger's paintings, we see ourselves as crawling embryos, as fetal, larval creatures protected by the membranes of our egos, waiting for the moment of our metamorphosis and new birth."[73] Giger's work focused on the alien, sexual, and deviant aspects of the psyche, creating dystopian landscapes that synthesized biology and technology. With a fondness for darkness, he gave it unparalleled artistic expression in humanity, bringing to our visual field snapshots of humanity's collective shadow.

On using psychedelics to access the collective unconscious for creative purposes, Grof writes:

> An entire generation of Avant-garde young artists embraced them [psychedelics] as tools for finding deep inspiration in the perinatal domain and in the archetypal realm of the collective unconscious. They portrayed with extraordinary artistic power a rich array of experiences originating in these deep and ordinarily hidden recesses of the human psyche . . . Many of them documented in their art their own spiritual and philosophical quest.[74]

A couple of such artists are the Wachowski siblings, who are best known for writing and directing *The Matrix* film series and *V for Vendetta*, which have brought many elements of psychedelic and integral culture into the mainstream. *V* became the face of the Occupy movement and still stands as a cultural symbol for revolution toward a less oppressive

---

[72] Grof, *Modern Consciousness Research*.

[73] Leary as cited in Grof, *Modern Consciousness Research*, 166.

[74] Grof, 32.

socioeconomic system. The *Matrix* trilogy brought breakthrough special effects while integrating many mystical ideas into the films. For the special collector's edition box set, the Wachowskis hired Ken Wilber to give a commentary on all three movies, totaling hours of analysis of the *Matrix* films from a nondual and integral perspective. During the commentary Wilber points out Stan Grof's BPMs several times as the movie expresses their archetypal themes. Most notably, Wilber continues to point out that fundamentally the humans and AI are both part of the same being, a unitive cosmic consciousness, and this is the context that underlies the whole trilogy, as Neo and Agent Smith each represent opposites in a universal polarity.[75] For many in both psychedelic and pop culture, *The Matrix* has been a metaphor for the process of awakening and describing a foundational layer of a collective consciousness beneath society. In 2021, more than twenty years after the first film, a new *Matrix* movie, *The Matrix Ressurections*, with original star Keanu Reeves was released.

The Wachowskis also created the Netflix show *Sense8*, which ran from 2015 to 2018 and dealt with many of the key concepts I have explored in this book. The premise of *Sense8* is that a separate evolutionary line of humans, called "*Homo sensorium*," coevolved parallel to *Homo sapiens* for the last hundreds of thousands of years. What distinguishes *Homo sensorium* is that they are telepathically linked to one another. Like *Homo sapiens*, these individuals are biologically born, but they then go through a second birth, a psychic one, at a maturation point in their lives, when they connect to seven other individuals who were born at the same time. The members in the *Homo sensorium* species empathically connect through a psychic substrate called psycellium. The Wachowskis have stated that fungi mycelium was the perfect metaphor to convey this psychic web that connects people. The word *psycellium* is the integration of the words *psilocybin*, *psychic*, and *mycelium* and represents a living network that connects all the people within the system.

---

[75] Silver and the Wachowskis, *The Matrix*.

The show presents several integral themes, notably that of the relations between autonomy, communion, and transcendence. These integral principles of evolution are expressed in the series within the structural dynamics of the sensate cluster, which is the grouping of eight individuals who are psychically linked. Each individual in the cluster is first and foremost an autonomous being, with their own consciousness; they live in different countries and bring with them their own culture and biography. These autonomous beings are irresistibly pulled toward one another, resulting in a communion of consciousness. Four people in the cluster form two separate couples. Aside from these four individuals in the cluster, another is a transgender woman in a lesbian relationship; another is a gay man who has a male lover, and they form a triad with a female model that becomes a close friend; and each of the other two cluster members find lovers with potentials of a long-term relationship. The show is an example of how communion transcends socially constructed boundaries, such as heteronormative monogamous relationships.

Aside from the one-to-one attraction of communion in the show, these individuals are transcendentally pulled, beyond their individuality, toward their eight-member cluster as a whole. There are moments when the cluster functions as a single organism and the individuals operate in synchronization; they share not only their thoughts as one but also their pain and motivation. The theme of transcendence is explicitly expressed in the series as the dissolving of divisions between individuals, genders, and cultures. The forces of autonomy, communion, and transcendence become most apparent in the orgy scenes, in which love and unity transcend their bodies as they are gravitationally attracted to telepathically meet in a shared imagination to have sex as a whole. These orgiastic scenes beautifully show the experience from the perspective of both individual and collective consciousness. The polyamorous orientation of the cluster also mimics the sexual practices of our ancestral tribes, where the focus was more on the whole of the tribe rather than on couples. In the orgy scenes, the lines between self and other, monogamy and polyamory, male and female, individual and whole, dissolve, leaving the audience with greater examples of how love and connection can be shown.

Another way the mycelial mind is integrating into popular culture is through the new series *Star Trek: Discovery*. For decades, *Star Trek* has been one of Western popular culture's leading narratives that presents possible future scenarios by integrating the latest scientific knowledge and technologies, as well as social and political issues. This time, in *Discovery*, which aired its first season in 2017–2018, mycelium sets the context of the series. *Discovery* is the ship's name, and the ship's chief science officer is named Paul Stamets, in honor of the real-life mycologist. The real-world Paul Stamets, though he has won several scientific awards, claimed in a recent presentation that having a lead character in the new *Star Trek* series is his greatest public honor. His greatest private honor was curing his mom's terminal cancer through a turkey mushrooms regimen.[76]

In the show, Paul Stamets is an astromycologist. Humans recently discovered that all places in the universe, and all the parallel universes, are connected through mycelial webs. In episode 3, called "Context Is for Kings," Stamets describes the universal mycelial structure in detail: "Imagine a microscopic web that spans the entire cosmos. An intergalactic ecosystem, an infinite number of roads leading everywhere. The veins and muscles that hold our galaxies together." This context also implies that the universe is fundamentally alive. Officer Stamets goes on to share that, with mycelium, physics and biology converge. The ship travels the mycelial network through spores grown onboard, creating an organic propulsion system. By traveling the mycelial web, the ship is able to travel a light year in 1.3 seconds and even move into alternate universes. For a while the team does not know how to navigate through the network—until they find a large tardigrade; though in real life tardigrades are microscopic animals, the one in the show is the size of an SUV. The science team learns that the tardigrade evolved to form a symbiotic relationship with the mycelium and is able to control navigation through the network at will. Paul Stamets integrates the tardigrade's

---

[76] Stamets, *Fantastic Fungi*, 78.

DNA into his own body, allowing him to travel space and time through the mycelial network.

The work of mycologist Paul Stamets has also influenced another cultural masterpiece, *Avatar*, which for ten years was the highest-grossing movie at the international box office. Louie Schwartzberg, award-winning producer and director of the film *Fantastic Fungi*, writes about the science and spirit behind it:

> The Mother Tree concept and underground internet idea—pioneered by Paul Stamets and Suzanne Simard—was the foundational science for concepts filmmaker James Cameron used in *Avatar*. Without that spiritual core, *Avatar* would never have become one of the top box office films of all time.[77]

Another group of artists who embraced psychedelics as tools for finding deep inspiration is the rock band Tool. The three-time Grammy award–winning band has been spreading awareness of psychedelics through their art for almost three decades to millions of fans. Their albums feature skits of the comedian Bill Hicks promoting psychedelics, as well as antiauthoritarian remarks from psychedelic rebel Timothy Leary. Lead singer Maynard James Keenan speaks in his autobiography, *A Perfect Union of Contrary Things*, of the impact a peyote ceremony with the Native American Church had on him. It allowed him "to face his vulnerabilities head-on, to face the roots of that anger and move from the abstract to the grounded."[78] He also frequently refers to the great influence psychologist Carl Jung and mythologist Joseph Campbell have on his work:

> In order to write effectively, you have to write from the spot you're standing in. You have to tap into the pure emotion of where you are, but also the broader picture, the Joseph Campbell of it all . . . Every

---

[77] Schwartzberg, "Afterword," 175.

[78] Jensen and Keenan, *Perfect Union of Contrary Things*, 216.

five minutes of a life is a story if you tap into the archetype that transcends the individual and connects to everybody.[79]

Jungian concepts are clearly present in Tool's work: they named an
album *ÆNIMA* (after the Jungian concept of the anima); an entire song,
"46&2," is an exploration of Jung's concept of the shadow. Their cerebral,
multilayered music, which the band states is inspired by the concept of
synesthesia that can be experienced more commonly with psychedelics,
generally deals with large spiritual and philosophical concepts. Tool's
music alone, which often attempts to translate highly transpersonal
states, is enough to help spread a spiritually inspired psychedelic paradigm, but it is also accompanied by the artwork of visionary artist Alex
Grey, who has designed art for Tool for the last fifteen years, including
album cover art and large-scale backdrop pieces for their live sets.

A rapidly growing number of artists are devoting their work to the
expression of psychedelic states, following in the footsteps of the movement's founder, Alex Grey. There is perhaps one work that stands out
as a defining masterpiece of the visionary art movement and captures
the complex unfolding of the relationship between humans and psychedelics—a painting by Alex Grey titled "The New Eleusis," named after
the Greek Eleusinian Mysteries, the annual multiday festival of Ancient
Greece during which citizens took a psychedelic brew called kykeon.
The painting was unveiled at Bicycle Day 2018 in San Francisco, cel-
ebrating the seventy-fifth anniversary of the creation of LSD by hon-
oring Albert Hofmann's discovery and commemorating the first LSD
journey where Hofmann rode his bicycle from a pharmaceutical chemistry lab and began an unexpected LSD experience. At the unveiling of
the painting, Alex Grey told the audience that studying the history of
psychedelics is his obsession. Each section of the painting presents a
piece of psychedelic history, most of which I have covered in this book.
I will describe the scenes in the painting starting with the center and
moving to the top left and around counterclockwise.

---

[79] Jensen and Keenan, 142.

At center of the painting is the LSD molecule. In it are eyes symbolizing awareness. Underneath the molecule we see the temple in which the Eleusinian Mysteries were held. Over the molecule is the chemist Albert Hofmann, with a halo around him representing the gills that are found underneath a mushroom cap, with the Burning Man symbol at its top. Over him, we see the sun coming up around Earth. Hofmann has a crown with the word "Eleusis" written on it. He also has light coming out of the area of his third eye and in one hand is holding a chemical beaker with the atomic symbol inside it, presenting the power of LSD, which was created the same year as the atomic bomb. In the other hand Hofmann holds mushrooms that produce psilocybin, which he was also first to synthesize.

For those of us who have purchased a print of the painting, Alex Grey includes a quote at the bottom from Hofmann, in which he stresses the importance of consciousness change to humanity:

> Alienation from nature and the loss of the experience of being part of the living creation is the greatest tragedy of our materialistic era. It is the causative reason for ecological devastation and climate change. Therefore I attribute absolute highest importance to consciousness change. I regard psychedelics as catalyzers for this. They are tools which are guiding our perception toward other deeper areas of our human existence, so that we again become aware of our spiritual essence. Psychedelic experiences in a safe setting can help our consciousness open up to this sensation of connection and of being one with nature. LSD and related substances are not drugs in the usual sense, but are part of the sacred substances, which have been used for thousands of years in ritual settings. The classic psychedelics like LSD, Psilocybin and Mescaline are characterized by the fact that they are neither toxic nor addictive. It is my great concern to separate psychedelics from the ongoing debates about drugs, and to highlight the tremendous potential inherent to these substances for self-awareness, as an adjunct in therapy, and for fundamental research into the human mind. It is my wish that a modern Eleusis will emerge, in which seeking humans can learn to have transcendent experiences with sacred substances in a safe setting. I am convinced that these soul-opening,

mind-revealing substances will find their appropriate place in our society and our culture.

Albert Hofmann was one hundred years old when he shared this perspective.

In the top-left quadrant of the painting we see the words "Soul Medicine for the Betterment of Well People" as well as "Healing Addiction, Trauma, & Depression." Underneath is a depiction of a client undergoing psychedelic psychotherapy with Stan Grof, who has been a guide for tens of thousands of participants undergoing holotropic experiences. To the left we see the mycologist Paul Stamets, and under him Terence and Dennis McKenna, who created the first psilocybin mushroom growing technique. Underneath them is a picture of a body and a brain, likely symbolizing the mushroom theory of human evolution that the McKenna brothers presented. To the right of them is a picture of Rick Doblin, who founded the Multidisciplinary Association of Psychedelic Studies and is now bringing MDMA into legalization. Beneath him is Roland Griffiths, who leads the Johns Hopkins Psilocybin Studies and underneath him Walter Pahnke, who conducted the Good Friday Psilocybin Harvard experiment, with the words "65% had mystical experience" to the right of him.

In the lower-left quadrant, we see the Mexican medicine woman Maria Sabina, with the words "Oaxaca, Mexico 1955," giving mushrooms to Gordon Wasson for the first time. Underneath them, we see the mushroom stones found throughout Mexico and Central and South America, with the date 1000 BCE. To the right of them, we see a scene of an Aztec mushroom ritual. Above them is a shaman with mushrooms growing on him (a picture from the Tassili, Africa, cave painting) with the date 10,000 BCE. Lower, we see a microscopic view of ergot, from which we derived LSD, which looks like little mushrooms growing on wheat and rye. Beneath them is a symbol, found in Eleusis, of a lady with snakes (serpents are commonly seen on mushrooms) holding wheat and surrounded by mushroom people (symbols found in caves in Europe and Asia). Beneath them, we see more images of ergot and wheat with the words "Triptolemus receives the Mysteries of Agriculture from Demeter + Persephone."

In the lower-right quadrant, we see a woman sitting with wheat, and to the right of her is a depiction of an actual Greek sculpture of people handing each other mushrooms in a sacramental fashion. The words "Persephone Abducted Underground by Hades" with a picture of Hades abducting Persephone are seen there as well. To their left is a woman having an insight with the caption "Persephone Springing Out." Socrates is drinking kykeon, with the text:

> Socrates—Idealist Philosophy was based on Visionary Experience— Greek Philosophers were Initiates of the Mysteries who drank the *Kykeon*, a Psychedelic brew, "the race of Gods and the Limits of All things can be seen even with closed eyes"—Proclus

Hermes, the archetypal messenger of the Gods, is whispering to Socrates. Over them is the geometric Flower of Life, which to many represents unity and interconnectedness.

In the upper-right quadrant, we see the philosopher and novelist Aldous Huxley with the psychologist Humphrey Osmond and a line— "To fathom hell or soar angelic, take a pinch of psychedelic"—from one of their letters in which the word *psychedelic* was coined. Above them is Ken Kesey and the bus called Further with an ecstatic Timothy Leary and his words "Tune in, Turn on, Drop out" over the bus. To his right is the book *Be Here Now* by Ram Dass, one of Leary's Harvard colleagues, which had a big impact on spirituality and psychedelic culture. To the left we see David Nichols, the chemist, and Amanda Feilding, founder of the Beckley Foundation, who together began taking MRI scans of brains on psychedelics. Over them is a phoenix, the symbol for death and rebirth, coming out of the chemical beaker. Above the phoenix, we see a depiction of the 5HT-2A receptor that most psychedelic molecules dock into. Lastly, to the right of it are the words "Neurogenesis" and "Neuroplasticity," showing what a brain looks like with LSD and with a placebo—showing a hyperconnected, actively growing brain while taking a psychedelic.

Soon the world will see the creation of the Entheon, a museum of visionary art, designed by Alex and Allyson Grey and located on their property in New York. The word *Entheon* means a place to discover the god within. The building itself is three stories tall and serves as both a temple and 12,000-square-foot gallery and exhibit space, with sculptures of enormous faces, deities, and the story of human evolution painted on the building. Construction of Entheon has been in the works since 2014 and is almost complete. It is a part of a larger project of the Greys called the Chapel of Sacred Mirrors (CoSM), an interfaith spiritual community whose mission "is to build an enduring sanctuary of visionary art to inspire a global community."[80] CoSM frequently hosts events and has its own journal showcasing the latest movements in visionary art.

In *The New Psychedelic Revolution: The Genesis of the Visionary Age*, James Oroc states that after Alex Grey, Andrew "Android" Jones has the greatest potential for mainstream success. Trained academically in traditional art, he went on to work for both George Lucas's Industrial Light & Magic, which creates special effects for major motion pictures, and as a concept artist for Nintendo. Jones eventually left to focus on his own projects. Kotler and Wheal write, "Combining a classical fine arts education with the power of digital software, Jones creates images that defy easy categorization: archetypal deities overlaid with fractal geometries, cosmic lovers projected across giant galaxies, and ornate masks stretched across crystalline hillsides."[81] On his website Android Jones states that the focus of his work is "spirituality and altered states of consciousness" and shares that "I have seen things in this life that I am incapable of translating into words. In my practice I have visited realms where the imagination ends, and the terrifying beauty of infinity unfolds over and over again."[82] Fitting well into the definition of a visionary artist, he attempts to translate these multidimensional states through two-dimensional mediums and fully immersive virtual reality environments.

---

[80] www.CoSM.org

[81] Kotler and Wheal, *Stealing Fire*, 143.

[82] www.AndroidJones.com/About/Statement, para. 1.

One of Android's projects is called Microdose VR. In his talk titled "The Future of Art" at the Lightning in a Bottle festival, on May 25, 2018, he said that he and his team practice what they preach—that psychedelic microdosing and full-dose journeys are integral parts of their creative process. Android states he has fully bet on, with both time and money, virtual reality becoming a prominent form of art in the future. When an audience member asked him about his creative process and spirituality, he disclosed that at times he experiences all of us as one being, and while making art in these moments, he feels in greater alignment with this living entity. In these precious moments, he experiences states of flow and surges of creative energy, and if he gets out of the way, this larger entity moves through him to create art. Android also creates art live on stage for many prominent DJs, as well as making designs for their album covers. He integrated much of his body of work into his film *Samskara* and constructed a 360-degree projection dome for the film. *Samskara*, and the dome it shows in, has traveled the globe. It has found a permanent home in Wisdome LA, the world's first fully immersive art park, in Los Angeles.[83]

Psychedelics, and the work of Terence McKenna, have inspired the work of another artist, Marloes Messemaker. Messemaker illustrated and authored a graphic novel titled *Five Dried Grams: A Graphic Novelty Meme* on the life of Terence McKenna. "To save the world . . . don't just take piss ant amounts . . . take . . . FIVE DRIED GRAMS" is the quote she used to open the book.[84] It is followed by a beautifully colored two-page scene of Terence McKenna giving a public talk where he says: "These mushrooms saved me, straightened me out. With their help we can transform society, find solutions we would never find while unstoned."[85] The exquisitely illustrated comic book shows the journey of McKenna discovering psilocybin mushrooms in the Amazon, lecturing

---

[83] www.wisdome.la

[84] Messemaker, *Five Dried Grams*, 1.

[85] Messemaker, 3–4.

about their wisdom throughout his adult life. Filled with popular quotes of Terence, the graphic novel is a delight to McKenna fans.

Mushrooms have also played a central role in the creative work of Adam Strauss, specifically his one-man show *The Mushroom Cure*. The play tells the real-life experience of Strauss treating his obsessive-compulsive disorder (OCD) with the help of psilocybin mushrooms.[86] Dynamic and funny, the play conveys the debilitating struggles that come with OCD and Adam's search to find mushrooms after reading about the scientific research on psilocybin healing people with OCD. The show, which originally started on the East Coast, has been sponsored by MAPS and has now made its way across the United States several times. Strauss is working on new material that continues his OCD saga through philosophical reflections and endorsements of psychedelics treatments.

Another comedian who has made psychedelics a centerpiece of his work is Shane Mauss. In 2018 Mauss released the documentary *Psychonautics*, which chronicles the life and work of the bipolar comedian.[87] He explains how psychedelics have influenced his psychology, as well as some of the struggles he has undergone because of them. In the documentary he also interviews some of the leading researchers in the field. The film, which is told through the personal story of Shaun Mauss, is not only a great resource for entertaining information on psychedelics, but it also stands as an art piece aside from being a documentary, using artistic filmmaking techniques to depict and evoke the psychedelic experience.

Psychedelic culture is perhaps most clearly represented in transformative festivals, which serve as a modern-day Eleusis that initiates many into psychedelic consciousness. Festivals such as Burning Man, Lightning in a Bottle, Symbiosis, and Boom attract hundreds of thousands of participants. The role of these festivals for many is that of a ritual—requiring enormous preparation, intention, initiation, endurance, and

---

[86] www.themushroomcure.com

[87] Mauss and Bellinkoff, *Psychonautics*.

integration. Kotler and Wheal write about a particular moment of research into transformation that took place at Burning Man:

> In 2015, a team of scientists led by Oxford neuropsychologist Molly Crockett joined forces with the Black Rock City Census to take a closer look at the festival's power. In their study, 75 percent of attendees reported having a transformative experience at the event, while 85 percent of those reported that the benefits persisted for weeks and months afterward. That's an incredibly high batting average. Three out of four people who attend the event are meaningfully changed by it.[88]

For those who have undergone such initiations, it is common to have this experience. Some of these festivals have even begun to purchase land, like the Burning Man organization purchasing Fly Ranch in northern Nevada, to begin creating permanent settlements.

Festivals presented by Take 3 Productions have been brewing in Northern California and Nevada. To attend one of their festivals, one must be invited by a previous participant, which creates a curated crowd. The festivals have had a maximum capacity of about 1,500 attendees, ensuring a tight community. Those who have gone, including myself, claim these festivals are the cream of the crop of the psychedelic festival scene. The core team of Take 3—Annie Oak, Chris Pezza, Benja Juster, and Mischa Steiner—have been long-time contributors to psychedelic culture and all met at Burning Man. Annie Oak cofounded the Women's Visionary Congress, a women-centered conference about psychedelics that has taken place both in Los Angeles and Oakland, California. In an anthology titled *Psychedelic Mysteries of the Feminine* she writes of the Women's Visionary Congress:

> As we address the challenges and possibilities ahead, presented by the renaissance of psychedelic cultures around the world, many members

---

[88] Kotler and Wheal, *Stealing Fire*, 143.

of our community continue to find balance and strength through their connection with the divine forces of the natural world.[89]

Chris Pezza used to run the Palenque Norte Burning Man talks, where well-known psychedelic researchers, authors, and artists presented; it was named after an inspired series of talks given by Terence McKenna—the Palenque Ethnobotany Seminars in 1999. Benja Juster creates interactive environments and immersive experiences and has directed the creation of such spaces for Google and other large festivals. Mischa Steiner is CEO of Stage Presence, a virtual talent agency that connects performers to remote team meetings. The Take 3 team meets weekly to work on the narrative for the two festivals they annually hold. Each festival unfolds within a cohesive story, with actors roaming the multiday event in character. All attendees are encouraged to participate. In between music sets are well-coordinated plays that carry along the story of the festival, which is usually a parody with a psychedelically inspired theme.

The art, immersive activities based on the story line, and tickets only handed out to friends of friends create what can be described as a curated version of Burning Man—which has become so large that it has attracted crowds of people who just want to party. The crowd at Take 3 events is largely composed of cultural creatives—researchers working on artificial intelligence, engineers, scientists, artists, activists, programmers, philanthropists, psychedelic community leaders, and self-proclaimed misfits—both drawing from and reinforcing a well-connected community with shared values. The strong sense of individuality, communal bonding, and participatory creativity are essential aspects of what keeps this community thriving.

As psychedelic communities expand, so does their encouragement of self-actualization, freeing people from their unconscious assumptions about culture and therefore supporting them to grow into their unique autonomy. Psychedelics beckon creativity, a quality of the

---

[89] Oak, "Creating a Community of Wise Women," 239.

transcendence instinct, continuously enabling a wellspring of individual expression. Psychedelic art and culture will continue maturing as people gain greater, and safer, access to psychedelics. Artists of all kinds can serve to translate previously ineffable states of consciousness, and by carrying out this sacred work, a psychonaut's discoveries in these uncharted territories can also be shared as insights and inspiration for all.

Philosophy and Science

"Modern consciousness research has shown that visionary states have remarkable potential to provide not only extraordinary religious illumination and artistic inspiration, but also brilliant scientific insights that open new fields and facilitate scientific problem-solving," writes Stanislav Grof.[90] In addition to these spiritual, artistic, and scientific insights, human performance itself can be enhanced through the expanded states induced by psychedelics. The work of Steven Kotler and Jamie Wheal, packed with empirical data, offers a strong scientific backbone to strengthen the validity that altered states enhance both creativity and productivity. Kotler and Wheal write about these ideas becoming mainstream, even in US business culture:

> Psychedelics have begun moving from recreational diversion to performance-enhancing supplements. "A shift began about four or five years ago," author and venture capitalist Tim Ferriss told us. "Once Steve Jobs and other successful people began recommending the use of psychedelics for enhancing creativity and problem solving, the public became a little more open to the possibility."
>
> And, as Ferriss explains on CNN, it wasn't just the cofounder of Apple that made the leap. "The billionaires I know, almost without exception, use hallucinogens on a regular basis" . . . Consider the gains: 200 percent boost in creativity, 490 percent boost in learning,

---

[90] Grof, *Modern Consciousness Research*, 26.

and 500 percent boost in productivity . . . if they were merely the result of a few studies done by a couple labs, they would be easier to dismiss. But there is now seven decades of research, conducted by hundreds of scientists on thousands of participants, showing that when it comes to complex problem solving, ecstasis could be the "wicked solution" we've been looking for.[91]

. . .

Research shows that these ecstatic experiences lift us above normal awareness, and propel us further faster. Much of our conventional schooling, personal development, and professional training still miscalculate this fact. It's hard to fathom how much faster we can go, how much more ground we can cover, if we can only appreciate what high performance now looks like.[92]

What makes their book unique in the world of psychedelic literature is its focus on productivity and measurable outcomes; it is geared toward the CEOs, scientists, artists, inventors, and philosophers of the world, many of whom system theorist Donella Meadows would call "leverage points"—powerful points in a system that if transformed can cause the whole system to naturally self-organize.[93]

An academic field starting to feel the influence of psychedelics is philosophy. Futurist Jason Silva, well known as the host of the TV show *Brain Games* on the National Geographic channel, regularly presents on psychedelics and philosophy on his popular internet videos—some of which surpass more than a million views. He has been releasing weekly content online for years under his YouTube channel Shots of Awe, consisting of short artistic videos exploring his inspired philosophical insights with artistic editing. Silva has been consistently forthcoming about the role psychedelics play in his life and his belief that they may support the evolution of our collective consciousness.

---

[91] Kotler and Wheal, *Stealing Fire*, 50.

[92] Kotler and Wheal, 221.

[93] Meadows, *Thinking in Systems*.

The Atlantic described him as "'A Timothy Leary of the Viral Video Age' . . . part Timothy Leary, part Ray Kurzweil, and part Neo from 'The Matrix.'"[94] The intersection of science, psychedelics, and philosophy are the foundation of Silva's work.

Peter Sjöstedt-H, an Anglo-Scandinavian philosopher who taught philosophy of mind at London College, has taken advantage of psychedelic insights and brought them into academia. In *Noumenautics: Metaphysics—Meta-Ethics—Psychedelics*, Sjöstedt-H traces Western philosophy—from Kant, Schopenhauer, and Nietzsche through to Henri Bergson and Alfred North Whitehead—and shows how psychedelics can contribute to the academic field. Sjöstedt-H writes:

> For philosophers of mind, phenomenologists of any school, and indeed for all those interested in consciousness, the psychedelic experience offers the supreme impression. To deny philosophers of mind psychedelic substances is tantamount to denying instruments to musicians. If one is to study consciousness, one must involve its most wondrous manifestation.[95]

Sjöstedt-H goes on to introduce the term *psy-phen* to refer to "psychedelic phenomenology," and states that "of all academic disciplines, philosophy has foregone most potential gains by abnegating psy-phen."[96] He argues that behaviorism and empiricism, which have dominated Western philosophy and science, seem absurd after one undergoes a strong psychedelic experience.[97] He proposes that psychedelic mushrooms can serve as catalysts for novel ideas: "The fungus liberated my thoughts enabling seeds to be sown for development when the mind is less free but more focused."[98] Those familiar

---

[94] www.ThisisJasonSilva.com/AboutJason, para. 4.

[95] Sjöstedt-H, *Noumenautics*, i.

[96] Sjöstedt-H, 1, 33.

[97] Sjöstedt-H, 2.

[98] Sjöstedt-H, 18.

with the field of Western philosophy will enjoy Peter Sjöstedt-H's clear thinking and detailed knowledge of the movements that have historically unfolded within this tradition, as he presents and deconstructs the work of prominent philosophers from a psychedelically informed perspective.

A generation prior to Sjöstedt-H, three of the most influential thinkers on the subject of psychedelics and philosophy—Rupert Sheldrake, Terence McKenna, and Ralph Abraham—led events that were usually held at Esalen Institute in Big Sur, California, where they gathered annually to deconstruct and imagine new possibilities in the fields of both philosophy and science. These trialogues first began in private in 1982 and then became a public series at Esalen in 1989 and continued until 1998 at the University of California, Santa Cruz. Rupert Sheldrake received his master's degree in philosophy and history of science from Harvard before obtaining his PhD in biochemistry from Cambridge, where he was director of studies in biochemistry and cell biology for many years. Terence McKenna, mentioned throughout this book, graduated from University of California, Berkeley, with a distributed major in ecology and shamanism and presented on psychedelics widely until his death in April 2000. Ralph Abraham earned his PhD in mathematics from the University of Michigan before teaching at UC Berkeley, Columbia University, and Princeton University while doing pioneering work in nonlinear dynamics, chaos theory, and global analysis. The discussions between these three men were recorded and distributed online and eventually collected into two books: *Chaos, Creativity, and Cosmic Consciousness* and *The Evolutionary Mind: Conversations on Science, Imagination and Spirit*. The trio—who were experts in their fields and developed a deep friendship—explored a wide range of topics, such as the role of creativity and chaos in evolution, the imagination of the world soul, the nature of light, the ontological existence of mathematics and physics, entities that arise in psychedelic space, the collective unconscious, and the telos of the cosmos. Jean Houston, an author of twenty-six scholarly books focused on the humanities, writes in an introduction to one of the books:

The trialogues are surely a minefield of mind probes, a singular sapient circle of gentlemen geniuses at their edgiest of edges . . . They cut loose from whatever remains of orthodox considerations and become minds at the end of their tethers, who then re-tether each other to go farther out in their speculations. In so doing, they have figured out how to achieve one of the best of all possible worlds: the sharing of mental space and cosmic terrains over many years of deep friendship and profound dialogue.[99]

These individually brilliant thinkers came together in communion and in doing so transcended the limitations of their autonomous minds, allowing them to delve deeper into speculative inquiry than any one of them could have done on their own.

In his 2019 book *LSD and the Mind of the Universe: Diamonds from Heaven*, Christopher Bache, a professor who taught philosophy and religion for decades, lays out a protocol for people to use psychedelics as a viable method for philosophical inquiry. He writes that even though he used Grof's protocol as his spiritual practice, he "did this work as a philosopher" and that he "was not primarily seeking healing but an understanding of our universe . . . We are witnessing the birth of not just new insights into consciousness but a new way of doing philosophy."[100] He boils down his philosophical method to three basic steps:

- Systemically push the boundaries of experience in carefully structured psychedelic sessions.

- Make a complete and accurate record of your experience immediately following each session.

- Critically analyze your experience, bringing it into dialogue with other fields of knowledge and with the experiences of other psychedelic explorers.

---

[99] Houston in T. McKenna, Sheldrake, and Abraham, *Chaos, Creativity, and Cosmic Consciousness*, xiii.

[100] Bache, *LSD and the Mind of the Universe*, 10.

"It is difficult to overstate the significance of this historic transition. With psychedelics we are entering a new era in philosophy," writes Bache.[101]

So much of what has occurred in the field of psychedelics for the last fifty years owes a great debt to the work of Stanislav Grof. After forty years of researching holotropic states of consciousness, Grof released his book *The Cosmic Game: Explorations at the Frontier of Human Consciousness* in 1998 to present the philosophical insights he harvested as a consciousness researcher. He writes about the existential realization of our deep interconnectivity that arises in these states and how it resonates with the perennial philosophical perspective:

> This research also radically changes our conception of the human psyche. It shows that, in its furthest reaches, the psyche of each of us is essentially commensurate with all of existence and ultimately identical with the cosmic creative principle itself. This conclusion, while seriously challenging the worldview of modern technological societies, is in far-reaching agreement with the traditions of the world, which the Anglo-American writer and philosopher Aldous Huxley referred to as the "perennial philosophy."[102]

In working with psychedelics, Grof reached the same conclusion regarding the perennial philosophy that Ken Wilber reached after decades of researching higher states of consciousness explored by consistent long-term meditators—that there are core mystical insights and perspectives shared cross-culturally by all spiritual traditions.[103] Grof goes on to summarize the overall perspective he reached in his work—that humans at their depth share a unitive consciousness with all creation while on a more surface level experiencing a personal autonomy:

---

[101] Bache, 11.

[102] Grof, *Cosmic Game*, 3.

[103] Wilber, *Eye of Spirit*; Huxley, *Perennial Philosophy*.

We can now try to summarize the insights from holotropic states describing existence as a fantastic experiential adventure of Absolute Consciousness—an endless cosmic dance, exquisite play, or divine drama. In producing it, the creative principle generates from itself and within itself a countless number of individuals, split units of consciousness, that assume various degrees of relative autonomy and independence. Each of them represents an opportunity for a unique experience, an experiment in consciousness. With the passion of an explorer, scientist, and artist, the creative principle experiments with all the conceivable experiences in their endless variations and combinations.[104]

This perspective of a unitive intelligence is shared by many who have repeatedly ventured deep into psychedelic states. The holonic vision of reality as composed of beings with beings, as first described by Arthur Koestler in 1967 and expanded by Ken Wilber throughout his writing career, is also one that Grof shares.[105] That the universe primarily evolves through a creative principle also resonates with the process philosophy of Alfred North Whitehead and Terence McKenna's novelty theory.[106]

As exemplified by Grof's work, most perspectives that are psyche-delically inspired are compatible with the findings of science. What psychedelic experiences may challenge is the context from which the data is interpreted. Grof ends his book by stating:

> The cosmology described in this book is not incompatible with the findings of science, but with the philosophical conclusions that were inappropriately drawn from these findings. What the experiences and observations described in this book challenge is not science, but materialistic monism.[107]

---

[104] Grof, *Cosmic Game*, 100.

[105] Koestler, *Ghost in the Machine*; Wilber, *Religion of Tomorrow*; Grof, *Cosmic Game*, 63.

[106] Whitehead, *Process and Reality*; T. McKenna, *Archaic Revival*.

[107] Grof, *Cosmic Game*, 266.

Material monism is the pre-Socratic belief that the entire world can be fully explained away by reducing it to simple physical elements—like quarks, atoms, or genetics. It is a perspective that fails to include consciousness and complexity as part of the process.

Simon Powell, a British researcher who wrote three books on psychedelics and the self-organizing properties of nature, believes that psychedelics can help humanity better understand nature. In his book *Magic Mushroom Explorer: Psilocybin and the Awakening Earth* he shares a journal entry about a mushroom experience:

> As I sit once more under nature's psilocybentic spell, I am convinced that a new science is called for, a science that views life anew under the perceptual lens afforded by the mushroom. For it is only through psilocybin's perception-enhancing magnification power that we are able to apprehend, in full, the sheer beauty of the biosphere, this luxuriant film of frenzied biological activity that surrounds the globe and from which we have been born. I therefore decree a new science—the science of psilocybentics![108]

Powell believes psilocybin mushrooms grow so abundantly in nature because nature wants us to view her from this perception-enhanced lens that will allow us to take in more information from her.

Alan Watts, who played a critical role in bringing Eastern philosophy to the West, was also influenced by psychedelics. In his book *The Joyous Cosmology: Adventures in the Chemistry of Consciousness*, Watts writes that psychedelics offer a way to experience the deeper truths that science concludes:

> Is it possible, then, that Western science could provide a medicine which would at least give the human organism a start in releasing itself from chronic self-contradiction? The medicine might indeed have to be supported by other procedures—psychotherapy, "spiritual" disciplines, and basic change in one's pattern of life . . . Is there, in

---

[108] Powell, *Magic Mushroom Explorer*, 51.

short, a medicine which can give us temporarily the sensation of being integrated, of being fully one with ourselves and with nature as the biologists know us, theoretically, to be? . . . Relatively recent research suggests that there are at least three such medicines . . . I am speaking, of course, of mescaline (the active ingredient of the peyote cactus), lysergic acid diethylamide (a modified ergot alkaloid), and psilocybin (a derivative of the mushroom *psilocybe mexicana*).[109]

In addition to his many publications and audio and video works, Watts helped found the California Institute of Integral Studies, an academic institution on the forefront of training psychedelic psychotherapists.

The idea that psychedelics bring systemic ecological awareness and enhance cognition is found throughout psychedelic literature. In *Psychedelic Information Theory: Shamanism in the Age of Reason*, which looks at psychedelic states through the lens of systems theory and neuroscience, author James Kent writes: "The primary tenets of Psychedelic Information Theory dictate that hallucinogens generate information by destabilizing linear perception to promote nonlinear states of consciousness."[110] From this perspective, by opening our mind to nonlinear thinking, we are able to grasp more complex information than can normally be processed by a habitually linear mind. Thomas Roberts, professor emeritus of educational psychology at Northern Illinois University, echoes this belief in *The Psychedelic Future of the Mind: How Entheogens Are Enhancing Cognition, Boosting Intelligence, and Raising Values*, in which he writes: "Current research offers some tantalizing support for claims that psychedelics can be used to enhance cognition, improve intelligence, and strengthen cognitive studies."[111] He believes "The Sleeping Giant of Psychedelics' Future" to be "Innovative Problem Solving" and ends

---

[109] Watts, *Joyous Cosmology*, 10–11.

[110] Kent, *Psychedelic Information Theory*, 170.

[111] T. Roberts, *Psychedelic Future of the Mind*, 135.

the book by stating his hopes that psychedelics may enrich most fields of human knowledge:

> In addition to their uses in psychotherapy I hope you will see the importance of psychedelics for religion, for simplifying and enriching daily life, and for increasing our understanding of the human mind— both our own and others'. I hope you will savor the rich diet of ideas that produce new flavors of history, philosophy, art, and film criticism, all the humanities and arts, and most of the sciences.[112]

Many breakthroughs in human understanding have already occurred because of humanity's relationship with psychedelic substances, and the works of philosophers like Roberts, Powell, McKenna, Sheldrake, Abraham, Grof, Sjöstedt-H, Wheal, Kotler, Kent, and Watts are themselves evidence that psychedelics expand perception, increase cognition, and elevate.

In the realm of science, Kary Mullis attributes his invention of the polymerase chain reaction, which won him a Nobel Prize in genetics, to insights gained while on LSD and says he doubts he would have ever made his discoveries if not for LSD.[113] Francis Crick also claims that he first envisioned the spiral structure of DNA after he ingested LSD.[114] As Grof points out, knowledge of neuroscience was greatly expanded as scientists attempted to understand psychedelics.[115] An article from *Nature* presents one way that psychedelics contributed to expanding our understanding of the brain's processes:

> DW Woolley, Ph.D. was by any measure a gifted and unusual man. He believed that scientific progress could best be achieved by finding

---

[112] T. Roberts, 232.

[113] Powell, *Magic Mushroom Explorer*, 108; T. Roberts, *Psychedelic Future of the Mind*, 136.

[114] Kent, *Psychedelic Information Theory*, 17; Strassman et al., *Inner Paths to Outer Space*, 301.

[115] Grof, *Psychology of the Future*.

the unified meaning of apparently isolated and diverse facts. This is exactly what he did—by combining the work of Betty Twarog, showing serotonin existed in the brain, with Albert Hofmann's discovery of LSD, and his own work on LSD as an "antimetabolite" of serotonin, Dr. Woolley proposed a role for serotonin in mental illness.[116]

The creation of serotonin-based SSRI antidepressants owes much to early psychedelic research, which showcased the important role serotonin plays in regulating consciousness. Another contribution to neuroscience came from the neuroscientist John Lilly, who was the first to map the pleasure pathways in the brain and is well known for his experiences of taking LSD and ketamine in sensory-deprivation tanks, which he was the first to create.[117]

An important scientist deeply embedded in psychedelic history is the chemist Alexander "Sasha" Shulgin. Shulgin first tried mescaline in the 1950s, around the time he earned his doctorate in biochemistry from the University of California, Berkeley. In 1961 Shulgin produced a profitable product, the first biodegradable pesticide, for Dow Chemicals, which granted him financial freedom. He then decided to focus his time and energy on exploring psychedelics. Shulgin had deep ties to the Drug Enforcement Agency (DEA), wrote their definitive guide on controlled substances, and was honored with several awards by the DEA. They also granted him permission to freely research psychedelic substances—which he did from the 1970s to 1990s—and he created 230 new psychedelic compounds. After synthesizing a compound, he would first ingest it himself, then with his wife, Ann Shulgin (who was a therapist), and finally with a group of close friends. Shulgin is also partly credited with bringing MDMA into therapy during the 1970s by introducing it to Leo Zeff and letting him know that it can be therapeutic for his work with clients. He open-sourced his research with the books *PiHKAL: Phenethylamines I Have Known and Loved* and *TiHKAL:*

---

[116] Whitaker-Azmitia, "Discovery of Serotonin," para. 29.

[117] Lilly, *Scientist*.

Tryptamines I Have Known and Loved. Because he went public with his research, believing this awareness belonged to all of humanity, he lost his license to legally create and explore psychedelics.

The influence of psychedelics on the field of technology has recently received public attention. Echoing the nonlinear, complex perception-enhancing capabilities that psychedelics can provide, several of the early computer engineers relied on LSD in designing circuit chips, especially in the years before they could be designed on computers. Peter Schwartz, an engineer who is now the senior vice president for government relations and strategic planning at Salesforce (which built and owns the largest building in San Francisco), told Michael Pollan, "You had to be able to visualize a staggering complexity in three dimensions, hold it all in your head. They found that LSD could help."[118] Schwartz continues, "Problem solving in engineering always involves irreducible complexity. You're always balancing complex variables you can never get perfect, so you're desperately searching to find patterns. LSD shows you patterns."[119]

The impact of psychedelics on the computer revolution, especially in Silicon Valley, was probably best presented by John Markoff, a senior writer for the *New York Times*, researcher on technology for over twenty-eight years, and author of the book *What the Dormouse Said: How the Sixties Counterculture Shaped the Personal Computer Industry*. It was in an interview with Markoff in 2001 that Steve Jobs famously stated that he "believed that taking LSD was one of the two or three most important things he had done in his life."[120] In the book Markoff presents the vibrant counterculture from which Silicon Valley arose. By 1961 there were already three LSD research facilities specializing in creativity in the Silicon Valley area. One of these projects was the International Foundation for Advanced Study, run by Myron Stolaroff and James Fadiman. Stolaroff was a Stanford engineer, and Fadiman studied at

---

[118] Pollan, *How to Change Your Mind*, 182.

[119] Pollan, 182.

[120] Markoff, *What the Dormouse Said*, xix.

both Harvard and Stanford. For research participants "they specifically chose scientists, researchers, engineers, and architects as their test cases."[121] Fadiman and others administered a standard dose of LSD to these creative intellectuals, all of whom were stuck in a particular project at work. Subjects reported greater fluidity in their thinking, as well as an enhanced ability to both visualize a problem and recontextualize it.[122]

Among Fadiman's test subjects were some of the visionaries who would revolutionize computers, most notably Doug Engelbart, a pioneer in artificial intelligence research.[123] He created the computer mouse and contributed to the development of hypertext, networked computers, email, videoconference calling, and precursors to graphical user interfaces. These were demonstrated in "the Mother of All Demos," a now legendary computer conference held in 1968 at the San Francisco Civic Auditorium. The presentation demonstrated nearly all the fundamental elements of personal computing. President Bill Clinton honored Engelbart with the National Medal of Technology, the United States' highest technology award, in December 2000.

John Markoff also presents the sociopolitical climate that spurred the personal computer revolution and explains that countercultural values inspired the creation of the personal computer. Previously, the computing establishment was on the East Coast and in Ivy League schools.[124] Markoff makes the case that it was the social climate in the West Coast, especially the idea of the empowered individual, that inspired the personal computer revolution. For example, Steve Wozniak and Steve Jobs were interested in hacking before launching Apple, and the personal computer was created with a similar liberal mindset;[125] the personal computer was launched as a tool for individual expression and freedom. Stewart

---

[121] Markoff, 65.

[122] Pollan, *How to Change Your Mind*, 179.

[123] Markoff, *What the Dormouse Said.*

[124] Markoff, xiv.

[125] Markoff, 272.

Brand—who participated in LSD research, became an MIT scientist, and organized conferences for AT&T and other technology corporations after organizing the Grateful Dead shows for the Silicon Valley community—wrote an article in a special issue of *Time* magazine in 1995 called "We Owe It All to the Hippies" where he says that "the counterculture's scorn for centralized authority provided the philosophical foundations of not only the leaderless Internet but also the entire personal-computer revolution."[126] This movement into a more decentralized social structure spurred by innovations in technology will be the focus of the next section.

In 2019 I attended the first Awakened Futures: Psychedelics, Technology, and Meditation summit, hosted by Consciousness Hacking, an organization focused on the intersection of technology and consciousness. The founder, Mikey Siegel, received his master's in robotics at MIT before starting Consciousness Hacking, which has spread from San Francisco to dozens of cities worldwide and holds over ten thousand members. The sold-out summit was the first event focused on the intersection of psychedelics and technology and created an inspirational space to deepen discussions about the potentials that can arise. This conversation will only continue to expand as people gain greater access to psychedelic experiences.

The creative breakthroughs discussed in this chapter originated in the imagination, expanded by psychedelics. Before anything is created by humans in this world, it first begins in one's vision. An area where this vision reveals itself, and where many scientific breakthroughs are first seen before being concretized in the physical world, is in the literary genre of science fiction. Slawek Wojtowicz, a scientist and science fiction writer, explores the relationship between psychedelics and science fiction in an essay titled "The Sacred Voyage: Beyond Science Fiction?", stating that sci-fi has continually predicted future discoveries:

> Science fiction has always been very good at predicting the future: from submarines and spaceships imagined by Jules Verne to communicators from Star Trek, we have seen many seemingly far-fetched inventions

---

[126] Markoff, xii.

and concepts come true—perhaps time travel (almost a thousand papers on this topic have recently been published in professional journals); travel in hyperspace or other dimensions; the discovery of multiple universes (string theory); the existence of antigravity (dark energy); teleportation (see the research on quantum entanglement); transport and communication with supraluminal speed (wormholes, signal non-locality); and even invisibility cloaks. The future promises to be very exciting indeed. Many of us are very impatient, however, and we can't wait much longer for these inventions to change our lives. We yearn to experience right now the taste of things to come. Yet is this possible?[127]

Psychedelics are imagination generators, churning creativity and enabling us to visualize novel possibilities. Many of these things mentioned by Wojtowicz, like traveling through both time and space, are experienced in the imagination of many people who take a decent dose of psychedelics. These experiences include going backward and forward in time—seeing humanity's past as well as what our personal and collective futures may look like. Just as psychedelic visions showed great thinkers the possibilities of computing and genetics, they may well show future minds ways to turn what is now science fiction into reality. We will explore how visionary explorations with psychedelics can lead us into the future in the last chapter.

Psychedelic Economics: Cryptocurrency, Blockchain, and Psychedelics

What she wants to see, says Danielle Negrin, executive director of the San Francisco Psychedelic Society, is not businesses selling psychedelics but instead psychedelically informed businesses.[128] There will likely be an acceleration of business expansion in the field of psychedelics once

---

[127] Strassman et al., *Inner Paths to Outer Space*, 299.

[128] Archetypal View, "Psychedelic (R)Evolution."

these medicines are legalized, and there is much care being taken by those who have been in the field for years to maintain the values psychedelics themselves promote. As presented in chapter 3, psychedelics may play an important role in ecological homeostasis, represented by the lower-right/interobjective quadrant, including the systemic structures that most affect our current social-ecological situation. Economic systems fall into this category and are arguably the hardest to transform. The current social structures that dominate this quadrant are economic structures, particularly capitalism. Our ecological crisis is intimately tied to our economics—we are destroying our environment for profit. Every large-scale problem humanity faces can be traced to someone's economic gain. A discussion on the transformation of our world and the evolution of humanity must involve a conversation about economics, because in our modern world it is the system that directly affects all other systems. And the development of new frameworks of social-economical organization may involve new technologies.

Humanity has evolved through several epochs of social organization. Robert Bellah, an internationally recognized sociologist, states that the social power structures in societies developed according to their spiritual belief systems.[129] After tribal life, agriculture enabled a political-religious-military elite to emerge, creating a two-class system within society. A priesthood eventually evolved, and the king was seen as the divine link to the gods. As the sociologist Jeremy Rifkin argues, social structures also organize according to their technology;[130] the advent of writing led to our historical religions, and it enabled further structures in society to form, including record keeping of transactions and a new legal order. Technology will likely continue to bring possibilities that reorganize societies. According to Bellah, the era of modern religion, which owes much to the advent of writing and then the printing press, is represented by the majority of today's societies—which are more pluralistic

---

[129] Bellah, *Religion in Human Evolution.*

[130] Rifkin, *Empathic Civilization.*

than past societies.[131] In many countries, there is a separation between church and state, which favors individual freedom. A shadow of this is that it created a society that is more materialistic than ever before and generally values material wealth over spiritual and personal development.

Capitalism, favoring autonomy of the individual, arose in response to cultures in which hierarchical elites, such as monarchies and clergy, held power in society. In such cultures, kings ruled the land, and even ideas were censored by dogmatic religious and patriarchal leaders. Due to events in Europe such as the Reformation and the Scientific Revolution, individuals fought for freedom of expression, thought, and markets.[132] Individual reason, rather than collective dogmatic beliefs, became the mark of intelligence. The philosophers of the Scientific Revolution, such as Rene Descartes (1600s), John Locke (1600s), and David Hume (1700s), laid the groundwork for the philosophical movement known as the Enlightenment, which included thinkers like Adam Smith (1700s), who directly influenced the mindset of modern economics.[133] Jeremy Rifkin, who has written twenty books on economics, notes that the capitalistic mentality, embodied in the first and second industrial revolutions, is best represented by the Enlightenment movement, from which many of the capitalistic ideals arose. The movement stated that freedom predominately meant autonomy: that is, the freedom from others, the freedom to own property, and the freedom to exist as an independent individual free from collective impositions like religion and government. Freedom meant being an island unto one's own.

In a world where authoritarian leaders hold the ability to dictate ideas and both economically and intellectually oppress people, autonomy certainly means freedom. Unfortunately, fully empowering individuals without contextualizing them within our larger systemic dynamics

---

[131] Bellah, *Religion in Human Evolution.*

[132] Tarnas, *Passion of the Western Mind.*

[133] Descartes, *Discourse on Method*; Locke, *Essay Concerning Human Understanding*; Hume, *Enquiry Concerning Human Understanding*; Tarnas, *Passion of the Western Mind*; A. Smith, *Wealth of Nations.*

is disastrous and creates serious consequences for our world. We are part of a planetary system—and capitalism focuses on the parts at the expense of the whole. Capitalism focuses on individual (autonomous) gain at the expense of other people (communion) and our evolution (transcendence). "Remember the definition of capitalism: an economic system in which the employers—the owners of capital—hire workers to produce goods and services for the owners' profit," writes James Speth, who held several positions in the United Nations and the United States government, in *America the Possible: Manifesto for a New Economy*.[134] This also leads to ego inflation. The patriarchal paradigm from which capitalism arises creates a hierarchy. There is a boss with a pyramid of workers under him. Some CEOs in today's societies make billions, more than they can ever spend in a lifetime. Today the bottom 40 percent of Americans hold only 0.3 percent of the wealth.[135] Besides the oppression of people inherent in our economic model, perhaps its greatest effect is environmental devastation. According to Speth, who founded the World Resources Institute, a Washington, DC-based think tank, "We know that environmental deterioration is driven by the economic activity of human beings."[136]

As a response to the 2007–2008 economic crisis, a new technology emerged that holds the power to reorganize the informational and economics systems of our time. That technology is blockchain—a decentralized hyper-ledger of trusted data. The Blockchain Council defines blockchain technology as "a peer-to-peer decentralized distributed ledger technology that makes the records of any digital asset transparent and unchangeable and works without involving any third-party intermediary."[137] The Council and other advocates of blockchain assert that the technology has a capability to reduce the risks of fraudulent financial

---

[134] Speth, *America the Possible*, 99.

[135] Jackson, *Occupy World Street*, 146.

[136] Speth, *America the Possible*, 6.

[137] Blockchain Council, "What Is Blockchain."

transactions in a way that scales. Blockchain keeps a virtually unhackable record of all activity on the network, and trust is placed on a transparent protocol rather than on another person.

Satoshi Nakamoto, an anonymous figure, released the first blockchain, Bitcoin, into the world in 2009. Cryptocurrencies, though, existed before blockchain technology. Most notable was BitGold. Nick Szabo, the creator of BitGold, was a computer science major working in the field of cryptography. He created the concept of the "smart contract," a programmable transaction within a currency that could be used for legal processes, and he went on to get a degree in law to more fully understand and implement the technology he conceived. He released BitGold in 1998, after thinking about the project for a decade. BitGold never grew to full realization as a globally used currency, as Szabo hoped, but it was a direct precursor to Bitcoin's architecture.

Bitcoin became the world's first fully digital and democratic currency—it is an open-source peer-to-peer cryptocurrency system with no central organization. For the first time in history, a currency is set using a transparent programmed mathematical protocol, and the ability to create new money is not held by an authoritative power. Programmed into the Bitcoin code is the creation of a total of twenty-one million Bitcoins. That is all the Bitcoins that will ever exist. Every ten minutes all Bitcoin transactions are recorded into the blockchain. This information is held by every miner—nodes in the blockchain system that process the information. Miners compete for who gets to create a block, the packaging of the information of the transactions within the network over the last ten minutes. The miners compete by attempting to solve complex mathematical equations. The more miners there are competing, the more complex the equations become. The system is designed so that the increasing complexity allows the equation to be steadily solved every ten minutes. The winner is rewarded by the creation of new Bitcoins, and the current reward for miners is 6.25 Bitcoins per block. Roughly every four years the rewards are cut in half, taking into account the increasing value of Bitcoins. The last halving occurred in May 2020.

Once a block is created, it is attached to the larger chain of blocks (that's why it's called blockchain) held in a decentralized fashion by the nodes on the network. This is akin to how the same DNA is contained in every cell in a body. Just as one cell contains all the genetic information of the entire body, each node holds the entire history of the network and its transactions—and therefore the whole system can come back online as long as one node exists. The only way the information on the block can change is by a 51 percent vote from all the nodes in a system. The technology is virtually unhackable, as someone would have to hack millions of systems across the planet, each with their own unique security protocols, and almost at the same time. These characteristics make Bitcoin the most resilient network system on the planet.

The programmable capability within blockchain offers the opportunity to create a more resilient backbone for a new internet—as is being done with projects such as Ethereum. Vitalik Buterin created Ethereum in 2014, when he was nineteen years old. Buterin realized that the blockchain technology behind Bitcoin can also exist as an underlying layer that carries programmable coding on top of it. He saw that in the transactions one can program in "smart contracts," agreements between people that can be verified by all the involved parties and written into the blockchain for permanent and safe record keeping. This simple realization is nothing short of revolutionary. Every legal agreement—from automobile titles and real estate ownership to notaries and all business transactions—can be recorded, distributed, and preserved in a tamperproof ledger. This offers more security and trust to all economic and legal proceedings. The potential of Ethereum supersedes just transactions by serving as a base on which to run programs. Buterin made Ethereum an open-source general platform on which all programmers can code and create their own projects. This enables the creation of decentralized applications, called Dapps, that can exist within the ecosystem. Theoretically all applications we use on our phones and computers can exist as a Dapp. This distributes power within a system, away from a central authority, and can function more powerfully and resiliently as an interconnected whole.

Bitcoin, in its current form, uses a lot of energy (though arguably not as much as the major banks, which have deep ties to oil companies). The technology, still in its infancy, needs time to develop to reach its potential, and many people have been focused on solving its technical challenges, such as energy usage and scalability. Even with its own set of challenges, blockchain offers many improvements upon our current economic system. "Blockchain could represent the very first time that human society has a system for creating an unbroken historical record," write Michael Casey and Paul Vigna of the *Wall Street Journal* in their book *The Truth Machine: The Blockchain and the Future of Everything*.[138] Casey and Vigna state:

> Blockchain is seen as capable of supplanting our outdated, centralized model of trust management, which goes to the heart of how societies and economies function . . . The broad idea is that to defer the management of trust to a decentralized network guided by a common protocol instead of relying on a trusted intermediary.[139]

They continue:

> We encourage people to reflect on these alternative visions for a post-capitalistic society, to imagine these technologies as the platform for a future that is neither mired in the failed, collectivist ideas of socialism, nor trapped by the centralized, exclusionary political economy of state-protected, big business monopolies. These ideas offer a way out, but a way that requires a change in thinking about how value is created. Rather than framing the exchanges that define our lives—of labor, asset, and ideas—as a means to acquire a particular form of money that's defined by a symbolic banknote, we should explore new value models, whether tokens or something else, that incentivize collaboration for the betterment of all.[140]

---

[138] Casey and Vigna, *Truth Machine*, 260.

[139] Casey and Vigna, 6–7.

[140] Casey and Vigna, 120.

As we will soon see, many people in the psychedelic space have taken on a similar perspective.

In the early months of 2018, the nonprofit Multidisciplinary Association for Psychedelic Studies (MAPS) was still millions of dollars short in raising the necessary funds to complete Phase III of the clinical trials needed to gain FDA approval for MDMA-assisted therapy. Unexpectedly, the money came to MAPS through cryptocurrency. An anonymous individual using the name Pine created the Pineapple Fund, a philanthropic project that gifted over $55 million in donations in the form of Bitcoin to sixty charities.[141] Pine donated more than $5 million of Bitcoin to MAPS, which allowed their MDMA research to continue.

Pine has said that he suffers severely from bipolar disorder. In his quest to ease the pain in his life, he came across ketamine therapy. Just one experience with ketamine made his life more manageable. Under the influence of a ketamine treatment, Pine decided to donate a portion of his Bitcoin. Later, he came across the work of MAPS and their MDMA research and decided to transfer some of his cryptocurrency to support their work.[142]

The first major users of Bitcoin were online black markets such as Silk Road, which was known as a platform for selling illegal substances. Many people looking for psychedelics online, whether to self-medicate in order to overcome their depression or anxiety or for recreational use, became aware of Bitcoin in the process. Since the original Bitcoin code was released in 2009, a growing number of companies have emerged to provide services to Bitcoin users in above-ground economies. Some who work for these companies have been outspoken about the connections between Bitcoin and psychedelics.

The Pineapple Fund's contribution to psychedelic research is just one example of how psychedelic and cryptocurrency communities overlap. Out of this intersection emerged the CryptoPsychedelic Summit, a

---

[141] www.PineappleFund.org

[142] Pine, "Bitcoin, Ketamine, and Pineapples."

conference in Tulum, Mexico, in February 2018.[143] Leaders in the fields of both psychedelics and cryptocurrencies converged to present their ideas on the symbiosis of these movements. Participants at the conference examined how psychedelics encourage us to expand our definition of how healing takes place, while cryptocurrencies allow us to question money and how financial systems work.[144]

Sterlin Lujan, former communications ambassador for Bitcoin.com, a company that developed a Bitcoin wallet (an app to hold, send, and receive Bitcoins), talked at the conference about a life-defining transformative experience that psychedelics catalyzed for him. In 2009 he was involved in the rave scene and an MDMA experience catalyzed "what the Zen Buddhists refer to as an experience of satori," says Lujan. "I was completely shaken to my core by MDMA because it allowed me to look at myself from a bird's-eye perspective."[145]

Months later Lujan was arrested for selling MDMA. The experience empowered him to become an activist focused on expanding social freedom. While delving into Libertarian culture, he became aware of Bitcoin and cryptocurrencies. "Blockchain technology, cryptocurrency in general, this trend towards decentralization is extremely important, because in my opinion, the greatest impediment to healing and health and wellness are these government bureaucrats," said Lujan at the summit.[146]

Three years after the CryptoPsychedelic Summit, Psychedelic Seminars and Tam Integration kicked off a three-part CryptoPsychedelic Flashback series.[147] They released the videos of the 2018 summit and brought back panelists for live roundtable discussions to reflect on

---

[143] Tulum.CryptoPsychedelic.com

[144] See my article for Lucid News: Khamsehzadeh, "CryptoPsychedelic Conferences Examine Links."

[145] Psychedelic Seminars, "CryptoPsychedelic 2018 #5," at 00:10:30.

[146] Psychedelic Seminars, at 00:15:00.

[147] www.Crowdcast.io/e/CryptoPsychedelic

how the psychedelic and cryptocurrency fields have evolved in the last three years. Ismail Ali, policy and advocacy counsel at MAPS, said, "The things preventing both of these movements . . . from reaching maximum potential is the social-political limitations."[148] Matt McKibbin, a cofounder of the CryptoPsychedelic Summit and founder of DecentraNet, an investment and advisory firm specializing in blockchain technology, said during the 2018 event that he believes psychedelics and blockchain are very intertwined. "Over the last six years I think there are a lot of people that can think outside the box because of psychedelics and thinking about new systems of money and new systems of governance and how we build incentive structures and things you can't be thinking inside the box about," said McKibbin.[149] At the summit McKibbin also said that blockchain technology and cryptocurrencies could be used as a new way to fund and direct resources to psychedelics, which he believes have great potential to positively impact humanity and provide effective healing from trauma.[150] Another way blockchain can support the integration of psychedelics into society is by keeping track of the supply chain, from the manufacturing of psychedelics to the distribution process—enabling greater quality control. Merete Christiansen, associate director of development at MAPS, states: "Blockchain technology has the potential to help us in the regulation and control of substances" and that it would allow users to see the supply chain and control of custody of these medicines.[151]

"The decentralized networks created by blockchain are interestingly analogous to the way researchers have described psychedelics as decentralizing the brain," says Mike Margolies, cofounder of the CryptoPsychedelic Summit and founder of Psychedelic Seminars.[152] Neuroscientists

---

[148] CryptoPsychedelic Flashback, "Psychedelic Research and Advocacy."

[149] Psychedelic Seminars, "CryptoPsychedelic 2018 #6," at 00:04:30.

[150] Psychedelic Seminars.

[151] Psychedelic Seminars, at 00:42:30.

[152] Margolies in Khamsehzadeh, "CryptoPsychedelic Conferences Examine Links."

like Robin Carhart-Harris believe that psychedelics disengage the default-mode network in the brain, the neurological representation for our experience of a central self. Carhart-Harris told the NPR radio show *Science Friday* in 2018 that "as the brain develops and we develop and mature, our thinking becomes more sophisticated, more specialized, more analytical. And all the systems start to parcellate off and specialize. What happens on psychedelics is that there's a kind of de-specialization in a way, and the brain sort of operates in this more sort of rudimentary, freer, more hyper-associative and plastic kind of way."[153]

Some of these subsystems within the default-mode network appear to be overdeveloped in people with severe depression and anxiety. The dissolution of the default-mode network, correlated with the hyperanalytical and more repressive part of the self, allows more information to arise from different systems within the brain and encourages creation of new neural networks between these systems. In a similar way, blockchain, as a decentralized system, encourages the creation of new financial structures. According to the *Harvard Business Review*, "The blockchain will do to the financial system what the internet did to the media."[154]

The World Economic Forum's Global Future Council on Cryptocurrencies believes that "Bitcoin, for example, is more than just a technology—it is a powerful social, political and cultural movement that asks us to imagine money, banking and payments in new and novel ways."[155] Currently, money is created from debt. There now exists three times more debt globally than there is money. Debt will continue to increase in our society, creating more stress, pushing us into our autonomy instinct through stress, and further supporting a self-destructive capitalistic mentality until the society can no longer take the pressure. Whether it be the increasing debt of student loans, the rising costs of rent and food, or the reduction of the middle class, the fact is: the math does not add up within

---

[153] Flatow, "Consciousness, Chemically-Altered."

[154] Ito, Nerula, and Ali, "Blockchain Will Do to the Financial System."

[155] World Economic Forum, *Crypto, What Is It Good For?*

our financial system, and this will have its inevitable culmination. The ever-growing sense of scarcity that our financial system creates engenders cognitive dissonance. As we are currently seeing in the United States, as the stress of debt builds, people will want to find someone to blame, and this will increase racism, xenophobia, and nationalism as the blame is placed on "outsiders."

Ninety-seven percent of the financial wealth in the world is already digital. Economic systems need currencies based on this fact. The encrypted ledger that blockchain provides also unifies the entire economic ecosystem throughout the globe, across both cultures and governments. A global currency would allow a common global economic language. Money would not be lost in translation, as businesses charge for converting one currency to another. If massively adopted, cryptocurrencies can provide standard global units of financial measurement that potentially offer greater stability worldwide, though currently most cryptocurrencies are at a stage of speculation and are highly volatile.

The current narrative surrounding Bitcoin is that it functions as a store of digital value, serving a similar financial function as gold.[156] As governments increasingly continue minting fiat, government-backed currencies, these traditional currencies begin to lose value. According to *Newsweek*, "Bitcoin appears to be a good hedge against inflation because, unlike government-issued fiat currencies such as the U.S. dollar, the British pound, and the euro, the supply of crypto-currency is limited."[157] *Forbes* reports that Bitcoin is the best-performing asset over the last decade.[158] If cryptocurrencies reach widespread adoption, it's possible that they could provide standard global units of financial measurement

---

[156] K. Smith, "How Is Money Created?"; Chu, "Global Debt"; Oswald, *97% Owned*; Zigah, "Is Bitcoin Really Digital Gold?"

[157] Reeves, "Bitcoin May Trump the Dollar."

[158] Torpey, "Bitcoin Price Has Outperformed."

and potentially offer greater worldwide financial stability in comparison to inflating fiat currencies.

The *European Business Review* notes five advantages cryptocurrencies have over fiat currency including low storage and transfer cost, support for small transactions, global reach, and strong barriers to government interference and the ability to falsify.[159] As there will never be more than twenty-one million Bitcoins in existence, since a limit of twenty-one million Bitcoins is encoded into its basic structure, supporters say this cryptocurrency cannot be used to support a debt-driven financial system. Bitcoin won't solve all problems with current financial systems. Unlike banks or credit card companies, Bitcoin currently has no easy way to reverse a purchase. Because Bitcoin is being used as a store of value, like a savings account, it may encourage hoarding of wealth instead of currency circulation. Cryptocurrencies other than Bitcoin that are better designed for moving money through economies may better serve day-to-day transactions.

According to Futurism, blockchain can make "Universal Basic Income a reality."[160] Universal basic income, an idea first put forth by American revolutionary Thomas Paine, asserts that a government, in service to residents of a nation, can disperse funds needed for basic economic survival of its citizens. In such a world, all citizens in a country are guaranteed the money for basic requirements of existence, such as food and rent. This may support greater equality and social stability.

The World Bank notes that about 1.7 billion adults worldwide are unbanked.[161] Without an account at a financial institution or mobile money provider, most of these people are disqualified from receiving government benefits or participating in our global economy. IBM believes that blockchain can help this significant portion of the human population and writes that "blockchain is more than capable of creating

---

[159] "Top 5 Advantages."

[160] Galeon, "Universal Basic Income Could Become a Reality."

[161] World Bank, "The Unbanked."

an environment that can finally bring inclusivity to banking."[162] According to Nasdaq, two-thirds of the unbanked own a smartphone.[163] People could use their phones or a public terminal to begin building verifiable data to receive cryptocurrencies that may enable them to live a life with less suffering.

Blockchain may have a profound impact in almost every industry as we move toward an internet of things (IoT) society. Jeremy Rifkin, who serves as an economic advisor to European governments and China, writes about the third industrial revolution now underway.[164] The third industrial revolution, allowed by digital platforms, emerged from digital networking. Society is evolving toward an IoT where all digital technologies are becoming interconnected and sharing information between platforms. This is the basis for the sharing economy that is developing, in which communities rent out automobiles and utilities on a need-by-need basis, instead of ownership, which wastes resources. Subscription technologies, like Netflix and Spotify, have already redefined industries such as movies and music. Even movie theaters are moving toward monthly subscriptions. The sharing economy that is enabled by a digital architecture is further supported and made more secure by blockchain technology. Rifkin believes that we can create the global infrastructure of a smart economy, based on renewable energy, in as little as thirty years.[165]

The networking of all digital information systems, the IoT, can also be seen as the fourth industrial revolution (with automatization being the third). In such a world, information will be shared between platforms, allowing greater coordination between systems, enabling them to work in unison. This allows movement toward a more consciously interconnected, unified world—an external expression of the internal

---

[162] Spilka, "Blockchain and the Unbanked."

[163] Gupta, "From Exclusion to Empowerment."

[164] Rifkin, *Third Industrial Revolution.*

[165] Rifkin.

realizations of a deep interconnected and unified consciousness that can be experienced in psychedelic states. The coming of an electronic and informationally unified world is the integral representation of the right quadrants of what one finds when they look deep into the domains represented by the left quadrants. At the root of the psychedelic insight is a realization of unity, of a supreme interconnectedness, where all information is shared. This would also eventually evolve to manifest itself structurally and physically in our world. The following quote from Casey and Vigna explains how blockchain can move us in that direction:

> A "global brain" can't really come into existence in an economy dominated by the centralized trust model . . . World Economic Forum founder Klaus Schwab says we're moving into a "fourth industrial revolution," not because one particular new line of products is coming but because a variety of technologies are combining to create whole new systems: mobile devices, sensors, nanotechnology processors, renewable energy, brain research, virtual reality, artificial intelligence, and so forth.
>
> Linking billions of data-gathering and processing nodes to a global, ubiquitous networked computer architecture will have a profound impact on how we interact with our world. It means that our *material* existence, both within the worlds of natural resources and of human-made manufactured objects, will be far more comprehensively measured, analyzed, and explained, creating an omnipresent, *dematerialized* understanding of that existence.
>
> New, interconnected computing and sensor systems will soon give us a far deeper understanding of how that material world functions . . . This expanded, more up-to-date, and more accurate information could have a huge impact on how we manage the planet's desperately stretched resources and on how we might improve our economic process to produce more, or at least better, things—such as food and tools—to widen the net of comfort and prosperity for all humanity.[166]

Blockchain may help bring more structural unity to our complex world.

---

[166] Casey and Vigna, *Truth Machine*, 122–23.

As presented in chapter 3, psychedelics expand ecological awareness. After reviewing thousands of psychedelic experiences for his book, professor and author Richard Doyle suggests in *Darwin's Pharmacy* that a common signature in these rich and varied experiences is what he calls the *ecodelic* insight: "the sudden and absolute conviction that the psychonaut is involved in a densely interconnected ecosystem for which contemporary tactics of human identity are insufficient."[167] This awareness includes not only care for the environment but also compassion for all the organisms in the environment, including humans. The lack of distribution of resources to the majority of our species might be the greatest single cause of suffering that we face, and this directly and indirectly affects all of humanity.

The founders of capitalism intentionally molded economic theory to resemble Newtonian physics, currently an outdated view of physics.[168] This makes our economic system based on an outdated view of reality. Society can improve by integrating a more holistic and interconnected economic system (one where there is a greater relationship between the parts and the wholes of a network), which reflects the larger reality that psychedelics help awaken one to. At a foundational level, blockchain can affect every realm of collective organization, from the movement of resources and identity, to government and the exchange of energy that is represented by money. Whether intentionally or not, blockchain has a degree of biomimicry, resembling resilient natural holistic patterns that took billions of years to evolve. Like the DNA found in all life, blockchain is a decentralized structure, in which information is distributed throughout the entire system.

Supporters of blockchain technology have pointed out some of the similarities between blockchain, psychedelics, and structures found in nature. In his article "Bitcoin Is the Mycelium of Money," entrepreneur Brandon Quittem writes at length about the similarities between fungi and cryptocurrency.[169] One the many commonalities he points to is that

---

[167] Doyle, *Darwin's Pharmacy*, 20.

[168] Nadeau, *Environmental Endgame*.

[169] Quittem, "Mycelium of Money."

fungi and blockchain technologies like Bitcoin are decentralized intelligence networks. This means that like mycelium, cryptocurrencies have no centralized points of failure. Any individual part can be removed, and the system still survives. Quittem also notes that like mycelium, the structure of blockchain makes cryptocurrencies less fragile than traditional financial systems.

Quittem likens Bitcoin's fluctuations in perceived and financial value to that of fungi reproduction. The majority of fungal life exists underground as mycelium, and most observers do not see the consistent growth happening behind the scenes. It is only when the conditions are right that a mushroom quickly forms above the ground and spreads its spores before disappearing again from most observers.

Bitcoin appears to follow a similar pattern. Months go by and, for most people, nothing big is happening with cryptocurrencies. Then, relatively quickly, Bitcoin appears to hijack public consciousness as the price quickly mushrooms and the cryptocurrency spreads like spores to a larger environment of adopters. The Bitcoin mushroom may fade, but it has already reached into a larger territory, allowing greater growth and awareness for the next cycle.

Quittem points out that as mycelium acts as a resource transport layer and communications network connecting organisms in an ecosystem, blockchain technology provides similar services. He believes that both mycelium and Bitcoin are catalysts of human consciousness and that they evolve through symbiotic relationships that can further evolve entire ecosystems.

At the CryptoPsychedelic Summit Liana Sananda Gillooly, development officer at MAPS, expanded on the similarities between blockchain and psychedelics. "There's something extremely psychedelic about the way in which the blockchain works," said Gillooly. "It's borderless. It's virtual. It's decentralized. It's distributed trust. It's all of these things that we find in the psychedelic experience naturally."[170] Like both blockchain and mycelium, the psychedelic movement and culture

---

[170] Psychedelic Seminars, "CryptoPsychedelics, Health and Healing."

is decentralized. Psychedelics are boundary dissolving and blockchain dissolves economic borders between nations. The United Nations writes, "Blockchain . . . is truly cross-border; it knows no national boundaries as either a currency or technology a unified, multilateral approach."[171] There are currently 180 fiat currencies, which largely work only within national regions. Blockchain could potentially help create more resilient and globally interconnected economic systems, supporting more fluent economic communications between markets and nations.

In June 2021, El Salvador become the first country to announce the adoption of Bitcoin as a national currency. Other countries that also are tending toward failing national currencies may follow suit. Their options are to tie themselves to the currency of another country—and then have their fate controlled by what happens in that country and what that government chooses—or tie themselves to a global ubiquitous decentralized currency. By choosing the Bitcoin network, the most resilient network in the world, we are really all in this together. Like psychedelics, cryptocurrencies may also have a unifying effect, dissolving ethnocentric ego-identification between nations and governments.

Researchers, including those at the *Harvard Business Review*, believe that blockchain encourages the distribution of power and information, allowing all people to act on the same data.[172] Openly distributed data and resources, as supported by blockchain, can unleash unforeseen collective creativity. Kotler and Wheal write:

> It's for this reason that so many Prometheans we've met in this book have taken a stand for open sourcing. When the government came knocking, John Lilly demanded his ideas remain declassified. When Sasha Shulgin got that first hint of a DEA crackdown, he published all his pharmacological recipes. It's there in the democratizing effect of Mikey Siegel's consciousness-hacking meet-ups, it's why OneTaste

---

[171] Mulligan, "Blockchain and Sustainable Growth."

[172] Lansiti and Lakhani, "Truth about Blockchain."

has built an Orgasmic Meditation app downloadable anywhere in the world, it's what fuels the volunteers of the Burning Man diaspora. Open-sourcing ecstasis remains one of the best counterbalances to private and public coercion. And once we do take those freely shared ideas and use them to unlock nonordinary states for ourselves, what do we find? A self-authenticating experience of selflessness, timelessness, effortlessness, and richness. In short, all the ingredients required for a rational mysticism. It cuts out the middlemen, and remains rooted in the certainty of the lived experience. This ability to continually update and advance our own understanding, ahead of anyone else's attempts to constrain or repurpose them may be the key to breaking the stalemate.[173]

Psychedelics enable people to draw from untapped potentials of creativity. This creativity can be better expressed when individuals have their base needs met, like those presented by Maslow's hierarchy. Blockchain allows a greater allocation and distribution of resources through a more trusted and resilient network and can be a platform in which to implement universal basic income, freeing individuals from the shackles of focusing on personal survival

According to Maslow's hierarchy of needs, human beings cannot collectively reach a level of self-actualization and self-transcendence until their basic requirements for resources and safety are widely met. When these needs are met, people might have more freedom to move toward greater expressions of creativity and sense of purpose—and more fully receive the benefits psychedelics can offer. One fundamental problem people encounter on that journey is access to resources. Blockchain can be one of our greatest allies in solving this problem.

Once we collectively establish physical security, which must involve the transformation of our economic systems, then we can further explore the imagination, including mining the deepest riches within psychedelic experiences, and make a quantum leap in human evolution. This is the focus of the next chapter.

---

[173] Kotler and Wheal, *Stealing Fire*, 200.

7

STRANGE ATTRACTORS

P sychedelics expand consciousness and, in doing so, bring our focus to the big picture. The potential of our collective future is the focus of this chapter. The first section presents how the future, seen through the lens of the evolution of complexity, is created. The second section shares visions that individuals have experienced about the future in psychedelic states, and it offers a model of how content from the collective unconscious may arise to allow these visions. The last section ties up this work as a whole and offers a possibility—that humanity can once again come into alignment with the planet and accelerate its evolution by rediscovering its ancient connection with psychedelics.

Complexity of Novelty

At a time when our species needs them most, awareness of psychedelics is spreading. Humans are now causing unparalleled pain on our planet, but the consequences of our actions are also waking us up to our interconnection. The premise of Jeremy Rifkin's *The Empathic Civilization: The Race to Global Consciousness in a World in Crisis* is that, as entropy is building through destruction and the loss of natural resources, humanity's capacity for empathy is also increasing.[1] In *LSD and the Mind of the Universe: Diamonds from Heaven,* Christopher Bache describes this correlation between pain and awareness in a chapter titled "The Ocean of Suffering," stating that if one does not resist pain in psychedelic states and stays with the process, it can act as a purification and lead to deep insight.[2] Our ecological devastation is setting the condition for an entire generation to be raised to see the long-term and domino-effect consequences of our actions. This process of coming to awareness can be painfully slow, but fortunately, Earth itself creates plants and fungi that allow us to expand our consciousness to see and feel the whole.

Part of my intention with this work was to provide a systemic and evolutionary framework for our understanding of psychedelics. A key concept in this understanding is complexity. Peter Russell, who earned degrees in both theoretical physics and computer science at the University of Cambridge, notes that complexity seems to have three characteristics. The first is *quantity/diversity*: "the system contains a large number of different elements." The second is *organization*: "The many components are organized into various interrelated structures." The third is *connectivity*: "The components are connected through physical links, energy interchanges, or some form of communication. Such connectivity maintains and creates relationships and organizes activity within the system."[3] Psychedelics emerge out of the diversity of their ecology. These plants and fungi bond with the nervous systems of animals, creating greater biological and ecological connections. This in turn leads to greater organization, both within the biology of the animal and in their behavior in the environment. From this perspective, psychedelics not

---

[1] Rifkin, *Empathic Civilization.*

[2] Bache, *LSD and the Mind of the Universe.*

[3] Russell, *Global Brain Awakens,* 90.

only arise from complexity, they also increase complexity within several systems.

The perspective of a collective evolution that situates development within the context of larger holons, such as an ecological environment or the biosphere itself, needs to be recognized in order to fully make sense of the existence of psychedelics. Howard Bloom, in *Global Brain: The Evolution of Mass Mind from the Big Bang to the 21st Century*, makes a strong case that evolution is primarily collective rather that individualistic, and this is the lens needed to understand the psychedelic and symbiotic plants and fungi. The book serves as a powerful rebuttal to Richard Dawkins's *The Selfish Gene*, which emphasizes evolution primarily as a process of competition rather than cooperation. From Bloom's perspective, it is the entire environment that evolves, not just a particular being; an entire network is engaged in an interlocked process of ever-evolving feedback loops. Bloom presents numerous examples of group selection, showing that entire species evolve, not just individual members, which resonates with theoretical biologist Rupert Sheldrake's concept of "morphogenetic fields," in which natural systems, including species, inherit a collective memory and evolve as a group.[4] Noting that many similar behavioral patterns emerge throughout several different species, Bloom proposes that we are all part of a larger, global mind:

> The global brain is not just human, made of our vaunted intelligence. It is webbed between all species. A mass mind knits the continents, the seas, and the skies. It turns all creatures, great and small, into probers, crafters, innovators, ears and eyes. This is the real global brain, the truest planetary mind.[5]

The understanding of time and of an ongoing evolution can be seen through the lens of complexity. Ralph Abraham, a mathematician who focused on complexity, says during a trialogue with Rupert Sheldrake

---

[4] R. Sheldrake, *Morphic Resonance*.

[5] Bloom, *Global Brain*, 207.

and Terence McKenna that "the future is created by the emergence of forms of increasing complexity (according to Rupert) and increasing integrity (according to Terence)."[6] The way one can track evolution is by seeing the increase of complexity—of interconnection and organization taking place—within the cosmos. As living systems grow in complexity, the depth of their consciousness expands. In *Coming Home: The Birth and Transformation of the Planetary Era*, Sean Kelly traces cycles of history, pointing toward an acceleration in the expansion of consciousness. Richard Tarnas, in *Cosmos and Psyche: Intimations of a New World View*, tracks the evolution of consciousness in history through the lens of archetypal dynamics. "Another popular proposal for a common element in all forms of evolution," writes Steve McIntosh in *Evolution's Purpose: An Integral Interpretation of the Scientific Story of Our Origins*, "is increasing complexity—the idea that unfolding evolution results in forms of organization with more parts, or more complex behaviors."[7]

The idea that we are part of a larger living consciousness—a larger holon—has likely been a part of humanity since its emergence. A unified living world is the primary perspective in shamanism, the first form of religion in humanity.[8] In the East there is the Tao, an intelligent organizing force, and in Hinduism there is Atman, the one universal consciousness within every being. In the West, we see the perspective of larger orders of intelligence with Plato, who in the *Republic* wrote: "What about the city that is most like a single person? For example, when one of us hurts his finger, the entire organism that binds the body and soul together into a single system under the ruling part within it is aware of this, and the whole feels the pain together with the part that suffers."[9] Plotinus later expanded the focus of a collective consciousness

---

[6] T. McKenna, Sheldrake, and Abraham, *Chaos, Creativity, and Cosmic Consciousness*, 18.

[7] McIntosh, *Evolution's Purpose*, 7.

[8] Narby and Huxley, *Shamans through Time*.

[9] Cooper and Hutchinson, *Plato: Complete Works*, 1089.

in his mystical orientation of the One, the supreme system of intelligence that choreographs all the parts within itself: "When Idea enters in, it groups and arranges what, from a manifold of parts, is to become a unit; contention it transforms into collaboration, making the totality one coherent harmoniousness because Idea is one and one as well must be the thing it informs."[10] Romanticism, influenced by philosophers and poets (Wordsworth, Shelley, Coleridge, Schelling, Blake, Hegel), emerged in response to the disenchanted mechanistic paradigm that arose out of the Scientific Revolution and the Enlightenment. The Romantics were largely impacted by Plotinus's work.[11] The movement, which saw the universe as a living organism, has been skillfully presented by M. H. Abrams in *Natural Supernaturalism: Tradition and Revolution in Romantic Literature.* The title intentionally states the Romantic desire to ground what is considered supernatural phenomenon through the lens of reason, focused on the oneness and unity of reality. They believed that both Mind and Nature were a part of the same phenomenon. In psychology, a similar holonic perspective of everyone held within a larger container of Mind was articulated by Carl Jung in his concepts of the collective unconscious and the self. In *Confrontation with the Unconscious: Jungian Depth Psychology and Psychedelic Experiences*, Jungian scholar Scott Hill writes:

> Jung classifies the unconscious into the *personal* and the *collective* unconscious. The personal unconscious contains "all the acquisitions of personal life," all ideas, sensations, perceptions, images, and emotions that are derived from personal experience, but which one had forgotten, repressed, or didn't notice in the first place. The collective unconscious consists of the psychological contents and "the patterns of life and behavior" that each of us has inherited from our evolutionary past and therefore shares with all other human beings. That is, underneath the personal, individual, or subjective unconscious, lies

---

[10] O'Brien, *Essential Plotinus*, 36.

[11] Abrams, *Natural Supernaturalism*.

an unconscious layer that Jung usually calls the *collective unconscious,* "which has nothing to do with our personal experience." He occasionally calls this deeper level the *objective psyche,* the *personal unconscious,* or the *transpersonal unconscious.*[12]

Hill goes on to present how valuable a Jungian approach can be to interpreting a psychedelic experience, since one confronts both the personal and collective unconscious in psychedelic states. Francoise Bourzat, after three decades of exploring and guiding people in expanded states of consciousness through working with the Mazatec people, also writes that psychedelics open people up to the collective unconscious:

> As the collective unconscious becomes available to us, we sometimes find we are able to have the experience of someone far away in place and time. It becomes possible to access different realities and connect with ancient creation myths, rituals, languages, and histories we may not know anything about. I have observed, after witnessing many experiences in expanded states on consciousness, including my own, that the content that emerges is coherent with Jung's maps of the unconscious. Experiencing life as a mythic journey complete with various archetypes, the presence of the anima and animus, masculine and feminine forces, as well as the theme of shadow, are powerful experiences to draw self-knowledge from.[13]

Ultimately, one deals with the same structures of our psyche whether on psychedelics or not. Psychedelics expand our consciousness, enabling the exploration of larger terrains, and many times this includes access to material found in the collective unconscious.

Another Jungian concept that is helpful in understanding psychedelic experiences is that of synchronicity. Jung defines synchronicity as a meaningful event that occurs beyond the chance of coincidence or as an acausal connecting principle, relating by meaning rather than

---

[12] Hill, *Confrontation with the Unconscious,* 30.

[13] Bourzat and Hunter, *Consciousness Medicine,* 152.

causation. In integral theory terms, synchronicity involves the alignment of a smaller holon within a larger one. For instance, when one's internal experience is in alignment with one's environment, one's ego (and probably default-mode network) begins to dissolve, and space arises internally for one to be sensitive to information from the whole. At the same moment, as thoughts and feelings arise within oneself, similar content perhaps arises within other people in the environment. This can create a feeling of flow and connection, a Tao-like experience, in which a fluid state of consciousness within oneself is harmoniously congruent with what is also happening in the environment. Because we are ultimately one being, as described by many who have undergone psychedelic breakthroughs, then ultimately we are each sharing and gathering information from one another and the whole universe. Those personally exploring psychedelics know synchronicities are almost constant in psychedelic states. For many, synchronicity may become a part of their daily sober life as they become more sensitive to their intuition and environment after psychedelically inspired expansive states. The title of Stanislav Grof's autobiographical work, *When the Impossible Happens: Adventures in Non-Ordinary Realities*, explores the changes one can experience in life after one's consciousness has been transformed by psychedelic experiences. Though he cautions against blindly following synchronicities, he presents personal experiences of synchronicity arising in his life. A student of Grof, Christopher Bache, also writes in *The Living Classroom: Teaching and Collective Consciousness* about the increase of synchronicity in his classroom and life due to his psychedelic work.

Grof and Bache both situate their work within a context of systems theory, and systems theory includes the idea that living systems naturally strive to achieve equilibrium.[14] When living systems are pushed far past equilibrium, they reach what is called a bifurcation point.[15] Either the system collapses into a lower level of complexity or reorganizes and

---

[14] Capra and Luisi, *Systems View of Life*.

[15] Capra, *Hidden Connections*.

achieves a greater degree of novelty and equilibrium. In *Dark Night, Early Dawn: Steps to a Deep Ecology of Mind,* Bache writes:

> Chaos theory tells us that when a system is driven beyond equilibrium, the subtle interconnectedness that lies latent beneath its surface can sometimes emerge to reshape the system itself . . . It is as if nature reaches into herself and draws forth higher orders of self-organization that are latent within the system, hidden and quiescent until their potential is actualized.[16]

As the dissolution instinct becomes active and the structures dissolve, especially if they are not in harmony with the larger holon, more interconnected patterns are given the opportunity to arise and become embodied:

> If matter has new properties when pushed far beyond its equilibrium state, might not the same be true of mind? I want to suggest that the global eco-crises may push the field of the species-mind so hard that it may draw forth new structures from itself, structures that reflect its inherent capacity for higher degrees of self-organization. Under the stress of so much suffering, the balance of the collective unconscious might shift. If this were to happen, synergistic tendencies that are latent within the species-mind may become manifest, exerting a coordinating influence within seemingly disparate human activities. Synchronicities may increase. Realities that are unconscious to all, but a few may become available to many. The ground of "common sense" may shift as the floor of the collective unconscious rises into awareness.[17]

The cracks we are seeing in our world might be the portals through which a higher form of complexity, with deeper interconnectivity and integrity, may arise.

---

[16] Bache, *Dark Night, Early Dawn*, 241.

[17] Bache, 242.

In *The Global Brain Awakens: Our Next Evolutionary Leap*, Peter Russell has a similar vision to Bache of what may happen. He presents that this planetary shift may come about by an "emergence through emergency"—that our ecological crises might awaken a planetary consciousness in humans that he terms the Gaiafield. He writes: "The Gaiafield will not be a property of individual beings any more than consciousness is a property of cells. The Gaiafield will occur at the planetary level, emerging from the combined interactions of all minds within the social superorganism."[18] Russell also speculates that as we move into a more synergistic, interwoven society, synchronicities in society will begin to increase:

> What we regard as curious chains of coincidence might likewise be
> the manifestation, at the level of the individual, of a higher organizing
> principle at the collective level, the as yet rudimentary social organism.
> As humanity becomes more integrated, functioning more and more
> as a healthy, high-synergy system, we might expect to see a steady
> increase in the number of supportive coincidences.[19]

Russell continues by offering the possibility that "if humanity were to evolve into a healthy, integrated, social superorganism, this transformation could signal the maturation and awakening of the global nervous system."[20] The book ends with Russell pondering if greater levels of unity can evolve after planetary consciousness, "or rather is it possible that the whole universe, like Gaia, is somehow organized so that living systems can evolve? If so, could the universe as a whole be headed towards becoming a single universal being?"[21]

That greater unity through complexity leads to diversity may, at face value, appear as a paradox. As new connections form, however,

---

[18] Russell, *Global Brain Awakens*, 150.

[19] Russell, 197.

[20] Russell, 315.

[21] Russell, 324.

emergent properties arise.[22] This leads to formation of new holons.[23] The more relationships there are in a system, the more synergy and creative potentials for expression exist. As cultures evolve, more potential exists for humans to find their unique identities through the increased possibilities of expression. Developing new mediums for art as well as new technological innovations enables even more creative expressions to emerge from one's imagination. Thus, complexity enables the emergence of novelty.

Terence McKenna spent decades working on his novelty theory, which states that as evolution moves forward so does the emergence of novelty.[24] McKenna believed that the two fundamental forces in the cosmos were habit and novelty. Similar to Rupert Sheldrake's morphic fields, which hold the memory of a species, habit always strives to maintain patterns. Novelty breaks patterns, brings in complexity, and moves evolution forward. Physiological mutations are a form of biological novelty that lead to adaptation and evolutionary transformation among species over generations. According to McKenna, psychedelics are novelty generators. This perspective is shared by the philosopher Peter Sjöstedt-H, a research fellow at the University of Exeter, who writes:

> Psy-phen [psychedelics] can present to us novelties, not combined actualities of the past. We are apprehending the delimited potentials of cognition. In entering the mind of "God" in this way, we access the infinite bank of possibility that conditions the advance of creativity in the universe. *The common ineffability of these experiences indicate their novelty: words are not created for phenomena that are never considered.*[25]

---

[22] Swimme and Tucker, *Journey of the Universe.*

[23] Wilber, *Brief History of Everything.*

[24] McKenna and McKenna, *Invisible Landscape.*

[25] Sjöstedt-H, *Noumenautics,* 52.

As he points out, the ineffability that many people experience on psychedelics is due to the fact that the subject is undergoing a novel experience. They do not have the words to describe the experience because the evolution of human language has yet to develop to encompass these domains of consciousness, a phenomenon which could support the idea that psychedelics are evolutionary catalysts of consciousness. Sjöstedt-H is in agreement with this view when he writes: "Assuming Whitehead's cosmology, it would seem difficult to deny that psychedelic experiences would be the greatest means by which God's aesthetic adventures of growth could be attained."[26] What both Sjöstedt-H and McKenna present is that there exists a correlation between novelty and evolution, and that psychedelics can play a critical role in these processes.

The model I have presented so far is of an entangled, evolving universe that is increasing in complexity and synchronicity (which tends to be a self-organizing process that potentially leads to greater wholeness), which leads to the creation of novel structures and expressions. Psychedelics, from the perspective I have offered, serve as an intermediary between our consciousness and the rest of the cosmos. The connections they manifest and catalyze connect us to the larger holons we are a part of—that of our environment, the Gaian mind, and that of the universe as a whole. Our very consciousness grows out of these larger holons, similar to the way new cells arise within a body. Just as the cells of our body rely on the networks they are a part of in order to exist, so does our mind rely on the larger mind. Our very experience emerges from these larger networks. Consciousness is born out of consciousness. This includes our innate instincts, such as autonomy, communion, transcendence, and dissolution, as well as the deepest part of the unconscious. If this is so, then might our individual psychedelic visions be expressions of a much larger, collective vision of our encompassing and shared minds?

---

[26] Sjöstedt-H, 48.

Teleological Visions

"The role of the attractors seems central to understanding what chaos dynamics is offering that is new," Terence McKenna states in *Chaos, Creativity, and Cosmic Consciousness*.[27] In chaos mathematics—a branch of mathematics focused on studying chaos—dynamics systems that appear irregular and as random states of disorder are actually governed by underlying patterns; an attractor is a point toward which the system tends to evolve. In the 1970s, with the invention of high-speed computers, mathematicians were able to compute models of networks and construct the equations comprising complexity theory (also known as nonlinear dynamics). From the roots of these equations branched out chaos theory and fractal geometry. Not only could mathematicians now construct nonlinear equations, but the new computers also allowed them to see the visual patterns that emerge when these equations are graphed, revealing the beauty of fractal geometry, patterns also commonly seen in psychedelic states. The mathematicians began to notice that specific points within a system held a special type of attraction, which, when reached, reoriented the movement of the system. These points were categorized as three basic types of attractors: point attractors (points in the system that pulled the motion toward equilibrium), periodic attractors (corresponding to the rhythmic, periodic oscillations within the system), and strange attractors (unique points in chaotic systems that dramatically changed the pattern, while still maintaining a coherent shape).[28] A strange attractor is one that pulls the system toward a fractal nature.[29] Many of these contain nonrepeating, and therefore novel, fractal patterns that evolve out of the shape that came before. When a strange attractor is present, the system may locally appear chaotic and yet be globally stable. A strange attractor is thus a point of power emerging from a collective pattern.

---

[27] T. McKenna, Sheldrake, and Abraham, *Chaos, Creativity, and Cosmic Consciousness*, 38.

[28] Capra and Luisi, *Systems View of Life*.

[29] T. McKenna, Sheldrake, and Abraham, *Chaos, Creativity, and Cosmic Consciousness*.

From an integral approach, the dynamics of the physical and mathematical world have correlations with our singular and collective experiences of consciousness. The internal world and external world are intrinsically connected, and common structures run deep in both the physical world and our minds. These structures have dynamic patterns. When an attractor enters our perception of reality, we perhaps begin to perceive that events are pulled from the future rather than pushed by the past. This idea, of causality based on complexity evolving in a particular direction toward an attraction point, runs deep in Western history. Aristotle identified four kinds of causes: material, efficient, formal, and final. The final cause, he said, was a movement toward a purpose in the future. The term *teleology*, originating with the writings of Plato and Aristotle, means the study of the final aim or purpose (*telos* in Greek, meaning "end, aim, or goal," and *logos,* meaning "explanation or study of"). Aristotle coined the word *entelechy* (from *telos*) to mean the complete realization of some potential concept or function. Rupert Sheldrake took Aristotle's concept and integrated it into his morphic field theory:

> The concept of morphic attractors in morphic resonance theory, like the concept of entelechy in Aristotle's notion of the soul, tries to deal with the fact that somehow the system, the person, the developing animal, the developing plant, or whatever is subject in the present to the influence of a potential future state is what directs and guides and attracts the development of the system in the present.[30]

Teleological models of reality have continued in Western culture long after Aristotle, showing up in many religions with the idea that the world is moving toward some perfect heavenly state, which may include going through an apocalyptic collapse before arriving to a new state of divine order. The Eastern concept of Nirvana describes a state that is the accumulation of work that one reaches that is perfect, ever present, and frees one's self from the process of birth and death. In the West, it

---

[30] T. McKenna, Sheldrake, and Abraham, 34.

is seen more as a moment of collective awakening. Pierre Teilhard de Chardin, who was both a Catholic priest and a paleontologist, describes this state in his influential book on evolution, *The Human Phenomenon*, as the omega point. The idea of the omega point is both a spiritual belief and a scientific speculation that everything in the universe is fated to spiral toward a final point of divine unification.[31]

A modern-day representation of a strange attractor is the Singularity as put forward by Ray Kurzweil, an American futurist and inventor who has received twenty honorary doctorates and honors from three US presidents. In *The Singularity Is Near: When Humans Transcend Biology*, Kurzweil lays out six major epochs of evolution. "Evolution," he writes, "is a process of patterns of increasing order."[32] These epochs are: (1) the realm of physics and chemistry, when the universe only consisted of atoms and molecules; (2) biology, when cells evolved self-replicating mechanisms and the ability to store information in DNA; (3) the evolution of the brain, where early animals began to recognize patterns; (4) technology, where humans now are able to store and process information externally through ever more efficient devices; (5) decades in the future, the merging of human technology with human intelligence, which will allow humans to transcend the human brain's intelligence; and (6) the universe will begin to wake up through a process of becoming embedded with technology and intelligence that allows it to reorganize matter and energy in the environment to provide an optimal level of computation. Kurzweil claims the Singularity will occur in the fifth epoch. He writes:

> The Singularity is an English word meaning a unique event with, well singular, implications. The word was adopted by mathematicians to denote a value that transcends any limitation, such as the explosion of magnitude that results when dividing a constant by a number that gets closer and closer to zero.[33]

---

[31] Teilhard de Chardin, *Human Phenomenon*.

[32] Kurzweil, *Singularity Is Near*, 14.

[33] Kurzweil, 22.

In describing the Singularity, Kurzweil states:

> In the half century that I've immersed myself in computer and related technologies, I've sought to understand the meaning and purpose of the continual upheaval that I have witnessed at many levels. Gradually, I've become aware of a transforming event looming in the first half of the twentieth-first century. Just as a black hole in space dramatically alters the pattern of matter and energy accelerating toward its event horizon, this impending Singularity in our future is increasingly transforming every institution and aspect of human life, from sexuality to spirituality.
>
> What, then, is the Singularity? It's a future period during which the pace of technological change will be so rapid, its impact so deep, that human life will be irreversibly transformed. Although neither utopian nor dystopian, this epoch will transform the concepts that we rely on to give meaning to our lives, from our business models to the cycle of human life, including death itself. Understanding the Singularity will alter our perspective on the significance of our past and ramifications for our future. To truly understand it inherently change's one's view of life in general and one's own particular life.[34]

Like most teleological interpreters of time, Kurzweil believes there is an event in our future that is leading us forward and is shaping the present. This strange attractor, the Singularity, will give an expanded context and sense of meaning to our evolutionary history.

Mathematician and philosopher Alfred North Whitehead proposed the idea that there exist eternal objects, much like Plato's concept of forms, that are pure potentials that the universe is always attempting to actualize.[35] Terence McKenna took Whitehead's concept further and spoke of a Transcendental Object at the End of Time that the universe is in the process of becoming.[36] In a 1998 talk titled "The Strange

---

[34] Kurzweil, 7.

[35] Whitehead, *Process and Reality*.

[36] We Plants Are Happy Plants, "Transcendental Object at the End of Time."

Attractor," Terence McKenna talks about the acceleration of novelty culminating in a singularity or Omega Point:

> Until very recently in scientific thought the idea has been that events are pushed by the causal necessity embedded in the events that preceded them. In other words, if you asked the question what is the most important event in terms of shaping this moment, the answer would be the moment just before this moment, because it hands on the energy, the space, the time. Recently, mathematicians have evolved what they call the notion of attractors, or strange attractors in some cases, and these are processes where a dynamic is not pushed by causal necessity from behind, but it's pulled by a point in the future . . . What the universe is doing is it's under the sway of what I call the Transcendental Object at the End of Time, and that is this domain of hyperconnectivity. That it would be perfect novelty, and all nature aspires for this state of perfect novelty. You can almost say that nature abhors habit, and so it seeks the novel by producing various kinds of phenomena at every level in biology, chemistry, and society. And so there really is a purpose to the universe. Its purpose is this state of hypercomplexification in which all of its points become related to each other, become what mathematicians call cotangent. And it gives the universe the feeling of being imbued with a caring presence. It makes it appear that nature is tending towards something, and it changes our own ethical position in the universe . . .
>
> If you take this point of view that process is under the influence of an attractor and that the value that the attractor is maximizing is novelty, then suddenly for the first time in 500 years human beings are moved back to the center of the stage, because we are the most novel thing on this planet. We are everything that biology is plus technology, language, politics, philosophy, art, so forth and so on. So suddenly human beings become important, not mere cosmic witnesses to a meaningless cosmos, but the cutting-edge of a cosmos that glories in order and is moving toward higher states of order, and at the present moment we are the carriers . . . The purpose of being a human is to complexify reality even more, to hand on a more diverse, more complicated, more multifaceted universe to our children. And when this process of complexification reaches the Omega Point, it will fulfill, I believe, the expectations of all of these religions, but will fulfill it in a

mature, scientific and universal way that all these religions lack because they all reflect patriarchal origins.[37]

It is worth noting that humans entering the center of the stage does not mean that they have power over other creatures. From this perspective, other creatures are also creators of novelty, and ultimately we are heading toward an interconnected unity. This idea of a supreme unity is what many people experience in the timeless states of the psychedelic journeys, meditation, and other holotropic states. It perhaps follows that when the individual self is deeply connected enough to this unity, visions of the strange attractors may arise.

Some who have experienced this unity claim that it is possible to have authentic visions of the future while in psychedelic states.[38] If one is truly dissolving into a larger mind—a mind holding the information and current intention of every being within its decentralized network—then this may indeed be plausible. The Aztecs, for example, used mushrooms to see the future. An Aztec prophecy, perhaps inspired by psilocybin visions, told of a god named Quetzalcoatl, portrayed as a bearded white man coming to claim his kingdom, in the same year Cortez landed.[39] This likely caused the Aztecs to lower their defenses, as the arrival of the conquistadors was seen as divine providence—proving that visions, like dreams, can be misinterpreted. They had no precedent for an attack by such a technologically advanced force; the Spanish invasion was a massacre.

Another notable experience of someone claiming to have seen the future with psilocybin is pioneer psilocybin researcher Stanley Krippner. Of this experience, he writes about how he envisioned the assassination of John F. Kennedy before it happened:

> Lincoln's features slowly faded away, and those of Kennedy took their place. The setting was still Washington D.C. The gun was still at the

---

[37] Evasius, "The Strange Attractor," at 00:00:26.

[38] Bache, *LSD and the Mind of the Universe*; T. McKenna, *Archaic Revival*.

[39] Letcher, *Shroom*, 74; DeKorne, *Psychedelic Shamanism*, 174.

base of the statue. A wisp of smoke seeped from the barrel and curled into the air. The voice repeated, "He was shot. The president was shot." My eyes opened; they were filled with tears . . . in 1962, when I had my first psilocybin experience, I gave this visualization of Kennedy relatively little thought, as so many other impressions came my way. However, it was the only one of my visualizations that brought tears to my eyes, so I described it fully in the report I sent to Harvard. Nineteen months later, on November 23, 1963, the visualization came back to me as I mourned Kennedy's assassination.[40]

To have envisioned such an emotional and concrete situation a year before it happened may seem like a mere coincidence from a purely materialistic perspective—but from the paradigm of a living and inter-connected world, one in which the larger ecological mind can, through the mediation of psychedelics, communicate to a subject information from the whole, it takes on much greater meaning.

Christopher Bache, a professor of philosophy and religion for three decades, experienced seventy-three high-dose LSD sessions with the intention of spiritual exploration over a twenty-year period while teaching his classes. He took meticulous notes and presents the harvest of the journeys in his books *Dark Night, Early Dawn* and *LSD and the Mind of the Universe*. Catalyzed by 500 micrograms of LSD, Bache claims to have been shown the future of our species, a vision that seemed to arise from the collective unconscious:

> If held properly, these experiences begin to function as "strange attractors," pulling us toward our future through the increased awareness they bring. We may not be able to fully actualize these experiences immediately after a session has ended, but they bend the trajectory of our lives.[41]

Following is an excerpt of an LSD session he shares in *Dark Night, Early Dawn* that presents his vision of the death and rebirth of our

---

[40] Krippner in Stafford, *Psychedelics Encyclopedia*, 276.

[41] Bache, *LSD and the Mind of the Universe*, 205.

species. It is a long quote but worth the read to fully grasp the transformation that takes place.

There was nothing personal about the state I was in, not even the residual personal of individual ecstatic experience. Instead, there was a wholeness that was species-wide; its movement was the movement of my kind . . . It was vast and beyond measure. Linear fixed-time opened to a holistic deep-time. As often happens, experience preceded understanding. I began to experience new things and only slowly did I get my bearings on what I was experiencing. I began to experience states of arousal, anxiety, crises, breakthrough, and a new beginning, but as a species experiences these things, not an individual person. It was how the entire human species would experience this if it was a single, integrated organism . . . The levels of arousal I was experiencing were ascending waves within the collective unconscious, and these waves were building up and breaking within me! It was like being able to experience a thunderstorm all at once, with every drop registering individually but subsumed into the patterns of the storm as a whole.

In time I began to realize that I was being allowed to experience some of the inner workings of the species that would be unfolding in response to events taking place over the next several decades, perhaps the next hundred years . . . The core scenario. Amidst a field of relative calm, a small anxiety began to grow. Slowly more and more persons were looking up and becoming alarmed . . . Conditions got worse and worse. People became more and more alarmed as the danger increased, forcing them to let go of their assumptions at deeper and deeper levels. The world as they knew it was falling apart. Decades were compressed into minutes, and I felt their alarm deepen and they lost more and more of what they had considered the normal and necessary structures of their world. Step by step, events were forcing a rapid re-assessment of everything in their lives . . . The level of alarm grew in the species field until eventually everyone was forced into the melting pot of mere survival. We were all in this together . . .

For a time it looked as though like we would all be killed, but just then, when the storm was at its peak . . . the danger slowly subsided. Though many had died, many were still alive. All the survivors began to find each other, new social units began to form. Parents and children from different families joined to form new types of families.

Everywhere new social institutions sprang into being that reflected our new reality—new ways of thinking, new values that we had discovered within ourselves during the crises. Every aspect of our lives was marked by new priorities, new perceptions of the good, new truths. These new social forms reflected new states of awareness that seemed to spread through the survivors like a positive contagion. These social forms then fed back into the system to elicit still newer states of awareness in individuals, and the cycle of creativity between individual and group spiraled.

The whole system was coming alive at new levels, and this aliveness was expressing itself in previously impossible ways. It was as if the eco-crises had myelinized connections in the species-mind, allowing new and deeper levels of self-awareness to spring into being. Repeatedly there was the message: "These things will happen much faster than anyone can anticipate because of the hyper-arousal of the species-mind." Thousands of fractal images drove this lesson home again and again. "Faster than anyone can anticipate." The pace of the past was irrelevant to the pace of the future. These new forms that were emerging were not temporary fluctuations but permanent psychological and social structures that marked the next evolutionary step in our long journey toward self-activated awareness. The entire process seemed to be driven by strange attractors that were rapidly drawing the system into new patterns of self-configuration. The time of rebuilding was suffused with an inner luminosity that signaled a profound awakening within the human heart. It was not the overwhelming brilliance of diamond luminosity that shines forth from individual awakening, but a softer luminosity that reflected the same reality but more gently present and more evenly distributed throughout the entire species.[42]

In Bache's experience, the ecological crises caused a bifurcation point within our global system, forcing humanity to reorganize at a higher degree of consciousness.[43] The bifurcation point involved dissolving old structures, both integrally within consciousness and those of

---

[42] Bache, 246–48.

[43] Bache, 243.

social structures, to ultimately make space for the development of new structures that would embody greater values based on a deeper love. In Bache's vision we see a permanent expansion of self-awareness (the upper-left/subjective quadrant) that correlates with changes in our brain (upper-right/objective quadrant) to anchor in these transformations, as well as an evolution of values (lower-left/intersubjective quadrant) and new social structures (lower-right/interobjective quadrant).

The apparent visions of the future that one can experience on psychedelics are best held lightly. It might be helpful to think of these visions as dreams with inspirational potential. Like anything in life, if held too tightly, one may lose attunement to their present moment and environment and may instead live in a fantasy. About this potential fixation on the future, the authors of *Stealing Fire* write:

> Contemporary psychonauts have even coined a term for this persistent
> distortion: eschatothesia—the perception of the Eschaton, or the end
> of the world. "It is not necessarily the absolute 'end of times,'" the
> Hyperspace Lexicon clarifies, "but can be a feeling of some huge event
> in the near future we are approaching, the end of an aeon, a marker in
> time after which nothing will be the same."[44]

Dennis McKenna, after decades of reflecting on his and Terence's ideas, reminds us, "Every person confronts their own Singularity at the end of time, the end of their own personal history. This is the only eschaton we can realistically look forward to."[45] Eventually, the dissolution instinct in us all becomes active enough that we dissolve back into the universe.

Many people, even without the use of psychedelics, have felt an important world-transforming moment lies just beyond the present, as generation after generation has believed in an imminent apocalypse or the coming of a messiah. What humanity can do is use the positive aspects of these visions as inspiration and let go of some of the shadow

---

[44] Kotler and Wheal, *Stealing Fire*, 204.

[45] D. McKenna, "Reflections in a Rear-View Mirror," 50.

potentials, such as ego inflation. There can be a tendency to put too much stock into one's visions, whether catalyzed by psychedelics or by one's imagination, as some kind of universal truth. Psychedelic visions, just as the content that organically arises from one's unconscious, can be archetypal and be used as a path to explore the collective unconscious, but even so, it is still the individual having them. As much as psychedelics break down the ego, it is not eradicated completely, and post-journey interpretation may run the risk of being viewed through an egoistic lens. Without time to properly integrate the experience, including receiving reflections by a community or integration specialist, one can even temporarily go into a psychotic break with reality.

In his 2021 book, *Recapture the Rapture: Rethinking God, Sex, and Death in a World That's Lost Its Mind*, Jamie Wheal focuses much of the work on analyzing rapture ideologies, those that prepare for "the end of history." Part 1 of the book is even titled "Choose Your Own Apocalypse." Wheal writes:

> Rapturists often fantasize that this Omega moment will be an eleventh-hour redemption that saves us from our impossible fate. It's a temptingly tidy fix for a bunch of wicked problems. Teilhard wasn't so optimistic. Even if we could solve the monkey puzzle of existence before we blow ourselves up, he wasn't sure everyone would come along for the ride …
>
> This notion of some people stepping up to the task, while others are unwilling or unable, fits neatly on top of psychologist Abraham Maslow's pyramid of development. His model begins with basic survival needs at the base, narrowing as it goes up through individuation, belonging, and actualization, all the way to Self-Transcendence—which reflects a return to simple service to others.
>
> Teilhard's notion of Christogenesis can really be seen as the final step of Self-Transcendent people coming together around a shared desire to help. In that light, the notion of a mythopoetic Omega Point is really just a final flourish on what are broadly accepted stages of human development. It only sounds magical because so few of us have gotten there yet.

This notion of a small group, "a faction of the noosphere," to effect transformational change is echoed in the political sciences. Erica Chenoweth at Harvard's Kennedy School has famously posited that historic civil rights movements have required 3.5 percent of a population to reach a tipping point of transformation. For current environmental and social justice movements that number has taken on almost mythical significance.[46]

From this perspective, not everyone needs to "wake up" to a greater unity, just a critical mass to catalyze a movement that cements in systemic transformation that embodies values of a larger consciousness. Psychedelics may play a key role in propelling this population into holotropic states, inspiring them to move humanity into a greater degree of wholeness.

Perhaps the best gift that teleological psychedelic visions can provide this population of leaders, and others, is to give our species direction, and vision, without which humanity wanders aimlessly into the future. We live in a world obsessed with progress, but the idea of progress is often chased without much consideration of destination. The aesthetics, values, and societal organizations we want to see in the world must first be visualized as a projection of a possible future before we can create and embody them in the present. Perhaps our collective unconscious contains visions of the future that we have the potential to access in psychedelic states. If psychedelic plants and fungi are creativity generators through which Earth most directly and consciously communicates with our consciousness, then perhaps she may share with us her visions of her self-actualization that dwell within her imagination.

What may aid one in comprehending that such a process can be possible is the idea that we are part of a shared imagination, which is something many venturing deep into psychedelic states continue to conclude. In *The New Science of Psychedelics: At the Nexus of Culture, Consciousness, and Spirituality*, David Jay Brown sees the possibility of evolution taking

---

[46] Wheal, *Recapture the Rapture*, 291–92.

us toward a much more self-transforming reality that is an extension of our imagination:

> I think DNA is ultimately trying to create a world where the imagination is externalized, where the mind and the external world become synchronized as one, so that basically whatever we can imagine can become a reality. Literally. And I think that everything throughout our entire evolution has been moving slowly toward that goal. In the past couple thousand years, it's been very steady. And through nanotechnology, through artificial intelligence, through advanced robotics, I think we're entering into an age where we'll be able to control matter with our thoughts and actually be able to create anything that our minds can conceive of. We're very quickly heading into a time where machines are going to be more intelligent than we are, and we're going to most likely merge, I think, with these intelligent machines and develop capacities and abilities that we can barely imagine right now, such as the ability to self-transform.[47]

Technology certainly won't solve all the world's problems or provide the shift in consciousness that humanity needs, but it will undoubtedly provide variables that we cannot conceive of today. Technology might catalyze a more bizarre and expansive world than is imaginable by most people today. Within a decade or two, we might have people walking around connected to the internet through their thoughts.[48]

Terence McKenna reached the same conclusion as Brown and states that history has been leading to full expression of imagination. At times he likened the Transcendental Object at the End of Time to a UFO but defines it as a synthesis of technology and consciousness. He sees this strange attractor moving us forward as the creation of pure novelty, that is to say, of infinite imagination:

> Finally, for me, imagination is the goal of history. I see culture as an effort to literally realize our collective dreams . . . Art as life lived in

---

[47] D. Brown, *New Science of Psychedelics*, 328.

[48] Metz, "Computer Chip in Your Brain"

the imagination is the great archetype that rears itself up at the end of history . . . We are on a journey to meet the great attractor, and as we close the distance it is more and more a multifaceted mirror of our own images of beauty. The journey is an ascending learning curve that is becoming asymptotic; at that point, we are face to face with a living mystery that is within each and all of us.[49]

The universe will continue to evolve into more complex novel forms through its ceaseless imagination, so that its ever-evolving beauty can continue to wow, inspire, and touch its subjects.

The Psychedelic (Re)Evolution

The word *revolution* can be thought of as "re-evolution." This means to re-evolve, to get back onto the trajectory of our evolutionary process, to reimagine humanity by recontextualizing our evolutionary journey— and in the process transforming the identity of humanity. As George Orwell points out in *1984*, changing one's understanding of the past shapes the trajectory of the future. It perhaps follows that forming an accurate explanation of human emergence, including our psychedelic origins, holds potential to shape the future of humanity. We are at a point in history when we have to dive deep into the past to integrate aspects of our human consciousness before we can really soar into the future. Currently, humanity as a whole does not have a complete and comprehensive understanding of how we evolved, nor do we have a clear vision of where we want to go. In our evolutionary past may lie the missing puzzle piece that could bring sense to our story here on Earth. Just like in an individual's psychotherapeutic process, healing our collective trauma may come from integrating the past, bringing the wholeness and understanding we desire. This is not purely a cognitive understanding,

---

[49] T. McKenna, Sheldrake, and Abraham, *Chaos, Creativity, and Cosmic Consciousness*, 48.

but as presented by the examples in the first chapter, the mushroom may bring us to a deeper understanding that transcends the cognitive realm.

Humanity's story needs to be integrally grounded both experientially and scientifically. As research delves deeper into humanity's origins, and as tests continue on the impacts of psilocybin on cognitive functioning, development, and creativity, it is likely that the mushroom theory of human origins may rise in status. Experiments on LSD and creativity have already been carried out, and experiments on creativity and psilocybin are underway.[50] If the findings are positive—which anecdotal evidence of individual self-experimentation has already shown in areas of art, philosophy, and science—they will be added to the body of supporting evidence in favor of this theory. Science has discovered that psilocybin, as well as other psychedelics, stimulates neurogenesis, and promotes neuroplasticity and a more interconnected brain.[51] This is affirmed by decades of experiential evidence and carefully controlled studies, which reveal that a single session of psilocybin can be one of the most important and insightful experiences of a person's life—even after a twenty-year follow-up.[52] For many modern people, psychedelics have been the catalyst of an authentic spiritual life.[53] Such experiences may have occurred in the lives of our ancestors, both accidentally and intentionally. Additionally, psychedelic fungi and plants may have helped develop the brain formations that allow one to experience mystical states and, therefore, they may be responsible for the original spark of religious thought in humanity.[54] This explanation is supported by historical evidence from cave art and religious texts, and it has been accepted by

---

[50] Fadiman, *Psychedelic Explorer's Guide*; Feilding, "Psilocybin and Depression."

[51] Renter, "Grow and Repair Brain Cells"; Ly et al., "Structural and Functional Neural Plasticity"; Ghose, "Magic Mushrooms Create a Hyperconnected Brain."

[52] Pollan, *How to Change Your Mind*; Doblin, "Note on Current Psilocybin Research Projects."

[53] Badiner and Grey, *Zig Zag Zen*.

[54] Hancock, *Divine Spark*.

anthropologists, who consider shamanism to be the oldest form of spirituality.[55] The idea that psilocybin-containing, consciousness-expanding fungi—simply chemicals that had been growing in the environment long before humanity evolved—caused a massive transformation in the consciousness and neurophysiology of our species epigenetically over many generations, stretching hundreds of thousands to perhaps millions of years, might be the most plausible explanation for human emergence, especially when compared to any other explanation.

At the dawn of human history may lie a mystery that sets us free. With this emerging understanding of human identity and evolution taking place through a symbiotic partnership, based on a shamanic worldview of unity and a living world within a living-systems context, we can grow into a deeper relationship with ourselves, each other, and our ecology—further embodying the processes of autonomy, communion, transcendence, and dissolution. While these instincts may appear to move in different directions, in reality they all support moving into deeper connection—with ourselves, others, and the whole. As the sociologist Jeremy Rifkin points out:

> The search for intimacy and universality at the same time continually forces the human mind to stretch itself in both directions. Although the two realms often appear at odds, the reality is that human beings are forever searching for "universal intimacy"—a sense of total belonging. What appears to be a strange confluence of opposites is really a deeply embedded human aspiration. It is our empathic nature that allows us to experience the seeming paradox of greater intimacy in more expansive domains. The quest for universal intimacy is the very essence of what we mean by transcendence.[56]

This journey toward transcendence may have at its root humanity's intimacy with nature. By eating the fruits of her mycelial web, which directly

---

[55] Lewis-Williams, *Mind in the Cave*; Wasson, *Soma*; Narby and Huxley, *Shamans through Time*.

[56] Rifkin, *Empathic Civilization*, 613.

and indirectly connects all life in the environment, humanity might have been given the capacities of increased cognition and language, allowing greater intimacy with the cosmos and one another.

As one's sense of self expands, characterized by shifts in paradigms, so do one's values, creating a radical reorganization in priorities.[57] As presented in chapters 3 and 6, many people influenced by the paradigm-transforming experiences of psychedelics have oriented toward a greater life of service. They express it through ecological and social activism, therapy, art, technology, and philosophy. We can only imagine the moral strength and creative breakthroughs that may arise from expanded hearts and minds as a greater portion of humanity undergoes a shamanic process of identity dissolution and rebirth that incorporates awareness of the whole.

As the systems theorist Fritjof Capra points out, most of our present systemic issues are results from a crisis of perception.[58] Our institutions are largely based on a fragmented perception of the world rather than one that sees interconnectivity. Our capitalist economic systems focus on profit for the privileged individual at the expense of other people, animals, and the environment. This leads to economic and ecological instability and injustice, creating strife for most of humanity as the majority of the population is forced to focus on survival. Technologies like blockchain and renewable energies that are based on whole-system thinking exist, as well as basic-income economic models and plant-based lifestyles that can lead to social and economic sustainability. There are solutions to our global problems. What is needed is a shift in worldview and values so that people choose optimal life *for everyone*. This can only happen when more people transform and expand their identity from an ego-self to an eco-self. Psychological evolution is best explained as an expansion of identity, as one moves from egocentric to ethnocentric to worldcentric to kosmocentric, as noted by Ken Wilber, who has spent

---

[57] Beck and Cowan, *Spiral Dynamics*.

[58] Capra, *Web of Life*.

a lifetime focused on understanding and describing personal development.[59] Peter Russell, who coined the term *global brain* in his eponymous 1980s best seller, writes, "At the very basis of this high-synergy society would be a widespread shift in personal identity,"[60] and this comes from acknowledging our interdependence. Realization of our interconnection and foundational unity is deepened by psychedelic experiences that continuously reveal how our consciousness is interwoven with all life.

Terence McKenna proclaimed that what today's society needs most is an Archaic Revival—the integration of tribal values and shamanic technologies.[61] This means the integration of today's scientific rationality with the recognition of a living, evolving planet and cosmos. The philosopher Jean Gebser believed an integral worldview would arise once we integrate the past paradigms into humanity's current perspective.[62] From the lens of a living, interconnected planet that communicates information through chemical transmissions, we can finally make sense of the existence of psychedelics and why they generate such elegant and complex patterns of experience in our consciousness. As McKenna states, psilocybin might be part of the self-organizing processes of the larger Gaian holon:

> Psilocybin has a unique relationship to the evolution of the human nervous system. In fact, it turns the human nervous system into an antenna for the Gaian mind, assisting people to behave appropriately in the same way that termites behave appropriately within the morphogenetic field of their termite nest. If this antenna is not present in human beings, then human beings have to think up their own program, and it's usually power crazed, lethal, shortsighted, and grabby.[63]

---

[59] Wilber, *Integral Spirituality*.

[60] Russell, *Global Brain Awakens*, 277.

[61] T. McKenna, *Archaic Revival*.

[62] Gebser, *Ever-Present Origin*.

[63] T. McKenna, Sheldrake, and Abraham, *Chaos, Creativity, and Cosmic Consciousness*, 137.

By aligning humanity back with Earth's most powerful evolutionary processes that were responsible for the creation of our species, we may participate more actively in the self-organizing and self-generating dynamics of the planet. Even simply microdosing these Gaian molecules and integrating them into our diet may attune our mental antennae. This may allow one to become more sensitive and to receive more subtle information from ourselves, each other, and the environment that can that powerfully affects our feelings, thoughts, and intuition, and transform our lives.

As the psychologist Richard Miller shares:

> Looking back at the past half century, and reading what the scientists in this book have brought us, it is abundantly clear that the American public has been denied access to medicines having potential to change the course of human history.[64]

Historian Paul Devereux reaches a similar conclusion after researching humanity's psychedelic history:

> But however the legal authorities and the scientific establishment finally decide to conduct themselves, the Long Trip will not be halted. The Long Trip is an essential part of the journey of the human mind in its quest for its full expression, and will continue even if it meets opposition.[65]

The war on mind-expanding drugs like psilocybin is a war on both consciousness and evolution, as made clear by UCLA pharmacologist Ronald Siegel's work, which shows that most of the animal kingdom uses plants and fungi to alter consciousness; the behavior is so predominant that he calls the instinct to alter consciousness the fourth evolutionary drive (after food, sleep, and sex).[66] This resonates with the understanding

---

[64] Miller, *Psychedelic Medicine*, 2.

[65] Devereux, *Long Trip*, 257.

[66] Siegel, *Intoxication*.

that, after meeting the needs for autonomy and communion, the next evolutionary instinct is transcendence. Kotler and Wheal point out just how popular psychedelic use is in the United States:

> Thirty-two million Americans use psychedelics on a regular basis (that's nearly one in ten) and report considered reasons for doing so. According to a 2013 study published in a journal of the National Institutes of Health, the most common motivations are to "enhance mystical experiences, introspection and curiosity." Transcendence, not decadence, appears to be driving use forward.[67]

The percentage of people using psychedelics may only increase as society moves toward medical legalization and decriminalization.

The Decriminalize Nature initiative, which decriminalized natural psychedelics—peyote, san pedro, ayahuasca, iboga, and psilocybin mushrooms—in Oakland, California, has gone nationwide. I personally testified in Oakland's hearing, and it was eye-opening to see that the city council was so supportive. The science, personal testimonies, and rich history collected by the organization are available to make the case worldwide for the decriminalization and integration of psychedelics. Representatives of over a hundred cities in the United States have reached out to Decriminalize Nature to support local movements.[68] In 2020 the people of Oregon voted to legalize psilocybin-assisted psychotherapy and decriminalize possession of all psychoactive substances. In 2021 the proposal for decriminalization of psychedelics across the entire state of California was initiated by state senator Scott Wiener.

Humans have an inherent drive to learn and grow and will forever venture into the unknown. Psychedelics perpetually reveal to us unexplored frontiers to discover. These sacred medicines provide unparalleled healing and accelerated learning while catapulting us into the ever-unfolding process through the nature of Being. They provide not only

---

[67] Kotler and Wheal, *Stealing Fire*, 177.

[68] www.decriminalizenature.org/

occasions for contemplative explorations, as traditionally done through philosophy and religion, but also the possibility for deep, experiential excursions that expand our imagination to unfathomable destinations. The states they activate are just as natural as the fungi and plants that mediate them. Psychedelics conjure novelty, never-ending creativity, and experiences that may activate our sense of aesthetic splendor while potentially opening our eyes to solutions to today's crises.

Shortly after his one hundredth birthday, Albert Hofmann said:

> In the future, I hope that LSD provides to the individual a new world-view, which is in harmony with nature and its laws.
>
> I am hopeful about the future evolution of the human species. I am hopeful because I have the impression that more and more human individuals are becoming conscious, and that the creative human spirit, which we call "God," speaks to us through his creation—through the endlessness of the starry sky, through the beauty and wonder of the living individuals of the plant, the animal, and the human kingdoms.
>
> We humans are able to understand this message because we possess the divine gifts of consciousness. This connects us to the universal mind and gives us divine creativity. Any means that helps to expand our individual consciousness—by opening up and sharpening our inner and outer eyes, in order to understand the divine universal message—will help humanity to survive. An understanding of the divine message—in its universal language—would bring an end to the war between the religions of the world.[69]

Psilocybin, readily found throughout nature and with a chemical composition closely resembling LSD, is likely finally integrating itself back into culture through the medical establishment. As we have seen in examples throughout history, these medicines hold incomprehensible transformative potential for our species.

These medicines may be key to healing many of today's psycho-emotional illnesses, our rapidly expanding epidemics of anxiety and

---

[69] Hofmann, *LSD: My Problem Child*, ii.

depression that stem from our sense of isolation, stress, and distorted perception of reality and ourselves. Near-end-of-life studies have repeatedly shown that therapeutic use of psilocybin helps patients shed their deepest anxieties, supporting them in facing the unknown with courage and a deep sense of peace. The greater sense of belonging and unity that can also occur can perhaps galvanize humanity toward becoming harmonious warriors who protect and cherish our Gaian family. As climate change threatens the collapse of ecosystems, and our economic systems continue to become unstable and affect billions of people across the planet, psychedelics can conjure in us the necessary hope and vision to take action instead of drowning in despair.

Psychedelics can awaken humanity into standing on the threshold of its greatest realization—the homecoming of its origins and spiritual identity. Thomas Berry, a scholar of both religion and evolution, writes in *The Great Work: Our Way into the Future*: "The historical mission of our times is to reinvent the human—at the species level, with critical reflection, within the community of life-systems, in a time-developmental context, by means of story and shared dream experience."[70] Psychedelic experiences and their explanation of our human origins have the potential to play a central role in this new shared story. The past may be the portal into our future. By reclaiming what made us human, by reestablishing our relationship with these plants and fungi, we may become more of who we integrally are.

The acclaimed sociologist Robert Bellah points out, after fifty years of research, that "evolution . . . is the only shared metanarrative among educated people of all cultures that we have."[71] The shared evolutionary story of our psychedelic origins has the potential to further globally unite us in our identity and propel us into a collective intelligence whose imagination may grace us with a never-ending novelty that continually awakens us through its beauty. In depth psychology, the spiral

---

[70] Berry, *Great Work*, 159.

[71] Bellah, *Religion in Human Evolution*, 600.

symbolizes the re-evolution toward a higher consciousness, expanding on each revolution as it circles back onto itself.[72] May we circle back into our past and grasp the deeper nature of our existence, and in doing so transform our present moment. As expressed by Tool in their song "Lateralus": "Swing on the spiral of our divinity and still be a human . . . We'll ride the spiral to the end and may just go where no one's been. Spiral out, keep going!"[73]

---

[72] Arrien, *Signs of Life.*

[73] Tool, *Lateralus,* track 9.

BIBLIOGRAPHY

Abrams, M. H. (1971). *Natural Supernaturalism: Tradition and Revolution in Romantic Literature*. New York, NY: Norton & Company.

Adams, C., Luke, D., Waldstein, A., Sessa, B., & King, D. (Eds.). (2013). *Breaking Convention: Essays on Psychedelic Consciousness*. Berkeley, CA: North Atlantic Books.

Allegro, J. (1970). *The Sacred Mushroom and the Cross*. Garden City, NY: Doubleday & Company.

Allen, J. (1997). *Maria Sabina: Saint Mother of Wisdom*. Psilly Publications and Raver Books.

American Association for the Advancement of Science. (1999, March 22). "Flatworms Are Oldest Living Ancestors to Those of Us with Right and Left Sides." *ScienceDaily*. www.sciencedaily.com/releases/1999/03/990322062150.htm

Anderson, A. (2016, April 13). "LSD May Chip Away at the Brain's 'Sense of Self' Network: Brain Imaging Suggests LSD's Consciousness-Altering Traits May Work by Hindering Some Brain Networks and Boosting Overall Connectivity." *Scientific American*. www.scientificamerican.com/article/lsd-may-chip-away-at-the-brain-s-sense-of-self-network/

Archetypal View. (2019, December 13). "Psychedelic (R)evolution: Past, Present, Future—PCC Forum" [Video]. https://youtu.be/KV6_HJbKL4A

Arrien, A. (1998). *Signs of Life: The Five Universal Shapes and How to Use Them (Paperback ed.)*. New York, NY: Tarcher Perigee.

Arthur, J. (2000). *Mushrooms and Mankind: The Impact of Mushrooms on Human Consciousness and Religion*. San Diego, CA: Book Tree.

Ausubel, K. (2007). "Preface." In J. Harpignies (Ed.), *Visionary Plant Consciousness: The Shamanic Teachings of the Plant World*. Rochester, VT: Park Street Press.

Bache, C. M. (2000). *Dark Night, Early Dawn: Steps to a Deep Ecology of Mind*. Albany: State University of New York Press.

Bache, C. M. (2008). *The Living Classroom: Teaching and Collective Consciousness*. Albany: State University of New York Press.

Bache, C. M. (2019). *LSD and the Mind of the Universe: Diamonds from Heaven*. Rochester, VT: Park Street Press.

Badiner, A. H., & Grey, A. (Eds.). (2002). *Zig Zag Zen: Buddhism and Psychedelics.* San Francisco, CA: Chronicle Books.

Ball, M. W. (2006). *Mushroom Wisdom: Cultivating Spiritual Consciousness with Entheogens.* Berkeley, CA: Ronin Publishing.

Barnhart, R. J. (Producer), & Dauber, R. (Director). (2019). *A New Understanding: The Science of Psilocybin* [Documentary]. www.anewunderstanding.org

Bateson, G. (1972). *Steps to an Ecology of Mind: The New Information Sciences Can Lead to a New Understanding of Man.* New York, NY: Ballantine Books.

Beach, H. (1996). "Listening for the Logos: A Study of Reports of Audible Voices at High Doses of Psilocybin." *Newsletter of the Multidisciplinary Association for Psychedelic Studies (MAPS)*, 7(1), 12–17. https://maps.org/news-letters/v07n1/07112bea.html

Beck, D., & Cowan, C. C. (1996). *Spiral Dynamics: Mastering Values, Leadership, and Change.* Cambridge, MA: Blackwell Business.

Bellah, R. (2011). *Religion in Human Evolution: From the Paleolithic to the Axial Age.* Cambridge, MA: Belknap Press of Harvard University Press.

Bergson, H. (1991). *Matter and Memory* (N. M. Paul & W. S. Palmer, Trans.). New York, NY: Zone Books.

Berry, T. (1999). *The Great Work: Our Way into the Future.* New York, NY: Bell Tower.

Berson, J. (2019). *The Meat Question: Animals, Humans, and the Deep History of Food.* Cambridge, MA: MIT Press.

Block, P. (2008). *Community: The Structure of Belonging.* San Francisco, CA: Berrett-Koehler.

Blockchain Council. (2019). "What Is Blockchain and How Does It Work?" www.blockchain-council.org/Blockchain/What-is-Blockchain-Technology-and-How-Does-It-Work

Bloom, H. (2001). *Global Brain: The Evolution of Mass Mind from the Big Bang to the 21st Century.* New York, NY: John Wiley and Sons.

Bourzat, F., & Hunter, K. (2019). *Consciousness Medicine: Indigenous Wisdom, Entheogens, and Expanded States of Consciousness for Healing and Growth.* Berkeley, CA: North Atlantic Books.

Brown, D. (2013). *The New Science of Psychedelics: At the Nexus of Culture, Consciousness, and Spirituality.* Rochester, VT: Park Street Press.

Brown, D., & Hill, R. (2018). *Women of Visionary Art.* Rochester, VT: Park Street Press.

Brown, J., & Brown, J. (2016). *The Psychedelic Gospels: The Secret History of Hallucinogens in Christianity.* Rochester, VT: Park Street Press.

Brown, M. (2004). "Dark Side of the Shaman." In J. Narby & F. Huxley (Eds.), *Shamans through Time: 500 Years on the Path to Knowledge* (pp. 251–256). New York, NY: Jeremy P. Tarcher/Penguin Books.

Browne, B. (2021). "Bitcoin Spikes 20% after Elon Musk Adds #Bitcoin to His Twitter Bio." CNBC. www.cnbc.com/2021/01/29/bitcoin-spikes-20percent-after-elon-musk-adds-bitcoin-to-his-twitter-bio.html

Buhner, S. H. (2014). *Plant Intelligence and the Imaginal Realm*. Rochester, VT: Bear & Company.

Buller, K., & Moore, J. (2018). *Navigating Psychedelics: Trip Journal*. Psychedelics Today.

Buller, K., & Moore, J. (2019). *Integration Workbook: Planting Seeds for Growth and Change*. Psychedelics Today.

Burns, J. (2018, June 7). "Study: Men Who Tried Psychedelics Are Less Likely to Be Violent toward Their Partners." *Forbes*. www.forbes.com/sites/janetwburns/2018/06/07/study-men-who-tried-psychedelics-are-less-likely-to-be-violent-toward-partners/

Cameron, J. (Director & Producer). (2009). *Avatar* [Motion picture]. 20th Century Fox, Lightstorm Entertainment.

Campbell, J. (Ed.). (1971). *The Portable Jung*. Harmondsworth, England: Penguin Books.

Capra, F. (1996). *The Web of Life: A New Scientific Understanding of Living Systems*. New York, NY: Bantam Doubleday Dell.

Capra, F. (2002). *The Hidden Connections: Integrating the Biological, Cognitive, and Social Dimensions of Life into a Science of Sustainability*. New York, NY: Doubleday.

Capra, F., & Luisi, P. L. (2014). *The Systems View of Life: A Unifying Vision*. Cambridge, England: Cambridge University Press.

Carhart-Harris, R. L., & Nutt, D. J. (2017). "Serotonin and Brain Function: A Tale of Two Receptors." *Journal of Psychopharmacology, 31*(9), 1091–1120. https://doi.org/10.1177/0269881117725915

Carhart-Harris, R. L., Roseman, L., Bolstridge, M., Demetriou, L., Pannekeok, J. N., Wall, M. B., Tanner, M., Kaelen, M., McGonigle, J., Murphy, K., Leech, R., Curran, H. V., & Nutt, D. J. (2017). "Psilocybin for Treatment-Resistant Depression: fMRI-Measured Brain Mechanisms." *Scientific Reports, 7*, Article 13187. https://doi.org/10.1038/s41598-017-13282-7

Caruana, L. (2010). *The First Manifesto of Visionary Art*. Paris, France: Recluse Publishing.

Casey, M. J., & Vigna, P. (2018). *The Truth Machine: The Blockchain and the Future of Everything*. New York, NY: St. Martin's Press.

Casimiro, J. N. (2007, January 1). "Doña Julia Julieta Casimiro." BOMB. https://bombmagazine.org/articles/do%C3%B1a-julia-julieta-casimiro/

Chalmers, D. J. (Ed.). (2002). *Philosophy of Mind: Classical and Contemporary Readings*. Oxford, England: Oxford University Press.

Cheung, T. (2018, August 22). "COMPASS Pathways Receives FDA Approval for Psilocybin Therapy Clinical Trial for Treatment-Resistant Depression." [Press release]. www.prnewswire.com/news-releases/compass-pathways-receives -fda-approval-for-psilocybin-therapy-clinical-trial-for-treatment-resistant -depression-868824616.html

Chu, B. (2018, January 5). "Global Debt: Why Has It Hit an All-Time High? And How Worried Should We Be about It?" *Independent*. www.independent .co.uk/news/business/analysis-and-features/global-debt-crisis-explained-all -time-high-world-economy-causes-solutions-definition-a8143516.html

Cooper, J., & Hutchinson, D. S. (Eds.). (1997). *Plato: Complete Works* (p. 1089). [The Republic, Book 5, 462 C]. Indianapolis, IN: Hackett Publishing. (Original work published ca. 375 BCE)

Cormier, Z. (2016, April 11). "Brain Scans Reveal How LSD Affects Consciousness." *Nature*. http://www.nature.com/news/brain-scans-reveal-how-lsd-affects -consciousness-1.19727

CryptoPsychedelic Flashback. "Live Roundtable/Q&A #1: Psychedelic Research & Advocacy" [Video]. www.crowdcast.io/e/cryptopsychedelic/4

Danforth, A. L., Grob, C. S., Struble, C., Feduccia, A. A., Walker, N., Jerome, L., Yazar-Klosinski, B., & Emerson, A. (2018). "Reduction in Social Anxiety after MDMA-Assisted Psychotherapy with Autistic Adults: A Randomized, Double-Blind, Placebo-Controlled Pilot Study." *Psychopharmacology*, *235*(11), 3137–3148. https://doi.org/10.1007/s00213-018-5010-9

Darwin, C. (2004). *The Descent of Man*. New York, NY: Penguin Putnam. (Original work published 1871)

Dass, R. (1971). *Be Here Now*. New York, NY: Crown Publishing Group.

Dawkins, R. (1976). *The Selfish Gene*. Oxford, England: Oxford University Press.

de Borhegyi, C., & de Borhegyi-Forrest, S. (2013). "The Genesis of a Mushroom/ Venus Religion in Mesoamerica." In J. A. Rush (Ed.), *Entheogens and the Development of Culture: The Anthropology and Neurobiology of Ecstatic Experience* (pp. 451–484). Berkeley, CA: North Atlantic Books.

de Laszlo, V. S. (Ed.). (1959). *The Basic Writings of C. G. Jung*. New York, NY: Random House.

DeKorne, J. (2011). *Psychedelic Shamanism: The Cultivation, Preparation, and Shamanic Use of Psychotropic Plants*. New York, NY: Penguin Books.

Descartes, R. (1993). *Discourse on Method and Meditations on First Philosophy*. (D. A. Cress, Trans., 3rd ed.). Indianapolis, IN: Hackett Publishing. (Original works published 16th century)

Devereux, P. (1997). *The Long Trip: A Prehistory of Psychedelia*. New York, NY: Penguin Books.

Doblin, R. (2005). "A Note on Current Psilocybin Research Projects." In R. Metzner, (Ed.), *Sacred Mushroom of Visions: Teonanácatl* (pp. 157–159). Rochester, VT: Four Trees Press.

Doblin, R. (2017). "The Science of the Sacred." In R. L. Miller (Ed.), *Psychedelic Medicine: The Healing Powers of LSD, MDMA, Psilocybin, and Ayahuasca* (pp. 179–186). Rochester, VT: Park Street Press.

Doblin, R., & Burge, B. (Eds). (2014). *Manifesting Minds: An Anthology from the Multidisciplinary Association for Psychedelic Studies: A Review of Psychedelics in Science, Medicine, Sex, and Spirituality*. Berkeley, CA: Evolver Editions.

Doyle, R. M. (2011). *Darwin's Pharmacy: Sex, Plants, and the Evolution of the Noösphere*. Seattle: University of Washington Press.

Dunbar, R. (1998). *Grooming, Gossip, and the Evolution of Language*. Cambridge, MA: Harvard University Press.

Evasius. (2012, January 17). "Terence McKenna—The Strange Attractor" [Video]. www.youtube.com/watch?v=Cget6JxSpfQ

Fadiman, J. (2011). *The Psychedelic Explorer's Guide: Safe, Therapeutic, and Sacred Journeys*. Rochester, VT: Park Street Press.

Feilding, A. (2017). "Psilocybin and Depression." In R. L. Miller (Ed.), *Psychedelic Medicine: The Healing Powers of LSD, MDMA, Psilocybin, and Ayahuasca* (pp. 160–165). Rochester, VT: Park Street Press.

Flatow, I. (Host). (2018). "Consciousness, Chemically-Altered." *Science Friday*. www.ScienceFriday.com/Segments/Consciousness-Chemically-Altered

Forte, R. (Ed.). (2012). *Entheogens and the Future of Religion* (Reprint ed.). Rochester, VT: Inner Traditions.

Freud, S. (1998). *The Basic Writings of Sigmund Freud* (A. A. Brill, Ed. & Trans.). New York, NY: Random House. (Original work published 1938)

Froese, T. (2013). "Altered States and the Prehistoric Ritualization of the Modern Human Mind." In C. Adams, D. Luke, A. Waldstein, B. Sessa, & D. King (Eds.), *Breaking Convention: Essays on Psychedelic Consciousness* (pp. 1–12). Berkeley, CA: North Atlantic Books.

G. F. (2018, July 9). "Why Bitcoin Uses So Much Energy." *The Economist*. www
.economist.com/the-economist-explains/2018/07/09/why-bitcoin-uses-so
-much-energy

Galeon, D. (2017). "Universal Basic Income Could Become a Reality, Thanks
to This Technology" Futurism. https://futurism.com/1-evergreen-the-best-
currency-for-a-universal-basic-income-could-be-digital

Gebser, J. (1986). *The Ever-Present Origin* (N. Barstad & A. Mickunas, Trans.).
Athens: Ohio University Press.

Ghose, T. (2014, October 24). "Magic Mushrooms Create a Hyperconnected
Brain." Live Science. www.livescience.com/48502-magic-mushrooms
-change-brain-networks.html

Gladwell, M. (2002). *The Tipping Point: How Little Things Can Make a Big Difference*. New York, NY: Little, Brown.

Goldsmith, N. (2010). *Psychedelic Healing: The Promise of Entheogens for Psychotherapy and Spiritual Development*. Rochester, VT: Healing Arts Press.

Graves, S., & Philips, D. (2021, July 16). "The 10 Public Companies with the Biggest
Bitcoin Portfolios." Decrypt. https://decrypt.co/47061/8-public-companies
-biggest-bitcoin-portfolios

Grey, A. (1990). *Sacred Mirrors: The Visionary Art of Alex Grey*. Rochester, VT:
Inner Traditions.

Grey, A. (1998). *The Mission of Art*. Boston, MA: Shambhala.

Grey, A. (2001). *Transfigurations*. Rochester, VT: Inner Traditions.

Grey, A. (2012). *Net of Being*. Rochester, VT: Inner Traditions.

Grey, A. (2015). "Foreword: Visionary Language." In D. R. Slattery, *Xenolinguistics: Psychedelics, Language, and the Evolution of Consciousness*. Berkeley, CA:
Evolver Editions.

Griffiths, R., & MacLean, K. (2017). "Spiritual Psychopharmacology." In R. L.
Miller (Ed.), *Psychedelic Medicine: The Healing Powers of LSD, MDMA, Psilocybin, and Ayahuasca* (pp. 139–153). Rochester, VT: Park Street Press.

Griffiths, R., Richards, W., McCann, U., & Jesse, R. (2006). "Psilocybin Can
Occasion Mystical-Type Experiences Having Substantial and Sustained Personal Meaning and Spiritual Significance." *Psychopharmacology*, *187*(3), 268–
283. https://doi.org/10.1007/s00213-006-0457-5, www.hopkinsmedicine
.org/press_releases/2006/griffithspsilocybin.pdf

Grob, C. (2017). "Seeking Solace for the Terminally Ill." In R. L. Miller (Ed.),
*Psychedelic Medicine: The Healing Powers of LSD, MDMA, Psilocybin, and Aya-
huasca* (pp. 154–159). Rochester, VT: Park Street Press.

Grof, S. (1985). *Beyond the Brain: Birth, Death and Transcendence in Psychotherapy.* Albany: State University of New York Press.

Grof, S. (1998). *The Cosmic Game: Explorations of the Frontiers of Human Consciousness.* Albany: State University of New York Press.

Grof, S. (2000). *Psychology of the Future: Lessons from Modern Consciousness Research.* Albany: State University of New York Press.

Grof, S. (2006). *When the Impossible Happens: Adventures in Non-Ordinary Realities.* Boulder, CA: Sounds True.

Grof, S. (2010). *The Ultimate Journey: Consciousness and the Mystery of Death.* Santa Cruz, CA: Multidisciplinary Association for Psychedelic Studies.

Grof, S. (2015). *Modern Consciousness Research and the Understanding of Art, Including the Visionary World of H. R. Giger.* Santa Cruz, CA: Multidisciplinary Association for Psychedelic Studies.

Grof, S. (2017). "Observations from 4,000 LSD Sessions." In R. L. Miller (Ed.), *Psychedelic Medicine: The Healing Powers of LSD, MDMA, Psilocybin, and Ayahuasca* (pp. 45–54). Rochester, VT: Park Street Press.

Grof, S. (2019). *The Way of the Psychonaut, Vol. 1: Encyclopedia for Inner Journeys.* Santa Cruz, CA: Multidisciplinary Association for Psychedelic Studies.

Grof, S. (2019). *The Way of the Psychonaut, Vol. 2: Encyclopedia for Inner Journeys.* Santa Cruz, CA: Multidisciplinary Association for Psychedelic Studies.

Gupta, S. (2020). "From Exclusion to Empowerment: How Crypto Could Hold Key to Financial Inclusion." Nasdaq. www.nasdaq.com/articles/from-exclusion-to-empowerment%3A-how-crypto-could-hold-key-to-financial-inclusion-2020-01-07

Hancock, G. (2015). *The Divine Spark: Psychedelics, Consciousness, and the Birth of Civilization.* San Francisco, CA: Disinformation Books.

Harari, Y. N. (2014). *Sapiens: A Brief History of Humankind.* New York, NY: Harper.

Harner, M. J. (Ed.). (1973). *Hallucinogens and Shamanism.* Oxford, England: Oxford University Press.

Harpignies, J. (Ed.). (2007). *Visionary Plant Consciousness: The Shamanic Teachings of the Plant World.* Rochester, VT: Park Street Press.

Harrison, K., Straight, J., Pendell, D., & Stamets, P. (2007). "Plant Spirit." In J. Harpignies (Ed.), *Visionary Plant Consciousness: The Shamanic Teachings of the Plant World.* Rochester, VT: Park Street Press.

Hartman, S. (2018, November 9). "Psilocybin Could Be Legal for Therapy by 2021." *Rolling Stone.* www.rollingstone.com/culture/culture-news/psilocybin-legal-therapy-mdma-753946/

Hawks, J. (2013, July 1). "How Has the Human Brain Evolved?" *Scientific American*. www.scientificamerican.com/article/how-has-human-brain-evolved/

Hendrix, H. (1988). *Getting the Love That You Want: A Guide for Couples*. Franklin, TN: Clovercroft.

Henriques, M. (2017, September 15). "Two Parents' Fight to Set up the Largest Ever Magic Mushroom Trial for Depression Is Nearly Over." *International Business Times*. www.ibtimes.co.uk/two-parents-fight-set-largest-ever-magic -mushroom-trial-depression-nearly-over-1639438

Hicks, B. (1997). *Rant in E-Minor* [Album]. Rykodisc.

Hill, S. (2013). *Confrontations with the Unconscious: Jungian Depth Psychology and Psychedelic Experience*. London, England: Muswell Hill Press.

Hofmann, A. (2009). *LSD: My Problem Child: Reflections on Sacred Drugs, Mysticism and Science*. Santa Cruz, CA: Multidisciplinary Association for Psychedelic Studies.

Holland, J. (Ed.). (2001). *Ecstasy: The Complete Guide: A Comprehensive Look at the Risks and Benefits of MDMA*. Rochester, VT: Park Street Press.

House of Representatives. (2018). *The 2018 Joint Economic Report* (Report 115-596). Washington, DC: U.S. Printing Office. www.congress.gov/115/crpt /hrpt596/CRPT-115hrpt596.pdf

Hume, D. (2007). *An Enquiry Concerning Human Understanding* (P. Millican, Ed.). Oxford, England: Oxford University Press.

Huxley, A. (1945). *The Perennial Philosophy*. New York, NY: Harper & Row.

Ito, J., Narula, N., & Ali, R. (2017, March 8). "The Blockchain Will Do to the Financial System What the Internet Did to Media." *Harvard Business Review*. https://hbr.org/2017/03/the-blockchain-will-do-to-banks-and-law-firms -what-the-internet-did-to-media

Jackson, R. (2012). *Occupy World Street: A Global Roadmap for Radical Economic and Political Reform*. Richmond, VT: Chelsea Green Publishing.

Jensen, S., & Keenan, M. (2016). *A Perfect Union of Contrary Things*. Milwaukee, WI: Backbeat Books.

Jesso, J. W. (2013). *Decomposing the Shadow: Lessons from the Psilocybin Mushroom*. Calgary, AB: Soulslantern Publishing.

Jones, A. (2018, May 25). "The Future of Art" [Lecture]. Talk delivered at Lightning in a Bottle Festival, Bradley, CA.

Jones, A. (2020). "Artist Statement." https://androidjones.com/about/statement/

Kegan, R. (1983). *The Evolving Self: Problem and Process in Human Development* (13th ed.). Cambridge, MA: Harvard University Press.

Keim, B. (2014, October 30). "How Magic Mushrooms Rearrange Your Brain." *Wired*. www.wired.com/2014/10/magic-mushroom-brain/

Kelly, S. (2010). *Coming Home: The Birth and Transformation of the Planetary Era*. Great Barrington, MA: Lindisfarne Books.

Kennedy, D. (2014). *Plants and the Human Brain*. New York, NY: Oxford University Press.

Kent, J. L. (2010). *Psychedelic Information Theory: Shamanism in the Age of Reason*. CreateSpace Independent Publishing Platform.

Khamsehzadeh, J. (2021) "CryptoPsychedelic Conferences Examine Links between Psychedelics and Blockchain Technology." Lucid News. www.lucid .news/cryptopsychedelic-conferences-examine-links-between-psychedelics -and-blockchain-technology/

Klein J. (2018, September 20). "On Ecstasy, Octopuses Reached Out for a Hug." *New York Times*. www.nytimes.com/2018/09/20/science/octopus-ecstasy -mdma.html

Koestler, A. (1967). *The Ghost in the Machine*. London, England: Hutchinson & Co.

Kotler, S., & Wheal, J. (2017). *Stealing Fire: How Silicon Valley, the Navy SEALs, and Maverick Scientists Are Revolutionizing the Way We Live and Work*. New York, NY: HarperCollins.

Krippner, S. (2017, March 1). "Salvador Roquet Remembered: An Innovative Psychedelic Therapist in 1960s Mexico." Chacruna. https://chacruna.net /salvador-roquet-remembered/

Krippner, S., & Luke, D. (2014). "Psychedelics and Species Connectedness." In R. Doblin & B. Burge (Eds), *Manifesting Minds: An Anthology from the Multidisciplinary Association for Psychedelic Studies: A Review of Psychedelics in Science, Medicine, Sex, and Spirituality*. Berkeley, CA: Evolver Editions.

Kurzweil, R. (2005). *The Singularity Is Near: When Humans Transcend Biology*. New York, NY: Penguin Books.

Lake, G. (2020). *Psychedelics in Mental Health Series: Psilocybin*. Self-published.

Lake, G. (2020). *The Law of Entheogenic Churches in the United States*. Self-published.

Lakoff, G., & Johnson, M. (1980). *Metaphors We Live By*. Chicago, IL: The University of Chicago Press.

Lakoff, G., & Johnson, M. (1999). *Philosophy in the Flesh: The Embodied Mind and Its Challenge to Western Thought*. New York, NY: Basic Books.

Lane, T. (2018). *Sacred Mushroom Rituals: The Search for the Blood of Quetzalcoatl*. Gainesville, FL: SolarWolf Publications.

Lansiti, M., & Lakhani, K. (2017, January–February). "The Truth about Blockchain: It Will Take Years to Transform Business, but the Journey Begins Now." *Harvard Business Review*. https://hbr.org/2017/01/the-truth-about-blockchain

Laszlo, E. (1972). *The Systems View of the World*. New York, NY: George Braziller.

Leary, T. (2005). "The Initiation of the "High Priest." In R. Metzner (Ed.), *Sacred Mushroom of Visions: Teonanácatl* (pp. 160–178). Rochester, VT: Four Trees Press.

Letcher, A. (2007). *Shroom: A Cultural History of the Magic Mushroom*. New York, NY: HarperCollins.

Levine, A., & Heller, R. S. F. (2012). *Attached: The New Science of Adult Attachment*. New York, NY: Tarcher Perigee.

Lewis-Williams, D. (2004). *The Mind in the Cave: Consciousness and the Origins of Art*. New York, NY: Thames and Hudson.

Lewis-Williams, D. (2010). *Conceiving God: The Cognitive Origin and Evolution of Religion*. New York, NY: Thames and Hudson.

Lieberman, D., & Long, M. (2018). *The Molecule of More: How a Single Chemical in Your Brain Drives Love, Sex, and Creativity—and Will Determine the Fate of the Human Race*. Dallas, TX: BenBella Books.

Lilly, J. C. (1997). *The Scientist: A Metaphysical Autobiography*. Berkeley, CA: Ronin Publishing.

Lipton, B. (2005). *The Biology of Belief*. Santa Rosa, CA: Mountain of Love/Elite Books.

Lobo, I. (2008). "Biological Complexity and Integrative Levels of Organization." *Nature Education*. www.nature.com/scitable/topicpage/biological-complexity-and-integrative-levels-of-organization-468/

Locke, J. (1993). *An Essay Concerning Human Understanding*. London, England: Dent.

Lovejoy, A. O. (1976). *The Great Chain of Being: A Study of the History of an Idea*. Cambridge, MA: Harvard University Press.

Lovelock, J. (1995). *The Ages of Gaia: A Biography of Our Living Earth*. New York, NY: W. W. Norton & Co.

Lovely, G. (2019, January–February). "Make America Trip Again." *Current Affairs*. www.currentaffairs.org/2019/04/make-america-trip-again

Luna, L. E. (2013). "Towards an Exploration of the Mind of a Conquered Continent: Shamanism, Sacred Plants and Amerindian Epistemology." In C. Adams, D. Luke, A. Waldstein, B. Sessa, & D. King (Eds.), *Breaking Convention: Essays on Psychedelic Consciousness* (pp. 13–29). Berkeley, CA: North Atlantic Books.

Ly, C., Greb, A. C., Cameron, L. P., Ori-McKenney, K. M., Gray, J. A., & Olson, D. E. (2018, June 12). "Psychedelics Promote Structural and Functional Neural Plasticity." *Cell Reports, 23*(11), 3170–3182. https://doi.org/10.1016 /j.celrep.2018.05.022

MAPS. (2017, May 11). "Paul Stamets: Psilocybin Mushrooms & the Mycology of Consciousness" [Video]. www.youtube.com/watch?v=vFWxWq0Fv0U.

Margulis, L. (1998). *Symbiotic Planet: A New Look at Evolution.* New York, NY: Basic Books.

Markoff, J. (2005). *What the Dormouse Said: How the Sixties Counterculture Shaped the Personal Computer Industry.* New York, NY: Penguin Books.

Maslow, A. H. (1962). *Toward a Psychology of Being.* Princeton, NJ: Insight Books.

Maslow, A. H. (1971). *The Farther Reaches of Human Nature.* New York, NY: Penguin

Maslow, A. H. (2013). *A Theory of Human Motivation.* Mansfield, CT: Martino Publishing.

Mason, N. L., Mischler, E., Uthaug, M. V., & Kuypers, K. P. C. (2019). "Sub-Acute Effects of Psilocybin on Empathy, Creative Thinking, and Subjective Well-Being." *Journal of Psychoactive Drugs, 51*(2), 123–134. https://doi.org/1 0.1080/02791072.2019.1580804

Masters, R. E. L., & Houston, J. (1966). *The Varieties of Psychedelic Experience.* New York, NY: Dell Publishing Co.

Maté, G. (1999). *Scattered: How Attention Deficit Disorder Originates and What You Can Do about It.* New York, NY: Dutton.

Maté, G. (2008). *In the Realm of Hungry Ghosts: Close Encounters with Addiction.* Toronto, ON: Knopf Canada.

Mauss, S. (Writer), & Bellinkoff, B. (Director). (2018). *Psychonautics: A Comic's Exploration of Psychedelics* [Documentary]. Gravitas Ventures. www .psychonauticsfilm.com

McAuliffe, K. (2011, January 19). "If Modern Humans Are So Smart, Why Are Our Brains Shrinking?" *Discover.* www.discovermagazine.com/the-sciences /if-modern-humans-are-so-smart-why-are-our-brains-shrinking

McIntosh, S. (2007). *Integral Consciousness and the Future of Evolution: How the Integral Worldview Is Transforming Politics, Culture, and Spirituality.* St. Paul, MN: Paragon House Publishers.

McIntosh, S. (2012). *Evolution's Purpose: An Integral Interpretation of the Scientific Story of Our Origins.* New York, NY: Select Books.

McKenna, D. (2014). "Foreword." In T. Wright & G. Gynn, *Return to the Brain of Eden: Restoring the Connection between Neurochemistry and Consciousness.* Rochester, VT: Bear & Company.

McKenna, D. (2015). "Reflections in a Rear-View Mirror: Speculations on Novelty Theory and the End Times." In G. Hancock (Ed.), *The Divine Spark: Psychedelics, Consciousness, and the Birth of Civilization*. San Francisco, CA: Disinformation Books.

McKenna, D. (2019). "Of Apes and Men." In Stamets, P. (Ed.), *Fantastic Fungi: How Mushrooms Can Heal, Shift Consciousness, and Save the Planet*. San Rafael, CA: Earth Aware.

McKenna, D., McKenna, T., & Davis, W. (2007). "Plant Messengers: Science, Culture, and Visionary Plants." In J. Harpignies (Ed.), *Visionary Plant Consciousness: The Shamanic Teachings of the Plant World* (pp. 63–74). Rochester, VT: Park Street Press.

McKenna, T. (1991). *The Archaic Revival*. New York, NY: HarperCollins Publishers.

McKenna, T. (1992). *Food of the Gods: The Search for the Original Tree of Knowledge: A Radical History of Plants, Drugs, and Human Evolution*. New York, NY: Bantam Books.

McKenna, T. (1993). *True Hallucinations: Being an Account of the Author's Extraordinary Adventures in the Devil's Paradise*. New York, NY: HarperCollins Publishers.

McKenna, T., & McKenna, D. (1993). *The Invisible Landscape: Mind, Hallucinogens, and the I Ching*. New York, NY: HarperCollins Publishers.

McKenna, T., Sheldrake, R., & Abraham, R. (2001). *Chaos, Creativity, and Cosmic Consciousness* (2nd ed.). New York, NY: Parker Street Press.

McKenna, T., Sheldrake, R., & Abraham, R. (2005). *The Evolutionary Mind: Conversations on Science, Imagination & Spirit* (2nd ed.). New York, NY: Parker Street Press.

Meadows, D. H. (2009). *Thinking in Systems: A Primer*. Sterling, VA: Earthscan.

Melchizedek, D. (1990). *The Ancient Secret of the Flower of Life*. Flagstaff, AZ: Light Technology Publishing.

Mesle, R. (2008). *Process-Relational Philosophy: An Introduction to Alfred North Whitehead*. West Conshohocken, PA: Templeton Foundation Press.

Messemaker, M. (2017). *Five Dried Grams: A Graphic Novelty Meme*. Utrecht, Netherlands: Drukkerij Libertas Pascal.

Metz, R. (2019, July 20). "Elon Musk Hopes to Put a Computer Chip in Your Brain. Who Wants One?" CNN. www.cnn.com/2019/07/20/tech/elon-musk-neuralink-brain-chip-experts/index.html

Metzner, R. (Ed.). (2005). *Sacred Mushroom of Visions: Teonanácatl*. Rochester, VT: Four Trees Press.

Metzner, R. (2015). *Allies for Awakening: Guidelines for Productive and Safe Experiences with Entheogens.* Berkeley, CA: Regent Press.

Miller, R. L. (Ed.). (2017). *Psychedelic Medicine: The Healing Powers of LSD, MDMA, Psilocybin, and Ayahuasca.* Rochester, VT: Park Street Press.

Montgomery, B. (2002). "Foreword: Evolution through Inebriation?" In G. Samorini, *Animals and Psychedelics: The Natural World and the Instinct to Alter Consciousness.* Rochester, VT: Inner Traditions/Park Street Press.

Moreno, F. A., Wiegand, C. B., Taitano, E. K., & Delgado, P. L. (2006). "Safety, Tolerability, and Efficacy of Psilocybin in 9 Patients with Obsessive-Compulsive Disorder." *Journal of Clinical Psychiatry, 67*(11), 1735–1740. https://doi.org/10.4088/jcp.v67n1110

Morgan, E. (1990). *The Scars of Evolution. What Our Bodies Tell Us about Human Origins.* New York, NY: Oxford University Press.

Mulligan, C. (2021). "Blockchain and Sustainable Growth." United Nations. www.un.org/en/un-chronicle/blockchain-and-sustainable-growth

Multidisciplinary Association for Psychedelic Studies. (2021, May 3). "MAPS' Phase 3 Trial of MDMA-Assisted Therapy for PTSD Achieves Successful Results for Patients with Severe, Chronic PTSD." https://maps.org /news/media/9122-maps-phase-3-trial-of-mdma-assisted-therapy-for-ptsd -achieves-successful-results-for-patients-with-severe-chronic-ptsd

Munn, H. (1973). "The Mushrooms of Language." In M. J. Harner (Ed.), *Hallucinogens and Shamanism.* Oxford, United Kingdom: Oxford University Press.

Muraresku, B. (2020). *The Immortality Key: The Secret History of the Religion with No Name.* New York, NY: St. Martin's Press.

Nadeau, R. L. (2006). *The Environmental Endgame: Mainstream Economics, Ecological Disaster, and Human Survival.* Piscataway, NJ: Rutgers University Press.

Narby, J. (2000). *The Cosmic Serpent: DNA and the Origins of Knowledge.* New York, NY: Jeremy P. Tarcher/Putnam.

Narby, J. (2005). *Intelligence in Nature: An Inquiry into Knowledge.* New York, NY: Penguin Books.

Narby, J., & Huxley, F. (Eds.). (2001). *Shamans through Time: 500 Years on the Path to Knowledge.* New York, NY: Penguin Books.

Noujaim, J., & Amer, K. (Producers & Directors). (2019). *The Great Hack* [Motion picture]. Netflix.

Nour, M., Evans, L., & Carhart-Harris, R. (2017). "Psychedelics, Personality and Political Perspectives." *Journal of Psychoactive Drugs, 49*(3), 1–10. https://doi .org/10.1080/02791072.2017.1312643

Oak, A. (2019). "Creating a Community of Wise Women: The Women's Visionary Congress." In M. Papaspyrou, C. Baldini, & D. Luke (Eds.), *Psychedelic Mysteries of the Feminine*. Rochester, VT: Park Street Press.

O'Brien, E. (Ed.). (1964). *The Essential Plotinus*. Indianapolis, IN: Hackett Publications.

Oroc, J. (2018). *The New Psychedelic Revolution: The Genesis of the Visionary Age*. Rochester, VT: Park Street Press.

Orsini, A. P. (2019). *Autism on Acid: How LSD Helped Me Understand, Navigate, Alter, and Appreciate My Autistic Perceptions*. Self-published.

Ortigo, K. (2021). *Beyond the Narrow Life: A Guide for Psychedelic Integration and Existential Exploration*. Santa Fe, NM: Synergetic Press.

Orwell, G. (1989). *1984*. London: Penguin Books. (Original work published 1949).

Oss, O. T., & Oeric, O. N. (1976). *Psilocybin Magic Mushroom Grower's Guide*. Oakland, CA: Quick American Publishing.

Oswald, M. (Director). (2012). *97% Owned* [Documentary]. Queuepolitely.

Ott, E. (2001). "Shamans and Ethics in a Global World." In J. Narby & F. Huxley (Eds.), *Shamans through Time: 500 Years on the Path to Knowledge*. New York, NY: Penguin Books.

Passie, T. (2005). "A History of the Use of Psilocybin in Psychotherapy." In R. Metzner (Ed.), *Sacred Mushroom of Visions: Teonanácatl: A Sourcebook on the Psilocybin Mushroom* (pp. 113–138). Rochester, VT: Park Street Press.

Pearson, A. (2011, May 4) "Out-of-Africa Migration Selected Novelty-Seeking Genes." *New Scientist*. www.newscientist.com/article/mg21028114 -400-out-of-africa-migration-selected-novelty-seeking-genes/

Petrovich, A. (2001). "The Shaman: A Villain of a Magician Who Calls Demons." In J. Narby & F. Huxley (Eds.), *Shamans through Time: 500 Years on the Path to Knowledge*. New York, NY: Penguin Books.

Pine. (2018, Winter). "Bitcoin, Ketamine, and Pineapples: Why I Donated $5 Million in Bitcoin to MAPS." *MAPS Bulletin,28*(3),36–37.https://maps.org /news/bulletin/articles/435-maps-bulletin-winter-2018-vol-28-no-3/7517 -bitcoin,-ketamine,-and-pineapples-why-i-donated-$5-million-in-bitcoin -to-maps-winter-2018

Pokorny T., Preller K. H., Kometer M., Dziobek I., & Vollenweider, F. X. (2017, September 1). "Effect of Psilocybin on Empathy and Moral Decision-Making." *International Journal of Neuropsychopharmacology, 20*(9), 747–757. https://doi.org/10.1093/ijnp/pyx047

Pollan, M. (2002). *The Botany of Desire: A Plant's-Eye View of the World*. New York, NY: Random House.

Pollan, M. (2018). *How to Change Your Mind: What the New Science of Psychedelics Teaches Us about Consciousness, Dying, Addiction, Depression, and Transcendence.* New York, NY: Penguin Press.

Pollan, M., & Davis, W. (2007). "The Garden of the Wild—Plants and Humans. Who's Domesticating Who?" In J. Harpignies (Ed.), *Visionary Plant Consciousness.* Rochester, VT: Park Street Press.

Powell, S. G. (2011). *The Psilocybin Solution: The Role of Sacred Mushrooms in the Quest for Meaning.* Rochester, VT: Park Street Press.

Powell, S. G. (2015). *Magic Mushroom Explorer: Psilocybin and the Awakening Earth.* Rochester, VT: Park Street Press.

Prestie, D., & Nichols, D. (2005). "Biochemistry and Neuropharmacology of Psilocybin Mushrooms." In R. Metzner (Ed.), *Sacred Mushroom of Visions: Teonanácatl: A Sourcebook on the Psilocybin Mushroom* (pp. 93–112). Rochester, VT: Park Street Press.

Prochazkova, L., Lippelt, D. P., Colzato, L. S., Kuchar, M., Sjoerds, Z., & Hommel, B. (2018). "Exploring the Effect of Microdosing Psychedelics on Creativity in an Open-Label Natural Setting." *Psychopharmacology, 235*(12), 3401–3413. https://doi.org/10.1007/s00213-018-5049-7

Psychedelic Seminars. (2020). "CryptoPsychedelic 2018 #5: CryptoPsychedelics, Health and Healing" [Video]. https://youtu.be/93RPxEl48bw

Psychedelic Seminars. (2020). "CryptoPsychedelic 2018 #6: Visioning the Future of Psychedelics and Blockchain" [Video]. https://youtu.be/r6Hxs3Fuv7E

Quittem, B. (2020) "Bitcoin Is the Mycelium of Money." www.brandonquittem.com/bitcoin-is-the-mycelium-of-money

Radin, D. (2009). *The Conscious Universe: The Scientific Truth of Psychic Phenomena.* New York, NY: HarperCollins.

Ramachandran, V. S., & Hubbard, E. M. (2001). "Synaesthesia—A Window into Perception, Thought and Language." *Journal of Consciousness Studies, 8*(12), 3–34. http://chip.ucsd.edu/pdf/Synaesthesia%20-%20JCS.pdf

Rätsch, C. (1998). *The Encyclopedia of Psychoactive Plants: Ethnopharmacology and Its Applications.* Rochester, VT: Park Street Press.

Reeves, S. (2021, January 27). "Bitcoin May Trump the Dollar as Hedge against Inflation." *Newsweek.* www.newsweek.com/bitcoin-may-trump-dollar-hedge-against-inflation-1564982

Renter, E. (2014, March 25). "Psychedelic Mushroom Compound Found to Grow and Repair Brain Cells." Natural Society. http://naturalsociety.com/research-suggests-psychedelic-mushrooms-offer-valuable-brain-treatments/

Reynolds, F. (2013). "Tracing Neolithic Worldviews: Shamanism, Irish Passage Tomb Art and Altered States of Consciousness." C. Adams, D. Luke, A. Waldstein, B. Sessa, & D. King (Eds.), *Breaking Convention: Essays on Psychedelic Consciousness* (pp. 13–29). Berkeley, CA: North Atlantic Books.

Riba, J. (2016) "Ayahuasca Stimulates the Birth of New Brain Cells: Latest Findings from the Beckley/Sant Pau Research Programme." Beckley Foundation. http://beckleyfoundation.org/2016/06/16/ayahuasca-stimulates-the-birth -of-new-brain-cells-latest-findings-from-the-beckleysant-pau-research -programme/

Richards, W. A. (2015). *Sacred Knowledge: Psychedelics and Religious Experiences.* New York, NY: Columbia University Press.

Riedlinger, T (2005). "The 'Wondrous Mushroom' Legacy of R. Gordon Wasson." In R. Metzner (Ed.), *Sacred Mushroom of Visions: Teonanácatl: A Sourcebook on the Psilocybin Mushroom* (pp. 76–92). Rochester, VT: Park Street Press.

Rifkin, J. (2009). *The Empathic Civilization: The Race to Global Consciousness in a World in Crisis.* New York, NY: Penguin Group.

Rifkin, J. (2011). *The Third Industrial Revolution: How Lateral Power Is Transforming Energy, the Economy, and the World.* New York, NY: Palgrave Macmillan.

Roberts, D. (2021). "Visa Has Quietly Warmed Up to Crypto, along with PayPal and Square." Yahoo Finance. www.yahoo.com/now/visa-has-also-quietly-warmed -to-crypto-along-with-pay-pal-and-square-200953910.html

Roberts, T. (2013). *The Psychedelic Future of the Mind: How Entheogens Are Enhancing Cognition, Boosting Intelligence, and Raising Values.* Rochester, VT: Park Street Press.

Rush, J. A. (Ed.). (2013). *Entheogens and the Development of Culture: The Anthropology and Neurobiology of Ecstatic Experience.* Berkeley, CA: North Atlantic Books.

Russell, P. (1995). *The Global Brain Awakens: Our Next Evolutionary Leap.* Palo Alto, CA: Global Brain.

Ryan, C. (2019). *Civilized to Death: The Price of Progress.* New York, NY: Avid Reader Press.

Ryan, C., & Jetha, C. (2010). *Sex at Dawn: The Prehistoric Origins of Modern Sexuality.* New York, NY: HarperCollins.

Sahlins, M. (2017). *Stone Age Economics.* New York, NY: Routledge Classics.

Samorini, G. (2002). *Animals and Psychedelics: The Natural World and the Instinct to Alter Consciousness.* Rochester, VT: Park Street Press.

Schultes, R. E., Hofmann, A., & Rätsch, C. (1998). *Plants of the Gods: Their Sacred, Healing, and Hallucinogenic Powers*. Rochester, VT: Healing Arts Press.

Schwartzberg, L. (2019). "Afterword." In P. Stamets, (Ed.), *Fantastic Fungi: How Mushrooms Can Heal, Shift Consciousness, and Save the Planet*. San Rafael, CA: Earth Aware.

Sedgwick, J. A., Merwood, A., & Asherson, P. (2019). "The Positive Aspects of Attention Deficit Hyperactivity Disorder: A Qualitative Investigation of Successful Adults with ADHD." *ADHD Attention Deficit and Hyperactivity Disorders, 11*, 241–253. https://doi.org/10.1007/s12402-018-0277-6

Sessa, B., & Nutt, D. (2015). "Making a Medicine out of MDMA." *British Journal of Psychiatry, 206*(1), 4–6. https://doi.org/10.1192/bjp.bp.114.152751

Sheldrake, M. (2020). *Entangled Life: How Fungi Make Worlds, Change Minds & Shape Our Futures*. New York, NY: Random House.

Sheldrake, R. (2009). *Morphic Resonance: The Nature of Formative Causation*. Rochester, VT: Park Street Press.

Sheldrake, R. (2012). *Science Set Free: 10 Paths to New Discovery*. New York, NY: Deepak Chopra Books.

Shubin, N. (2008). *Your Inner Fish: A Journey into the 3.5-Billion-Year History of the Human Body*. New York, NY: Pantheon Books.

Shubin, N. (2013). *The Universe Within: Discovering the Common History of Rocks, Planets, and People*. New York, NY: Random House.

Shulgin A., & Shulgin, A. (1991). *PiHKAL: A Chemical Love Story*. Berkeley, CA: Transform Press.

Shulgin A., & Shulgin, A. (1997). *TiHKAL: The Continuation*. Berkeley, CA: Transform Press.

Siegel, R. K. (2005). *Intoxication: The Universal Drive for Mind-Altering Substances*. Rochester, VT: Park Street Press.

Sifferlin, A. (2016, December 1). "Just One Dose of This Psychedelic Drug Can Ease Anxiety." *Time*. https://time.com/4586333/psilocybin-cancer-anxiety-depression/

Silva, J. (2019). "Who Is Jason Silva." www.thisisjasonsilva.com/aboutjason

Silver, J. (Producer), & The Wachowskis (Directors). (1999). *The Matrix* [Motion picture]. Warner Bros., DVD Limited Edition Collector's Set.

Sjöstedt-H, P. (2015). *Noumenautics: Metaphysics, Meta-ethics, Psychedelics*. Cornwall, England: Psychedelic Press.

Slattery, D. R. (2015). *Xenolinguistics: Psychedelics, Language, and the Evolution of Consciousness*. Berkeley, CA: Evolver Editions.

Smith, A. (1994). *An Inquiry into the Nature and Causes of the Wealth of Nations*. New York, NY: Modern Library.

Smith, H. (1999). *The World's Religions: Our Great Wisdom Traditions*. San Francisco, CA: HarperSanFrancisco.

Smith, K. (n.d.). "How Is Money Created?" How the Market Works. https://Education.HowTheMarketWorks.com/How-Is-Money-Created

Speth, J. G. (2012). *America the Possible: Manifesto for a New Economy*. New Haven, CT: Yale University Press.

Spilka, D. (2020, March 17). "Blockchain and the Unbanked: Changes Coming to Global Finance." IBM. www.ibm.com/blogs/blockchain/2020/03/blockchain-and-the-unbanked-changes-coming-to-global-finance/

Stafford, P. (1992). *Psychedelics Encyclopedia* (3rd ed.). Berkeley, CA: Ronin Publishing.

Stamets, P. (1996). *Psilocybin Mushrooms of the World: An Identification Guide*. Berkeley, CA: Ten Speed Press.

Stamets, P. (2005). *Mycelium Running: A Guide to Healing the Planet through Gardening with Gourmet and Medicinal Mushrooms*. Berkeley, CA: Ten Speed Press.

Stamets, P. (Ed.). (2019). *Fantastic Fungi: How Mushrooms Can Heal, Shift Consciousness, and Save the Planet*. San Rafael, CA: Earth Aware.

Stolaroff, M. (2004). *The Secret Chief Revealed*. Naples, Italy: Albatross Publishers.

Strassman, R. (2000). *DMT: The Spirit Molecule: A Doctor's Revolutionary Research into the Biology of Out-of-Body Near-Death and Mystical Experiences*. Rochester, VT: Bear & Company.

Strassman, R., Slawek, W., Luna, L. E., Wojtowicz, S., & Frecska, E. (2008). *Inner Paths to Outer Space: Journeys to Alien Worlds through Psychedelics and Other Spiritual Technologies*. Rochester, VT: Bear & Company.

Strauss, M. (2015, September 12). "12 Theories of How We Became Human, and Why They're All Wrong." *National Geographic*. http://news.nationalgeographic.com/2015/09/150911-how-we-became-human-theories-evolution-science/

Swan, T. (2018). *The Anatomy of Loneliness: How to Find Your Way Back to Connection*. London, England: Watkins Media Publishing.

Swimme, B. (2011). "The Powers of the Universe." *EnlightenNext*, issue 47, 28–41.

Swimme, B., & Berry, T. (1994). *The Universe Story: From the Primordial Flaring Forth to the Ecozoic Era—A Celebration of the Unfolding of the Cosmos*. San Francisco, CA: HarperCollins Publishers.

Swimme, B., & Tucker, M. (2011). *Journey of the Universe*. New Haven, CT: Yale University Press.

Tarnas, R. (1991). *The Passion of the Western Mind: Understanding the Ideas That Have Shaped Our World View*. New York, NY: Random House.

Tarnas, R. (2006). *Cosmos and Psyche: Intimations of a New Worldview*. New York, NY: Viking Books.

Teilhard de Chardin, P. (1975). *The Phenomenon of Man* (B. Wall, Trans.). New York, NY: Harper. (Original work published 1955)

Thevet, A. (2004). "Ministers of the Devil Who Learn about Secrets." In J. Narby & F. Huxley (Eds.), *Shamans through Time: 500 Years on the Path to Knowledge*. New York, NY: Penguin Books.

Tool. (1996). *AENIMA* [Album]. Zoo.

Tool. (2001). *Lateralus* [Album]. Volcano.

Tool. (2006). *10,000 Days* [Album]. Volcano.

Tool. (2019). *Fear Inoculum* [Album]. Volcano.

"Top 5 Advantages of Bitcoin Over Fiat Currency." (2020, September 5). *The European Business Review*. www.europeanbusinessreview.com/top-5-advantages-of-bitcoin-over-fiat-currency/

Torpey, K. (2020, April 13). "The Bitcoin Price Has Outperformed All Other Major Asset Classes over the Past Year." *Forbes*. www.forbes.com/sites/ktorpey/2020/04/13/the-bitcoin-price-has-outperformed-all-other-major-asset-classes-over-the-past-year

University of California, Irvine. (2002, January 9). "Attention-Deficit Hyperactivity Disorder Related to Advantageous Gene." ScienceDaily. www.sciencedaily.com/releases/2002/01/020109074512.htm

Upfront Ventures. (2018, February 21). "Thomas Lee Presents the Economics of Cryptocurrencies | Upfront Summit 2018" [Video]. www.youtube.com/watch?v=GGberGnxiJk

US Department of Veterans Affairs. (2020). *2020 National Veteran Suicide Prevention Annual Report*. www.mentalhealth.va.gov/docs/data-sheets/2020/2020-National-Veteran-Suicide-Prevention-Annual-Report-11-2020-508.pdf

Volk, T. (2003). *Gaia's Body: Toward a Physiology of Earth*. Cambridge, MA: MIT Press.

Von Bertalanffy, L. (1969). *General System Theory: Foundations, Development, Applications* (4th ed.). New York, NY: George Braziller.

Von Neumann, John. (2012). *The Computer and the Brain*. New Haven, CT: Yale University Press. (Original work published 1958)

Waldman, A. (2017). *A Really Good Day: How Microdosing Made a Mega Difference in My Mood, My Marriage, and My Life*. New York, NY: Anchor Publishing.

Walsh, R. (2007). *The World of Shamanism: New Views of an Ancient Tradition*. Woodbury, MN: Llewellyn Publications.

Wasson, R. G. (1968). *Soma: Divine Mushroom of Immortality*. New York, NY: Harcourt Brace Jovanovich.

Wasson, R. G., Hofmann, G., & Ruck, C. (2008). *The Road to Eleusis: Unveiling the Secret of the Mysteries*. Berkeley, CA: North Atlantic Books.

Watts, A. (1962). *The Joyous Cosmology: Adventures in the Chemistry of Consciousness*. New York, NY: Vintage Books.

Wayman, E. (2012, October 31). "Five Early Primates You Should Know." *Smithsonian*. www.smithsonianmag.com/science-nature/five-early-primates-you-should-know-102122862/

We Plants Are Happy Plants. (2014). "The Transcendental Object at the End of Time (Terence McKenna Movie)" [Video]. www.youtube.com/watch?v=aAlaRdrcQcY

Weil, A. (2019). "Counterpoint: The Stoned Ape Theory—Not." In P. Stamets (Ed.), *Fantastic Fungi: How Mushrooms Can Heal, Shift Consciousness, and Save the Planet*. San Rafael, CA: Earth Aware.

Weiser, B. (2015, May 29). "Ross Ulbricht, Creator of Silk Road Website, Is Sentenced to Life in Prison." *New York Times*. www.nytimes.com/2015/05/30/nyregion/ross-ulbricht-creator-of-silk-road-website-is-sentenced-to-life-in-prison.html

Weller, C. (2017, February 13). "Elon Musk Doubles Down on Universal Basic Income: 'It's Going to Be Necessary.'" Business Insider. www.businessinsider.com/elon-musk-universal-basic-income-2017-2

Wheal, J. (2021). *Recapture the Rapture: Rethinking God, Sex, and Death in a World That's Lost Its Mind*. New York, NY: HarperCollins.

Whitaker-Azmitia, P. M. (1999). "The Discovery of Serotonin and Its Role in Neuroscience." *Neuropsychopharmacology, 21*(Supplement 2), S2–S8. https://doi.org/10.1016/S0893-133X(99)00031-7

Whitehead, A. N. (1979). *Process and Reality: An Essay in Cosmology*. New York, NY: Free Press.

Whitehead, A. N. (1985). *Science and the Modern World*. London, England: Free Association Books. (Original work published 1925).

Wiener, N. (1961). *Cybernetics: Control and Communication in the Animal and the Machine*. Cambridge, MA: MIT Press.

Wighton, K. (2016, April 11). "The Brain on LSD Revealed: First Scans Show How the Drug Affects the Brain." Imperial College London. http://www3.imperial.ac.uk/newsandeventspggrp/imperialcollege/newssummary/news_11-4-2016-17-21-2

Wilber, K. (2000). *Integral Psychology: Consciousness, Spirit, Psychology, Therapy.* Boston, MA: Shambhala Publications.

Wilber, K. (2000). *Sex, Ecology, Spirituality: The Spirit of Evolution* (2nd ed.). Boston, MA: Shambhala Publications.

Wilber, K. (2001). *A Brief History of Everything* (2nd ed.). Boston, MA: Shambhala Publications.

Wilber, K. (2001). *A Theory of Everything: An Integral Vision for Business, Politics, Science, and Spirituality.* Boston, MA: Shambhala Publications.

Wilber, K. (2001). *The Eye of Spirit: An Integral Vision for a World Gone Slightly Mad.* Boston, MA: Shambhala Publications.

Wilber, K. (2006). *Integral Spirituality: A Startling New Role for Religion in the Modern and Postmodern World.* Boston, MA: Integral Books.

Wilber, K. (2007). *Integral Vision.* Boston, MA: Shambhala Publications.

Wilber, K. (2017). *The Religion of Tomorrow: A Vision for the Future of the Great Traditions.* Boulder, CO: Shambhala Publications.

Williams, J., & Taylor, E. (2005, December 1). "The Evolution of Hyperactivity, Impulsivity and Cognitive Diversity." *Interface, 3*(8), 399–413. https://dx.doi.org/10.1098%2Frsif.2005.0102

Winkelman, M. (2013). "Altered Consciousness and Drugs in Human Evolution." In J. A. Rush (Ed.), *Entheogens and the Development of Culture: The Anthropology and Neurobiology of Ecstatic Experience.* Berkeley, CA: North Atlantic Books.

Wittmann M., Carter O., Hasler F., Cahn B. R., Grimberg U., Spring P., Hell D., Flohr H., & Vollenweider F. X. (2007, January 21). "Effects of Psilocybin on Time Perception and Temporal Control of Behaviour in Humans." *Journal of Psychopharmacology, 21*(1), 50–64. https://doi.org/10.1177/0269881106065859

Wolfson, R. (2018, March 28). "Millennials Speak Out about Investing in Cryptocurrencies for Retirement Funds." *Forbes.* www.forbes.com/sites/rachelwolfson/2018/03/28/millennials-speak-out-about-investing-in-cryptocurrencies-for-retirement-funds/

World Bank. (2017). "The Unbanked." In *Findex 2017* (pp. 35–41). https://globalfindex.worldbank.org/sites/globalfindex/files/chapters/2017%20Findex%20full%20report_chapter2.pdf

World Economic Forum: Global Future Council on Cryptocurrencies. (2020). *Crypto, What Is It Good For? An Overview of Cryptocurrency Use Cases.* http://www3.weforum.org/docs/WEF_Cryptocurrency_Uses_Cases_2020.pdf

World Health Organization. (2020, January 30). "Depression." www.who.int/en/news-room/fact-sheets/detail/depression

Wright, T., & Gynn, G. (2014). *Return to the Brain of Eden: Restoring the Connection between Neurochemistry and Consciousness.* Rochester, VT: Bear & Company.

"Young v Old Votes for Bernie and Hillary in the 2016 Primaries." (2016, April 27). *The Economist.* www.economist.com/graphic-detail/2016/04/27/young-v-old-votes-for-bernie-and-hillary-in-the-2016-primaries

Zigah, X. (2020, May 11) "Is Bitcoin Really Digital Gold?" *Forbes.* www.forbes.com/sites/forbesfinancecouncil/2020/05/11/is-bitcoin-really-digital-gold

Ziv, I. (Producer & Director). *Capitalism: A Six-Part Series* [Motion picture]. Icarus Films.

INDEX

italic page numbers indicate figures

5-HT2A serotonin receptors, 18, 131,
160–161, 163
1984 (Orwell), 1–2, 289

A

Abraham, Ralph, 86, 142, 234–235,
240, 267–268
Abrams, M. H., 269
academia's lack of interest in
psychedelics, 170–171
acid. *See* LSD
Acid Tests, 40
Adderall, 210
addiction
MDMA, 204
nicotine, 32
ADHD (attention deficit
hyperactivity disorder), 125–126
agency (self-preservation). *See*
autonomy
Agricultural Revolution, 110, 118–121
decrease in brain size, 171–173
transition to agriculture, 109–121
Ali, Ismail, 254
Allegro, John, 177
Alpert, Richard (Ram Dass), 39–40
Amanita muscaria, 90, 175–176
*America the Possible: Manifesto for a
New Economy* (Speth), 248
American Indigenous cultures, 179–185

anamnesis, 157
anecdotes. *See* peak experiences
anima, 59, 222, 270
animals and psychedelics, living
systems theory, 88–94
*Animals and Psychedelics: The Natural
World and the Instinct to Alter
Consciousness* (Samorini),
89–90, 92
animistic worldview, 134
anthropology
anthropologists on shamanism,
190–191
prehistoric societies, 173–185
antidepressants
creation of serotonin-based SSRI
antidepressants, 241
MDMA, 204
anxiety, 296–297
brain scans, 160
cancer patients' anxiety treatment,
27–30
treating social anxiety with
MDMA, 203
Apple, 231, 243
archaeology
cave art, 137–138, 174
Irish tomb art, 140
Archaic Revival, 45, 137, 293
Aristotle, 177, 277
Armillaria ostoyae, 84

art. *See also* visionary art
  cave art, 137–138, 174
  evolution and expansion of mind,
    137–148
  mushroom sculptures, 175
Atman, 268
Atman Retreat, 212
attachment theory, 64–65
attention deficit hyperactivity disorder
  (ADHD), 125–126
attractors, 276–278
  connection to supreme unity, 281
  future visions, 281–287
  shared imagination, 287
  Singularity, 278–279
  three types of, 276
  Transcendental Object at End of
    Time, 279–281, 288–289
Ausubel, Kenny, 95–96
Autism on Acid (Orsini), 213
autonomy, 59–62, *60*, 82
  capitalism, 248
  language, 150
Avatar, 221
*Awakened Futures: Psychedelics,
  Technology, and Meditation
  summit*, 244
ayahuasca, 44
Aztecs, 180–181, 183
  Feast of Revelations, 181
  prophecy, 281
  teonanácatl, 35–36

B

Bache, Christopher, 70–71, 207–208,
  266, 271–272, 282–285
  protocol for philosophical inquiry,
    235–236
Badiner, Allan, 134

basic perinatal matrices (BPMs),
  206–207, 218
Be Here Now (Dass), 40, 225
Beach, Horace, 155
Beckley Foundation, 225
  brain imaging, 163, 166
  treatment-resistant depression
    study, 31
Bellah, Robert, 246, 297–298
Berry, Thomas, 297
*Beyond the Brain: Birth, Death and
  Transcendence in Psychotherapy*
  (Grof), 71
Beyond the Narrow Life (Ortigo),
  208–209
Big Bang, 104–106
Bioneers Conference, 95, 97
Bitcoin, 249–262
  advantages of cryptocurrencies
    have over fiat currency, 257
  El Salvador Bitcoin adoption, 262
  similarities between blockchain,
    psychedelics, and structures
    found in nature, 260–262
  store of value, 256–257
BitGold, 249
Block, Peter, 114
blockchain, 245, 248–263
  advantages of cryptocurrencies over
    fiat currency, 257
  benefit of a global currency, 256
  Bitcoin, 249–251
  BitGold, 249
  black markets, 252
  bringing inclusivity to banking,
    257–258
  CryptoPsychedelic Flashback,
    253–254
  CryptoPsychedelic Summit, 252–
    253, 261

Dapps (decentralized
applications), 250
definition of, 248
El Salvador Bitcoin adoption, 262
energy consumption, 251
Ethereum, 250
internet of things (IoT), 258–259
openly distributed data and
resources, 262–263
Pineapple Fund, 252
similarities between blockchain,
psychedelics, and structures
found in nature, 260–262
smart contracts, 250
store of digital value, 256–257
supporting integration of
psychedelics into society,
254–255
universal basic income, 257
Blockchain Council, 248
Bloom, Howard, 267
bonobos, 108–109, 112
Boom, 228
Botanical Preservation Corps, 92
*The Botany of Desire: A Plant's-Eye
View of the World* (Pollan), 85, 91
Bourzat, Francoise, 196, 270
BPMs (basic perinatal matrices),
206–207, 218
brain development, 139, 158–166
brain imaging studies, 32, 160,
163–166
decrease in brain size since
Agricultural Revolution,
171–173
default-mode ("me") network,
164–165
neurogenesis, 159
research, 159–160
serotonin, 160–161, 163

Brain Games TV show, 232
brain scans, 32, 160, 163–166
Brand, Stewart, 243–244
Brewer, Judson, 32, 164
Brown, David Jay, 216, 287–288
Brown, Jerry, 177
Brown, Julie, 177
Brown, Michael, 190–191
Buhner, Stephan, 160
Burning Man, 46, 147, 213, 223,
228–230, 263
business. *See* economics
Buterin, Vitalik, 250

C

California Institute of Integral
Studies, 46, 208, 239
Certificate in Psychedelic-
Assisted Therapies and
Research, 212
Cameron, James, 221
Campbell, Joseph, 221
cancer patients' anxiety treatment,
27–30
capitalism, 247–248
Capra, Fritjof, 76, 80, 292
Carhart-Harris, Robin, 32,
164–165, 255
Caruana, Laurence, 215–216
Casey, Michael, 251, 259
causality, 277
cave art, 137–138, 174
Center for Consciousness
Medicine, 212
Center for Mindfulness, University
of Massachusetts Medical
School, 32
chaos mathematics, 276
chaos theory, 142, 234, 272, 276

Chaos, Creativity, and Cosmic Consciousness (McKenna, T., Sheldrake, R., & Abraham, R.), 234–235, 276
Chapel of Sacred Mirrors (CoSM), 226
Chenoweth, Erica, 287
Christianity, 183–184
    Dark Ages, 178
    European perspective of shamanism, 191–192
    Reformation, 247
    role mushrooms in early Christianity, 177–178
    Spanish Church at time of Spain's conquest of the Americas, 180–183
Christiansen, Merete, 254
Christogenesis, 286
churches (legal churches), 212
climate change, 297
Clinton, Bill, 243
Coatlicue, 183
Cognitive Revolution, 119, 140
collective evolution, 273–274
collective unconscious, 51, 269–270
Coming Home: The Birth and Transformation of the Planetary Era (Kelly), 268
communion, 63–65, *63*
    capitalism, 248
    language, 150
    synchronicity, 271
Community: The Structure of Belonging (Block), 114
Compass Pathways, 33–35, 46
complexity, 265–275
    characteristics of, 266–267
    collective evolution, 267–268, 273–274
    equilibrium and chaos, 271–273

humanity as part of larger living consciousness, 268–270
    increasing complexity in unfolding evolution, 268
    novelty theory, 274
    psychedelics as novelty generators, 274–275
    synchronicity, 270–271
    time, 267–268
complexity theory, 276
computers
    cryptocurrency. *See* cryptocurrency
    influence of psychedelics, 242–244
Concord Prison Study, 24
Confrontation with the Unconscious: Jungian Depth Psychology and Psychedelic Experiences (Hill), 269–270
Congo River basin, 109–110, 145
connectivity, 266
    synchronicity, 271
consciousness
    evolution, 82
    humanity as part of larger living consciousness, 268–270
    instincts of. *See* instincts of consciousness
Consciousness Hacking organization, 244
Consciousness Medicine (Hunter), 196–197
CoSM (Chapel of Sacred Mirrors), 226
The Cosmic Game: Explorations at the Frontier of Human Consciousness (Grof), 57, 236–237
Cosmos and Psyche: Intimations of a New World View (Tarnas), 268
creativity, 59, 263
    enhancement due to altered states, 231–232

evolution and expansion of mind,
137–148
imagination, 145–146
Jung's disagreement with Freud, 59
neurodivergent individuals, and
novelty, 126
research, 147–148
symbiosis generates novelty, 83
transcendence instinct, 66–69, *66*
Crick, Francis, 240
Crockett, Molly, 229
cryptocurrency, 245, 249–263
advantages over fiat currency, 257
benefit of global currency, 256
Bitcoin, 249–251
BitGold, 249
black markets, 252
bringing inclusivity to banking,
257–258
CryptoPsychedelic Flashback,
253–254
CryptoPsychedelic Summit,
252–254, 261
Dapps (decentralized
applications), 250
El Salvador Bitcoin adoption, 262
energy consumption, 251
Ethereum, 250
internet of things (IoT), 258–259
openly distributed data and
resources, 262–263
Pineapple Fund, 252
similarities between blockchain,
psychedelics, and structures
found in nature, 260–262
smart contracts, 250
store of value, 256–257
supporting integration of
psychedelics into society,
254–255

universal basic income, 257
CryptoPsychedelic Flashback,
253–254
CryptoPsychedelic Summit,
252–254, 261
cultural bias against consciousness-
altering substances, 170
culture and visionary art, 214–231
Adam Strauss's *The Mushroom
Cure*, 228
Alex and Allyson Grey's Entheon
museum, 225–226
Alex Grey, 215–216
Alex Grey's "The New Eleusis",
222–225
Andrew "Android" Jones, 226–227
festivals, 228–230
H. R. Giger, 216–217
Laurence Caruana, 215–216
Marloes Messemaker's *Five Dried
Grams: A Graphic Novelty Meme*,
227–228
The Matrix film series, 217–218
Sense8 Netflix series, 218–219
Shane Mauss's *Psychonautics*
documentary, 228
Star Trek: Discovery, 220–221
Tool, 221–222
visionary art movement, 215–216
women artists, 216
curandera, 11, 36

D

Dapps (decentralized applications), 250
Dark Ages, 178
dark night of the soul, 70–71
*Dark Night, Early Dawn: Steps to a
Deep Ecology of Mind* (Bache),
70–71, 207, 272, 282–284

DARPA (Defense Advanced Research
Projects Agency), 17
Darwin, Charles, 79–81, 113–114
*Darwin's Pharmacy: Sex, Plants, and the
Evolution of the Noösphere* (Doyle),
75, 82, 97, 158, 260
Dass, Ram, 40, 225
Dawkins, Richard, 82, 267
de Bary, Heinrich Anton, 78
de Benavente, Toribio, 181
de Borhegyi, Carl, 180
de Borhegyi-Forrest, Suzanne, 180
de Chardin, Pierre Teilhard, 278, 286
de las Casas, Bartolome, 181
de Rios, Marlene Dobkin, 194
DEA (Drug Enforcement
Agency), 241
death
death instinct, 71
death-rebirth experiences, 207–208
dissolution instinct and our
Singularity at end of time, 285
Indigenous Mexican and Central
American cultures' perception
of, 183–184
DecentraNet, 254
decision-making process, 141
*Decomposing the Shadow: Lessons from
the Psilocybin Mushroom* (Jesso),
12–13, 204–205
decriminalization movements,
295–296
Decriminalize Nature, 213, 295
default-mode ("me") network,
164–165
dissolution of, 255
Defense Advanced Research Projects
Agency (DARPA), 17
DeKorne, Jim, 42–43

Denisova Cave, 111
depression, 31–35, 297
creation of serotonin-based SSRI
antidepressants, 241
research studies, 159–160
spinogenesis, 159
World Health Organization, 31
depth psychology, 269–270, 297–298
Descartes, Rene, 247
*The Descent of Man and Selection in
Relation to Sex* (Darwin), 113–114
Developing a Relationship with
Sacred Mushrooms group, 213
Devereux, Paul, 173–174,
214–215, 294
Diderot, Denis, 192
Diego, Juan, 183
diet of our ancestors, 108, 166–167, 169
Dikov, N. N., 174
dinosaurs, 106
dissolution, 69–73
dissolution instinct
arising of more interconnected
patterns, 272–273
Singularity at the end of time, 285
diversity, 266
*The Divine Spark: Psychedelics,
Consciousness, and the Birth of
Civilization* (Hancock), 138–139
Dixon, Roland, 192–193
DMT, 44, 142
DNA, 162
Doblin, Rick, 24–25, 34, 224
Dogrib, 175
dopamine, 125
dosage
heroic dose (five dried grams), 12,
19, 132, 214
lethal dose, 10

LSD, 214
microdosing, 18, 127
ritual use of psychedelics, 140
sexual arousal, 128–129
therapeutic index, 10
downloads, 156–158
anamnesis, 157
prehension, 60, 156
Doyle, Richard, 75, 82, 97, 158, 260
DRD4-7R (wanderlust gene), 125
Drug Enforcement Agency
(DEA), 241
Dunbar, Robert, 117, 149–151
Dunbar, Robin, 149
Dunbar's number, 117
Duran, Diego, 180–181
dynamic systems theory, 142

E

ecodelic insight, 75, 260
ecodelics, 97
ecological awareness, increase in,
238–239
ecodelic insight, 75, 260
ecological self, 94–99
economics, 245–263
blockchain & cryptocurrency,
248–263
capitalism, 247–248
global banking accessibility,
257–258
open sourcing, 262–263
universal basic income, 257
ecstasis, 31, 232, 263
ecstasy. *See* MDMA
Ecstasy: The Complete Guide (Holland),
202–203
ego dissolution, 132, 164

ego inflation, and capitalism, 248
El Salvador Bitcoin adoption, 262
Eleusinian Mysteries, 133, 176–178
Eleusis, 176
*The Empathic Civilization: The Race
to Global Consciousness in a
World in Crisis* (Rifkin), 115, 266
empathy, 115, 130–131
research, 147
*The Encyclopedia of Psychoactive
Plants: Ethnopharmacology and Its
Application* (Rätsch), 88–89
Encyclopédie, 192
Engelbart, Doug, 243
enhanced consciousness vs. expanded
consciousness, 209
Enlightenment, 192, 247, 269
Entangled Life (Sheldrake), 85–88
entelechy, 277
Entheogenic Research Integration
Education (ERIE), 212–213
Entheogenic Review, 42
*Entheogens and the Development of
Culture* (Rush), 135, 141
Entheon museum, 225–226
epigenetics, 162–163
equilibrium, 271–273
ergot, 18, 177
ERIE (Entheogenic Research
Integration Education), 212–213
eros (self-transcendence). *See*
transcendence
Esalen Institute trialogues, 86,
234–235
eschatothesia, 285
eternal objects, 279
Ethereum, 250
ethics, 211
guides, 211

ethics (*continued*)
  need for shaman code of ethics,
    194–195
ethnobotany, 89
evolution
  Big Bang to primates, 104–106
  brain development, 158–166
  collective evolution, 267–268,
    273–274
  competition/survival of the
    fittest, 82
  consciousness, 82
  consumption of mushrooms,
    123–125
  contrasts with established theories
    of evolution, 166–173
  decision-making and problem-
    solving process, 141
  diet, 108, 166–167, 169
  dosage and sexual arousal, 128–129
  expansion of mind (art, logic, and
    perception of time), 137–148
  extension of our imagination, 288
  fungi, 105–106
  fungi-directed evolution of
    ecosystems, 92–93
  group dynamics, 127–132
  impact of psilocybin on brain
    evolution, 127
  increasing complexity, 268
  infinite imagination, 288–289
  K/T extinction event, 106
  language, 149–158
  life in trees, 106–109
  mushroom theory of human
    origins, 167, 170, 172–173, 224,
    290–291
  neurodivergent individuals,
    125–126

primates, 129-130
psilocybin, 87–88
psychedelic re-evolution, 289–298
psychedelics as novelty generators,
  274–275
religion, 136–137
revisioning evolution, 80–83
ritual use of psychedelics, 140
serotonin, 160–161
sexual relationships, 111–117, 121,
  167–168
six epochs, 278
spirituality, 132–137
symbiogenesis, 79–80
transition to agriculture, 109–121
*Evolution's Purpose: An Integral
  Interpretation of the Scientific Story
  of Our Origins* (McIntosh), 268
*The Evolutionary Mind: Conversations
  on Science, Imagination and Spirit*
  (McKenna, T., Sheldrake, and
  Abraham), 234
expansion of mind in history, 137–148
experiences. *See* peak experiences
experiments, 22–35
  brain imaging, 32
  Concord Prison Study, 24
  creativity, 147–148
  empathy, 147
  FDA, 32
  fear of death in terminally ill
    cancer patients, 27–30
  Harvard Good Friday
    Experiment, 24
  Harvard Psilocybin Project, 23–24
  Johns Hopkins psilocybin
    experiments, 25–27
  LSD research in creativity in
    Silicon Valley, 242–243

nicotine addiction, 32
personality development, 29–31
treatment-resistant depression,
   31–35
University of Arizona OCD
   research, 27

F

Fadiman, James, 18, 148, 197–198,
   209–210, 242–243
families eating mushrooms together,
   209
Fantastic Fungi (movie), 17, 46, 221
*Fantastic Fungi: How Mushrooms Can
   Heal, Shift Consciousness, and Save the
   Planet* (McKenna), 123–124, 168
FDA (Food and Drug
   Administration)
   approved research, 32
   depression treatment studies, 33–35
   halting of psychedelic research in
      1966, 42
Feast of Revelations, 181
Feilding, Amanda, 31–32, 225
Ferriss, Tim, 231–232
festivals, 213, 228–230
fight, flight, freeze, and fawn, 61
Fireside Project, 213–214
The First Manifesto of Visionary Art
   (Caruana), 215–216
Fischer, Roland, 127–128
Fisher, Helen, 112
five dried grams (heroic dose), 12, 19,
   25, 132, 214, 227–228
*Five Dried Grams: A Graphic Novelty
   Meme* (Messemaker), 227–228
Flaring Forth, 104
flow, and synchronicity, 271

Flower of Life, 225
fMRI brain scans, 32, 160, 164–166
Food and Drug Administration.
   See FDA (Food and Drug
   Administration)
*Food of the Gods: The Search for
   the Original Tree of Knowledge*
   (McKenna), 85, 126, 128, 136, 150
fourth universal evolutionary drive of
   animals, 91
fractal geometry, 276
Frecska, Ede, 20
Freud, Sigmund, 50, 59
   death instinct, 71–72
   instincts of consciousness, 58
Froese, Tom, 140
fungi. *See also* mushrooms
   evolution, 105
   fungi-directed evolution of
      ecosystems, 92–93
   living systems theory, 83–88
Fungi Perfecti company, 17
future visions, 281–287

G

Gaia, 76–78, 92, 160–161, 184
   fungi-directed evolution of
      ecosystems, 92–93
   nitrogen cycle, 96–97
   self-organizing of Gaian holon,
      293–294
*Gaia's Body: Toward a Physiology of
   Earth* (Volk), 77
Gaiafield, 273
Gaian molecules, 97–99
Gebser, Jean, 293
The Ghost in the Machine (Koestler),
   52–56

Giger, H. R., 216–217
Gillooly, Liana Sananda, 261
Gladwell, Malcom, 117
Glide language, 153
global brain, 293
The Global Brain Awakens: Our Next Evolutionary Leap (Russell), 273
Global Brain: The Evolution of Mass Mind from the Big Bang to the 21st Century (Bloom), 267
glossolalia, 150–152
God
    Christianity, 184
    entering the mind of "God", 274
    Ground of Being, 15
    Hindu Rigveda, 176
    Logos, 157–158
    peak experiences, 19–21
Golding, William, 77
Goldsmith, George, 34
Goldsmith, Neal, 23–24, 189–190, 198–199
Good Friday Psilocybin Harvard experiment, 224
Grateful Dead, 40, 244
Graves, Robert, 36, 177
The Great Work: Our Way into the Future (Berry), 297
Greece (Ancient Greeks), 176–177
Grey, Alex, 45, 134, 155, 223, 226
    Entheon museum, 225–226
    "The New Eleusis", 222–225
    Secret Language, 154
    Tool art work, 222
    visionary art, 215–216
Grey, Allyson, 225–226
    Secret Writing, 154–155
Griffiths, Roland, 25–28, 32–33, 224

Grob, Charles, 27–28
Grof, Stanislav, 21, 53, 57, 59, 94, 115, 116, 205–207, 216–218, 224, 231, 236–237, 240, 271
    Alex Grey portrait, 216
    basic perinatal matrices (BPMs), 206–207
    death instinct, 71
    dissolution instinct, 72
    instincts of consciousness, 58
Grooming, Gossip, and the Evolution of Language (Dunbar), 149
Ground of Being, 15
group dynamics, 127–132
    dosage and sexual arousal, 128–129
    ego dissolution, 132
    empathy, 130–131
    Navy SEALs, 130
guides, 190–214
    anthropologists on shamanism, 190–191
    basic perinatal matrices (BPMs), 206–207
    benefits of, 195–197, 199
    Consciousness Medicine and expanded states of consciousness, 196–197
    dealing with shadow material, 204–207
    death-rebirth experiences, 207–208
    educational organizations and resources, 211–214
    ethics, 211
    European perspective of shamanism, 191–192
    Goldsmith's "Ten Lessons of Psychedelic Psychotherapy", 198–199
Inaura, 212

microdosing, 209–211
need for shaman code of ethics,
194–195
preparing subject for journey,
208–209
The Psychedelic Explorer's Guide,
197–198
relationship with explorers, 201–204
safety when using psychedelics, 198
similarity between shaman and
psychoanalyst, 193–194
titles of psychedelic psychotherapist
and medicine guide, 195
training, 200
view of shamanism in early
literature, 192–193
Guild of Guides training manual, 198
Guzman, G., 176
Gynn, Graham, 107–109, 129, 171–172

H

Haight-Ashbury, 43
Hakomi somatic psychotherapy, 2
Hancock, Graham, 138–139
Haoma, 176, 190
Harari, Yuval Noah, 110–111, 117–
120, 140, 149, 167, 172
Harpignies, J. P., 97
Harris, Marvin, 112
Hartman, Shelby, 34
Harvard Good Friday Experiment, 24
Harvard Psilocybin Project,
23–24, 39
health benefits of mushrooms, 124
Hericium erinaceus (lion's mane), 18, 211
Hermes, 225
heroic dose (five dried grams), 12, 19,
25, 132, 214, 227–228

Hicks, Bill, 19–20, 45, 221
The Hidden Connections (Capra), 76
Hill, Rebecca Ann, 216
Hill, Scott, 269–270
Hinduism
Atman, 268
Rigvedas, 134, 175–176, 190
*Historia general de las cosas de la Nueva
España* (de Sahagun), 180
history. *See also* evolution
expansion of mind in history,
137–148
modern history, 35–47
prehistoric societies, 173–185
Hofmann, Albert, 241, 296
Bicycle Day, 222
kykeon research, 133
microdosing, 210
"The New Eleusis", 223–224
trip to Mexico with Gordon
Wasson, 38–39
Holland, Julie, 202–203
holons, 52–57, 55
collective unconscious, 268–270
instincts of consciousness. *See*
instincts of consciousness
self-organizing of Gaian holon,
293–294
synchronicity, 270–271
holotropic, 53
Houston, Jean, 199–200,
234–235
How to Change Your Mind (Pollan),
16–17, 23, 41–42, 46, 148, 152,
161–162, 164
Human Genome Project, 162
The Human Phenomenon (de
Chardin), 278
Human Potential Movement, 200

humanity, evolution of. *See also*
  evolution
  Big Bang to primates, 104–106
  life in trees, 106–109
  sexual relationships, 111–117, 121,
    167–168
  transition to agriculture, 109–121
Hume, David, 247
Hunter, Kristina, 196–197
Huxley, Aldous, 225
Huxley, Francis, 136, 190–191

I

Igorot, 175
imagination, 145–146
  infinite, 288–289
  shared, 287
*The Immortality Key: The Secret History
  of the Religion with No Name*
  (Muraresku), 176, 178
Imperial College of London
  brain imaging, 163
  psilocybin research, 45–46
Inaura, 212
Indigenous
  Ancient Greeks, 176–177
  Aztecs, 181
  Dogrib, 175
  Igorot, 175
  Kiambi and Kuma, 175
  Mazatec, 10–11, 35–38, 175,
    182–183
  Mexican and Central American
    cultures, 179–185
  Ojibwa, 175
Industrial Light & Magic, 226
infinite imagination, 288–289
Inner Paths to Outer Space (Strassman
  et al.), 20–21

instincts of consciousness, 57–59
  autonomy, 59–62, 60
  communion, 63–65, 63
  dissolution, 69–73
  transcendence, 66–69, 66
Institute of Noetic Sciences, 197
Institute of Transpersonal
  Psychology, 197
*Integral Consciousness and the Future of
  Evolution* (McIntosh), 49
integral philosophy (integral theory), 49
  fourth universal evolutionary drive
    of animals, 91
  group bonding as example of
    universal instincts, 113
  holons, 52–57, 55
  instincts of consciousness. *See*
    instincts of consciousness
  quadrants, 50–52, 51
  tetra-prehension, 81
integral theory. *See* integral
  philosophy (integral theory)
Integration Communications, 212
International Foundation for
  Advanced Study, 197, 242–243
internet of things (IoT), 258
*Intoxication: The Universal Drive for
  Mind-Altering Substances* (Siegel),
  90, 91
IoT (internet of things), 258
Irish tomb art, 140
Islam, *Haoma*, 190

J

James, William, 26
Jesse, Bob, 27
Jesso, James, 12–13, 204–205
Jesus, 183
Jetha, Cacilda, 111, 113

Jobs, Steve, 231, 242–243
Johns Hopkins University School of
Medicine, 23
addiction studies, 32
psilocybin studies, 12, 27,
45–46, 224
study of treatment of anxiety with
cancer patients, 28–30
Johnson, Jean Bassett, 35–36
Johnson, Mark, 76
Jones, Andrew "Android",
226–227
Jonson, Ben, 53, 56
*The Joyous Cosmology: Adventures in the
Chemistry of Consciousness* (Watts),
238–239
Jung, Carl
anima, 59, 222
collective unconscious and the self,
51, 269–270
disagreement with Freud, 59
influence on rock band Tool,
221–222
shadow, 204, 222
synchronicity, 270–271
Juster, Benja, 229–230

K

K/T extinction event, 106
Keenan, Maynard James, 221–222
Kegan, Robert, 30, 50
Kelly, Sean, 268
Kennedy, David, 135–136, 165, 174
Kennedy, John F., assassination,
281–282
Kent, James, 239–240
Kesey, Ken, 40, 225
Kiambi tribe, 175
Koestler, Arthur, 52–56, 237

Kotler, Steven, 30–31, 130, 142, 177,
226, 229, 231–232, 240, 262–263,
285, 295
Krippner, Stanley, 98, 281–282
Kuma tribe, 175
Kurzweil, Ray, 278–279
kykeon, 133, 177–178, 225

L

Lake, George, 211-212
Lakoff, George, 76
Lane, Tom, 179
language, evolution of, 149–158
audible voices, 155, 158
autonomy, communion, and
transcendence, 150
connection with Logos, 155,
157–158
downloads/prehension, 60, 156–158
experiences with novel languages,
153–155
glossolalia, 150–152
research, 153
synesthesia, 151–153, 222
*The Law of Entheogenic Churches in the
United States* (Lake), 212
Leary, Timothy, 39, 41, 53, 217,
221, 225
Concord Prison Study, 24
Harvard Psilocybin Project,
23–24, 39
legality
decriminalization movements, 46,
295–296
FDA halting of psychedelic
research in 1966, 42
legal churches in U.S., 212
war on mind-expanding drugs,
294–295

Letcher, Andy, 9–10, 148
lethal dose, 10
leverage points, 232
Levi-Strauss, Claude, 193
Lewis-Williams, David, 137–138
Lieberman, Daniel, 125
Life magazine, 37
Lightning in a Bottle festival, 146,
213, 227–228
Lilly, John, 241, 262
lion's mane (*Hericium erinaceus*), 18,
211
Lipton, Bruce, 162
*The Living Classroom: Teaching and
Collective Consciousness* (Bache),
271
living systems theory, 75
animals and psychedelics, 88–94
ecological self, 94–99
fungi and plants, 83–88
Gaia, 76–78
revisioning evolution, 80–83
symbiosis, 78–80
Locke, John, 247
logic, development of, 142–143
Logos, 155, 157–158
*The Long Trip: A Prehistory of
Psychedelia* (Devereux), 173–174
Long, Michael, 125
Lovelock, James, 76–77, 92
LSD, 38–42
discovery of, 38–39
dosage, 214
kykeon, 133
microdosing, 18, 209–211
move from controlled environments
into recreational use, 39–42
"The New Eleusis", 223
Silicon Valley creativity research,
242–243

*LSD and the Mind of the Universe:
Diamonds from Heaven* (Bache),
235–236, 266, 282
LSD: My Problem Child (Hofmann), 39
Luisi, Pier Luigi, 80
Lujan, Sterlin, 253
Luke, David, 98
Luna, Luis, 20, 182

M

MacLean, Katherine, 29–30
The Magic Mushroom Explorer
(Powell), 134
*Magic Mushroom Explorer: Psilocybin
and the Awakening Earth* (Powell),
43, 98, 238
Malievskaia, Ekaterina, 34
MAPS (Multidisciplinary Association
for Psychedelic Studies), 24–25,
224, 228, 252
cryptocurrency gift, 252
Entheogeneration Speaker Series
at Burning Man 2019, 147
MDMA, 46, 202. *See also* MDMA
Zendo Project, 213
MAPS Psychedelic Science
Conference, 211
Margolies, Mike, 254
Margulis, Lynn, 77, 79, 83, 92
Markoff, John, 242–243
Mary (Mother Mary), 183–184
Maryland Psychiatric Research
Center, 12
Maslow, Abraham, 50, 263
general dynamic theory, 61
hierarchy of needs, 9, 61, 63, 66, 82,
114, 286
instincts of consciousness, 58
peak experiences, 8, 22

Masters, Robert, 199–200
material monism, 238
mathematics, 276
   chaos mathematics, 276
   mathematical capabilities,
     142–143
The Matrix film series, 217–218, 233
Mauss, Shane, 228
Maya, 183
Mazatec, 10–11, 35–38, 175,
   182–184, 196
   family journeys, 209
McIntosh, Steve, 49, 268
McKenna, Dennis, 44, 93–94, 145,
   168, 172, 224, 285
   brain development, 158
   devolution of human brain, 109
   time expansion, 144–145
McKenna, Terence, 42–45, 85–86,
   124, 128–130, 151–152, 165, 172,
   176–177, 201, 224, 227, 237, 240,
   268, 288, 293
   Archaic Revival, 137, 293
   chaos, 276
   emergence of language,
     150–152
   Esalen Institute trialogues, 86,
     234–235
   evolution of religions, 136–137
   heroic dose (five dried grams), 12,
     19, 132, 227–228
   impact of psilocybin on brain
     evolution, 126–127
   Logos, 155–157
   novelty theory, 68, 274
   Palenque Ethnobotany
     Seminars, 230
   psychedelics as novelty generators,
     274–275
   time expansion, 143–145

   Transcendental Object at End of
     Time, 279–281, 288–289
   verbal capacities, 153
McKibbin, Matt, 254
MDMA, 201–203
   addiction potential, 204
   developing trust between guides
     and explorers, 202–204
   introduction to therapy by
     Alexander "Sasha" Shulgin, 241
   MAPS research, 46, 252
Meadows, Donella, 232
medicine guides, 195. *See also* guides
meditation, 134
Mereschkowski, Konstantin, 79
Merry Pranksters, 40
Mesolithic shamanism, 173–174
Messemaker, Marloes, 227–228
Metaphors We Live By (Lakoff and
   Johnson), 76
Metzner, Ralph, 13–15, 39–40, 129,
   170, 179
Mexican and Central American
   cultures, 179–185
Microdose VR, 227
microdosing, 18, 209–211
   ancestors, during evolution, 127
   Stamets Stack, 17–18
Miller, Richard, 25, 294
The Mission of Art (Grey), 216
Modern Consciousness Research and
   the Understanding of Art (Grof),
   216–217
modern history, 35–47
   Albert Hofmann and LSD,
     38–39
   Dennis McKenna, 44. *See also*
     McKenna, Dennis
   FDA's halting of psychedelic
     research in 1966, 42

modern history (*continued*)
  Gordon Wasson and Maria Sabina,
    10–12, 36–38
  LSD, 39–42
  Michael Pollan's *How to Change
    Your Mind*, 41–42, 46
  Ralph Metzner, 39–40
  research on MDMA, 46
  research on psilocybin, 45–46
  Richard Alpert (Ram Dass), 39–40
  Terence McKenna, 42–45. *See also*
    McKenna, Terence
monogamous sexual relationships,
  121, 167–168
Montgomery, Bob, 92
Morgan, Elaine, 109–110, 145
morphic fields, 274, 277
morphogenetic fields, 267
Mother of All Demos, 243
Mt. Tam Integration, 212–213
Mullis, Kary, 240
Multidisciplinary Association for
  Psychedelic Studies. *See* MAPS
  (Multidisciplinary Association for
  Psychedelic Studies
Munn, Henry, 152, 209
Muraresku, Brian, 176–178
Museum of Anthropology (Mexico
  City), 183
The Mushroom Cure (Strauss), 228
mushroom sculptures, 175
mushroom theory of human
  evolution, 167, 170, 172–173, 224,
  290–291
mushrooms
  consumption during evolution,
    124–127
  edibility by primates, 123

health benefits, 124–125
mycelium, 83–84
psilocybin. *See* psilocybin
  mushrooms
similarities between fungi and
  cryptocurrency, 260–262
mycelial mind
  expansion of mind (art, logic, and
    perception of time), 137–148
  group dynamics, 127–132
  impact of psilocybin on brain
    evolution, 127
  language, 149–158
  neurodivergent individuals,
    125–126
  primate consumption of
    mushrooms, 123–125
  spirituality, 132–137
mycelium, 83–84
  similarity to cryptocurrency,
    260–262
*Mycelium Running: How Mushrooms
  Can Help Save the World* (Stamets),
  83–84
MycoRising, 212
Mysteries (Eleusinian Mysteries), 133,
  176–178

N

Nakamoto, Satoshi, 249
Narby, Jeremy, 89, 136, 190–191
National Institutes of Health, 17
*Natural Supernaturalism: Tradition and
  Revolution in Romantic Literature*
  (Abrams), 269
nature
  enhanced view of, 238–239, 260

Gaia. *See* Gaia
similarities between blockchain, psychedelics, and structures found in nature, 260–262
Navy SEALs, 130
Negrin, Danielle, 245
neuritogenesis, 159
neurodivergent individuals, 125–126
neurogenesis, 159, 290
neurotransmitters, 125
"The New Eleusis", 222–225
The New Psychedelic Revolution: The Genesis of the Visionary Age (Oroc), 44–45, 226
The New Science of Psychedelics (Brown), 287–288
New York University (NYU), 23, 27, 45–46
study of treatment of anxiety with cancer patients, 28–29
niacin (vitamin B3), 18, 211
Nichols, David, 25, 32, 225
nicotine addiction, 32
Nintendo, 226
Nirvana, 277
nitrogen cycle, 96–97
nonlinear dynamics, 276
North Star ethics pledge, 211
Noumenautics: Metaphysics—Meta-Ethics—Psychedelics (Sjöstedt-H), 233
novel languages, 153–155
novelty, 237, 265–275
collective evolution, 267–268, 273–274
culmination in a singularity/ . Omega Point, 280–281
equilibrium and chaos, 271–273

humanity as part of larger living consciousness, 268–270
infinite imagination, 288–289
neurodivergent individuals, 125–126
novelty theory, 274
psychedelics as novelty generators, 274–275
symbiosis generates novelty, 83
synchronicity, 270–271
novelty theory, 68
Nutt, David, 165
NYU (New York University), 23, 27, 45–46
cancer patient study, 28–29

O

Oak, Annie, 229–230
obsessive-compulsive disorder (OCD), 27, 228
Occupy movement, 217
OCD (obsessive-compulsive disorder), 27, 228
Oeric, O. N., 44
Ojibwa, 175
Omega Point, 278, 280–281, 286
On the Origin of Species (Darwin), 79
OneTaste Orgasmic Meditation app, 262–263
open sourcing, 262
openness, 29–30; 132, 167
organization, 266
Orgasmic Meditation app, 263
Oroc, James, 44–45, 226
Orsini, Aaron Paul, 213
Ortigo, Kile, 208–209
Orwell, George, 1–2, 289

Osmond, Humphrey, 225
Oss, O. T., 44
Ott, Eleanor, 194–195
overdose/lethal dose, 10

P

Pahnke, Walter, 24, 224
Paine, Thomas, 257
Palenque Ethnobotany Seminars, 230
Palenque Norte Burning Man
    talks, 230
Paleolithic shamanism, 173–174
panpsychism, 54
patterns
    chaos mathematics, 276
    collective evolution, 267
    collective unconscious, 269–270
    complexity and novelty, 272–274
    fractal geometry, 276
    strange attractors, 276–277
peak experiences, 8–22
    Abraham Maslow, 8–9, 22
    Ayelet Waldman, 18
    Bill Hicks, 19–20
    David S. (presented by Ralph
        Metzner), 13–14
    description of a general psilocybin
        experience, 9–10
    dosage, 10, 12
    friend of Slawek Wojtowicz,
        20–21
    Gordon Wasson and Maria Sabina,
        10–12
    James Jesso, 12–13
    Jason Serle, 14–15
    Maslow's hierarchy of needs, 9
    Paul Stamets, 16–18
    unity, 16, 19–22

A Perfect Union of Contrary Things
    (Keenan), 221–222
periodic attractors, 276
personal and unconscious, 270
personality development research,
    29–31
Petrovich, Avvakum, 192
peyote, 35
Pezza, Chris, 229–230
philosophy
    Bache's protocol for philosophical
        inquiry, 235–236
    influence of psychedelics,
        231–240
    integral philosophy. *See* integral
        philosophy (integral
        theory), 49
    philosophers of the Scientific
        Revolution, 247
    process-relational philosophy, 54
philosophy of organism, 54, 76
*PiHKAL: Phenethylamines I Have
    Known and Loved* (Shulgin), 241
Pineapple Fund, 252
plant-based diet, 108, 166–167
plants and fungi, living systems theory,
    83–88
Plants and the Human Brain
    (Kennedy), 165, 174
*Plants of the Gods: Their Sacred,
    Healing, and Hallucinogenic Powers*
    (Schultes, Hofmann, and Rätsch),
    179, 180
Plato, 177
    forms, 142, 279
    Republic, 268
    teleology, 277
Plotinus, 268–269
point attractors, 276

Pollan, Michael, 16–17, 23, 33, 41–42, 46, 85, 91, 146, 148, 152, 161–162, 242
  guided journeys, 195–196
  recent neuroscience research, 164
  spirituality, 68–69
  symbiotic relationship of humans and plants, 84–85
posttraumatic stress disorder (PTSD), MDMA treatment, 202–204
Powell, Simon, 43, 98, 134, 238, 240
prehension/downloads, 60, 156–158
  tetra-prehension, 81
prehistoric societies, 173–185
  Ancient Greeks, 176–177
  cave art, 174
  early Christianity, 177–178
  Indigenous Mexican and Central American cultures, 179–185
  Indigenous mushroom societies, 175
  mushroom sculptures, 175
  Paleolithic and Mesolithic shamanism, 173–174
  religious texts, 175–176
preparing for journeys, 208–209
primates
  evolution. *See* primates, evolution of
  ingestion of mushrooms, 168–169
  mushroom consumption, 123
  serotonin, 161
primates, evolution of, 104–106, 109, 129–130
  life in trees, 106–108
  sexual relationships, 111–117, 121, 167
  transition to agriculture, 109–121
problem-solving process, 141

Process and Reality (Whitehead), 59
process-relational philosophy, 54
Proclus, 225
productivity enhancement due to altered states, 231–232
prophecy, 281–287
psilocybentics, 238
psilocybin mushrooms, 1
  brain development. *See* brain development
  description of a general psilocybin experience, 9–10
  dosage. *See* dosage
  evolution of, 87–88
  impact on evolution of brain, 127
Psilocybin Magic Mushroom Grower's Guide (Oss and Oeric), 44
Psilocybin Mushrooms of the World (Stamets), 89
The Psilocybin Solution (Powell), 134
Psilocybin Summit, 213
Psychedelic Education and Continuing Care Program, 29
The Psychedelic Future of the Mind (Roberts), 28, 239–240
The Psychedelic Gospels: The Secret History of Hallucinogens in Christianity (Brown and Brown), 177
Psychedelic Healing (Goldsmith), 198–199
Psychedelic Healing: The Promise of Entheogens for Psychotherapy and Spiritual Development (Goldsmith), 24, 189–190
Psychedelic Information Theory, 239
Psychedelic Information Theory: Shamanism in the Age of Reason (Kent), 239
Psychedelic Medicine (Miller), 25

Psychedelic Mysteries of the Feminine
(Papaspyrou, Baldini, and Luke
(Eds.)), 229–230
psychedelic psychotherapists, 195. *See
also* guides
Goldsmith's "Ten Lessons of
Psychedelic Psychotherapy",
198–199
psychedelic re-evolution, 289–298
Archaic Revival, 293
decriminalization movements,
295–296
impact of war on mind-expanding
drugs, 294–295
journey toward transcendence,
291–292
mushroom theory of human
origins, 290–291
potential of psilocybin and
psychedelics, 296–297
psychological evolution, 292–293
search for universal intimacy, 291
self-organizing of Gaian holon,
293–294
spiral toward higher consciousness,
297–298
Psychedelic Seminars, 212, 253–254
Psychedelic Shamanism (DeKorne),
42, 43
Psychedelic Times, 211
psychedelics
animals and psychedelics, living
systems theory, 88–94
potential of psilocybin and
psychedelics, 296–297
*Psychedelics in Mental Health Series:
Psilocybin* (Lake), 212
Psychedelics Today, 211
psychoactive plants, 88–89

psychoanalysis' similarity to
shamanism, 193–195
psychological evolution, 292–293
Psychology of the Future (Grof),
205–206
Psychonautics (movie), 228
psychonauts, 46, 156
psychotherapy, 190–214
attachment theory, 64–65
Goldsmith's "Ten Lessons of
Psychedelic Psychotherapy",
198–199
psy-phen (psychedelic
phenomenology), 233, 274
PTSD (posttraumatic stress disorder),
MDMA treatment, 202–204
Pythagoras, 177

Q

quadrants, 50–52, *51*, 139
tetra-prehension, 81
quantity, 266
Quetzalcoatl, 281
Quittem, Brandon, 260–262

R

Ramachandran, V. S., 151
Rätsch, Christian, 88–89
A Really Good Day (Waldman),
18, 210
Recapture the Rapture (Wheal),
286–287
Reeves, Keanu, 218
re-evolution, 289–298
Archaic Revival, 293
decriminalization movements,
295–296

impact of war on mind-expanding drugs, 294–295
journey toward transcendence, 291–292
mushroom theory of human origins, 290–291
potential of psilocybin and psychedelics, 296–297
psychological evolution, 292–293
search for universal intimacy, 291
self-organizing of Gaian holon, 293–294
spiral toward higher consciousness, 297–298
Reformation, 247
Reich, Wilhelm, 115–116
Reko, Bras Pablo, 35
religion, 134–137, 246–247. *See also* Christianity; Hinduism
legal churches in U.S., 212
Omega Point, 280–281
Reformation, 247
societal evolution, 119–120
teleological models of reality, 277–278
texts, 175–176
Republic (Plato), 268
research, 22–35
brain development, 159–160
brain imaging, 32, 160, 163
Concord Prison Study, 24
creativity, 147–148
empathy, 147
FDA, 32
fear of death in terminally ill cancer patients, 27–30
Harvard Good Friday Experiment, 24
Harvard Psilocybin Project, 23–24
Johns Hopkins. *See* Johns Hopkins University School of Medicine
linguistics, 153
LSD research in creativity in Silicon Valley, 242–243
nicotine addiction, 32
personality development, 29–31
treatment-resistant depression, 31–35
University of Arizona OCD research, 27
Return to the Brain of Eden (Wright and Gynn), 107–109, 129, 171–172
"Return Trip to Nirvana", 53
Reynolds, Ffion, 140
Richards, William, 12
Rifkin, Jeremy, 115, 149, 246–247, 258, 266, 291
Rigvedas, 134, 175–176, 190
risk of overdose, 10
Ritalin, 210
The Road to Eleusis (Hofmann, Wasson, and Ruck), 177
Roberts, Thomas, 28, 239–240
Rolling Stone, 33–34
Romanticism, 269
Romantics, 269
Ross, Stephen, 29, 32–33
Ruck, Carl, 133
Rush, John, 134, 141, 171
Russell, Peter, 266, 273, 293
Ryan, Christopher, 111, 113

S

Sabina, Maria, 11–12, 36–38, 151–152, 184, 224
Sacred Knowledge: Psychedelic and Religious Experiences (Richards), 12

Sacred Mirrors: The Visionary Art of Alex Grey (Grey), 215–216

The Sacred Mushroom and the Cross (Allegro), 177

Sacred Mushroom of Visions: Teonanácatl (Metzner), 13–15, 40, 170, 179

Sacred Mushroom Rituals: The Search for the Blood of Quetzalcoatl (Lane), 179

Sahagun, Bernardino de, 180

Sahlins, Marshall, 112–113

Samorini, Giorgio, 89–90, 92

Samskara, 227

San Francisco Psychedelic Society (SFPS), 212–213, 245

Sapiens: A Brief History of Humankind (Harari), 110–111, 117–120, 149, 167

satori, 253

The Scars of Evolution: What Our Bodies Tell Us of Human Origins (Morgan), 109–110, 145

schizophrenia, MDMA treatment, 202

Schroeder, R., 176

Schultes, Richard Evans, 35–36

Schwab, Klaus, 259

Schwartz, Peter, 146, 242

Schwartzberg, Louie, 17, 46, 221

science
influence of psychedelics, 240–245
living systems theory. *See* living systems theory
philosophy of organism, 54, 76
productivity enhancement due to altered states, 231–232

Science and the Modern World (Whitehead), 60, 73, 76, 156

science fiction, 244–245

Scientific Revolution, 247, 269

The Secret Chief Revealed (Stolaroff), 201

Secret Writing, 154, 155

self
collective unconscious and the self, 269–270
ecological self, 94–99
self-adaption (communion). *See* communion
self-dissolution (thanatos). *See* dissolution

The Selfish Gene (Dawkins), 82, 267

self-preservation (agency). *See* autonomy

self-transcendence (eros). *See* transcendence

Sense8, 218–219

Serle, Jason, 14–15

serotonin, 131
5-HT2A receptors, 18, 131, 160–161, 163
brain function, 160–161, 163
SSRI antidepressants, 204, 241

Sex at Dawn: The Prehistoric Origins of Modern Sexuality (Ryan and Jetha), 111, 113

Sex, Ecology, Spirituality (Wilber), 50

sexual relationships
dosage and sexual arousal, 128–129
non-monogamous, 111–117
transition to monogamy, 121, 167–168

SFPS (San Francisco Psychedelic Society), 212–213, 245

shadow, 222
dealing with shadow material, 204–207

shamanism, 134, 136, 141. *See also*
  guides
  American perspective,
    192–193
  animistic worldview, 134
  anthropologists' perspective,
    190–191
  complexity, 268
  European perspective, 191–192
  need for code of ethics, 194–195
  Paleolithic and Mesolithic
    shamanism, 173–174
  similarity to psychoanalysis,
    193–195
  view of shamanism in early
    literature, 192–193
*Shamans through Time: 500 Years on
  the Path to Knowledge* (Narby and
  Huxley), 136, 190–191
shared imagination, 287
Sheldrake, Merlin, 85–88
Sheldrake, Rupert, 86, 234–235, 240,
  267–268
  morphic field theory, 274, 277
Shots of Awe YouTube channel, 232
*Shroom: A Cultural History of the Magic
  Mushroom* (Letcher), 9–10, 148
Shubin, Neil, 104–105, 107
Shulgin, Alexander "Sasha", 201,
  241–242, 262
Shulgin, Ann, 241
Siegel, Mikey, 244, 262
Siegel, Ronald, 90–91, 294
Silicon Valley, 242
Silva, Jason, 232–233
Simard, Suzanne, 221
Singularity, 104, 278–279
Sjöstedt-H, Peter, 233–234, 240,
  274–275

Slattery, Diana Reed, 45, 151–153, 156
smart contracts, 249–250
Smith, Adam, 247
social anxiety, treating with
  MDMA, 203
Socrates, 177, 225
soma, 134, 175–176
Spanish Church at time of Spain's
  conquest of the Americas, 180–183
Speth, James, 248
spinogenesis, 159
spiral toward higher consciousness,
  297–298
spirituality, 132–137
  dark night of the soul, 70–71
  Logos, 155, 157–158
  meditation, 134
  religion, 134–137
  shamanism, 134, 136
  transcendence, 66–69, 66
SSRI antidepressants, 241
  MDMA usage, 204
Stage Presence, 230
Stamets Stack, 17, 18
Stamets, Paul, 16–17, 45–46, 83–84,
  89, 92, 97–98, 123–124, 146–147,
  175, 224
  Avatar influence, 221
  microdosing, 211
  Star Trek: Discovery character,
    220–221
Star Trek: Discovery, 220
Stealing Fire (Kotler and Wheal),
  30–31, 130, 177, 226, 229, 231,
  232, 262–263, 285, 295
Steiner, Mischa, 229–230
Stolaroff, Myron, 201, 242–243
Stone Age Economics (Marshall),
  112–113

strange attractors, 276–278
connection to supreme unity, 281
definition of, 276
future visions, 281–287
shared imagination, 287
Singularity, 278–279
Transcendental Object at End of
Time, 279–281, 288–289
Strassman, Rick, 20, 42
Strauss, Adam, 228
Stropharia cubensis, 177
Swain, Fredrick, 151
Swimme, Brian, 104
symbiogenesis, 79–80
symbiosis, 78–80
humans and plants, 84–85
symbiosis generates novelty, 83
symborgs (symbiotic organisms), 88
Symbiosis festival, 228
*Symbiotic Planet: A New View of
Evolution* (Margulis), 79
synchronicity, 270–271, 273
synesthesia, 151–153, 222
*The Systems View of Life: A Unifying
Vision* (Capra and Luisi), 80
Szabo, Nick, 249

T

Take 3 Productions, 229
Tam Integration, 253
Tao, 268
Tarnas, Richard, 157, 268
technology
blockchain. *See* blockchain
future technology, 288
influence of psychedelics, 242–244
TED talks, 17
teleological visions, 276
connection to supreme unity, 281

eternal objects, 279
future visions, 281–287
shared imagination, 287
Singularity, 278–279
strange attractors, 276–278
teleological models of reality in
religion, 277–278
Transcendental Object at End of
Time, 279–281, 288–289
teleology, 277
teonanácatl, 35–36
tetra-prehension, 81
Tezozomoc, 179
thanatos (self-dissolution), 57,
69–73
The Molecule of More (Lieberman and
Long), 125
*The Psychedelic Explorer's Guide: Safe,
Therapeutic, and Sacred Journeys*
(Fadiman), 18, 197–198, 210
*The Singularity Is Near: When Humans
Transcend Biology* (Kurzweil),
278–279
theories of human evolution, 166–173.
See also evolution
the theory of everything. *See* integral
philosophy (integral theory)
Theory of Human Motivation
(Maslow), 63
therapeutic index, 10
Thevet, Andre, 191
*TiHKAL: Tryptamines I Have Known
and Loved* (Shulgin), 241–242
time
complexity, 267, 268
perception, 143–146
Time magazine, 28–29, 244
*The Tipping Point: How Little
Things Can Make a Big Difference*
(Gladwell), 117

Toltecs, 179–180, 183
Tool, 221–222, 298
Toward a Psychology of Being
  (Maslow), 22
transcendence, 66–69, 66
  capitalism, 248
  empathy, 115
  humanity's journey toward
    transcendence, 291–292
  language, 150
Transcendental Object at End of
  Time, 279–281, 288–289
trauma, PTSD and MDMA,
  202–204
treatment-resistant depression,
  31–35
tree of life, 16–17
trialogues at Esalen Institute and
  University of California, Santa
  Cruz, 86, 234–235
True Hallucinations (McKenna), 44,
  143–145
trust between guides and explorers,
  201–204
tryptamines, 159–161, 163
*The Truth Machine: The Blockchain and
  the Future of Everything* (Casey and
  Vigna), 251, 259

U

UCLA (University of California,
  Los Angeles), research, 23, 27,
  45–46
*The Ultimate Journey: Consciousness and
  the Mystery of Death* (Grof), 72
unconscious, 269–270
unity, 16, 19–22
universal basic income, 257
universal intimacy, 291

*The Universe Within: Discovering the
  Common History of Rocks, Planets,
  and People* (Shubin), 104
University of Arizona research, 27,
  45–46
University of California, Davis,
  Psychedelics Promote Structural
  and Functional Neural Plasticity
  study, 159–160
University of California, Los Angeles
  (UCLA) research, 23, 27, 45–46
Usona Institute, 33–35, 46

V

V for Vendetta, 217
The Varieties of Psychedelic
  Experience (Masters and
  Houston), 199–200
Vigna, Paul, 251, 259
Virgin Mary, 183–184
visionary art, 214–231
  Adam Strauss's *The Mushroom
    Cure*, 228
  Alex and Allyson Grey's Entheon
    museum, 225–226
  Alex Grey, 215–216
  Alex Grey's "The New Eleusis",
    222–225
  Andrew "Android" Jones, 226–227
  festivals, 228–230
  H. R. Giger, 216–217
  Laurence Caruana, 215–216
  Marloes Messemaker's *Five Dried
    Grams: A Graphic Novelty Mem*,
    227–228
  The Matrix film series, 217–218
  Sense8 Netflix series, 218–219
  Shane Mauss's *Psychonautics*
    documentary, 228

visionary art (*continued*)
   Star Trek: Discovery, 220–221
   Tool, 221–222
   visionary art movement, 215–216
   women artists, 216
Visionary Plant Consciousness
   (Harpignies, ed.), 97
vitamin B3, 18
voices, 155, 158
Volk, Tyler, 77

W

the Wachowskis, 217–218
Waldman, Ayelet, 18, 210
wanderlust gene (DRD4-7R), 125
war on mind-expanding drugs,
   294–295
Wasson, Gordon, 10–12, 36, 37–39,
   133, 155, 176–177, 224
Watts, Alan, 238–240
Weil, Andrew, 168
Weitlaner, Irmgard, 35–36
What the Dormouse Said (Markoff), 242
Wheal, Jamie, 30–31, 130, 142, 177,
   226, 229, 231–232, 240, 262–263,
   285–287, 295
When the Impossible Happens:
   Adventures in Non-Ordinary
   Realities (Grov), 271
Whitehead, Alfred North, 54, 59–60,
   73, 76, 156, 237, 279
   category of creativity, 68
Wilber, Ken, 31, 49–50, 52–54, 56–57,
   80–81, 94, 139, 208, 216, 218,
   236–237, 292

dissolution, 69
   relationship with Alex Grey, 216
Winkelman, Michael, 135, 161
Wojtowicz, Slawek, 20, 244–245
women artists, 216
Women of Visionary Art, 216
Women's Visionary Congress,
   229–230
Woolley, D. W., 240–241
World Bank, 257
World Economic Forum, 255, 259
World Resources Institute, 248
Wozniak, Steve, 243
Wright, Tony, 107–109, 129,
   171–172

X

Xenolinguistics: Psychedelics, Language,
   and the Evolution of Consciousness
   (Slattery), 45, 151–156

Y

Your Inner Fish: A Journey into the 3.5
   Billion-Year History of the Human
   Body (Shubin), 105, 107

Z

Zeff, Leo, 201, 241
Zen Buddhism, 253
Zendo Project, 213
Zig Zag Zen (Badiner and
   Grey), 134
Zoroastrian texts, 176

ABOUT THE AUTHOR

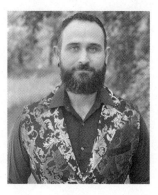

Jahan Khamsehzadeh, PhD, completed his dissertation work on psychedelics in the Philosophy, Cosmology, Consciousness Doctorate program at the California Institute of Integral Studies (CIIS). He earned his master's in Consciousness and Transformative Studies from John F. Kennedy University and his bachelor's from the University of Arizona with a major in philosophy and minors in both psychology and physics. Aside from his academic work, Jahan has undergone several multiyear trainings, including working within the Mazatec mushroom tradition, and is a graduate of the Hakomi Comprehensive Somatic-Psychotherapy Program. He assisted the Psychedelic-Assisted Psychotherapy Certificate Training at CIIS for two years and mentored for a year at the Center for Consciousness Medicine comprehensive guide training. He also works as a facilitator for legal psilocybin mushrooms ceremonies in Jamaica with Atman Retreats and serves as an advisor to psychedelic-focused organizations. Jahan leads a free monthly public online group called "Developing a Relationship with Sacred Mushrooms" with the San Francisco Psychedelic Society. You can learn more about his work and services at www.PsychedelicEvolution.org.

About North Atlantic Books

North Atlantic Books (NAB) is an independent, nonprofit publisher committed to a bold exploration of the relationships between mind, body, spirit, and nature. Founded in 1974, NAB aims to nurture a holistic view of the arts, sciences, humanities, and healing. To make a donation or to learn more about our books, authors, events, and newsletter, please visit www.northatlanticbooks.com.